Improving Therapeutic Communication

A Guide for Developing Effective Techniques

D. Corydon Hammond
Dean H. Hepworth
Veon G. Smith

Improving Therapeutic Communication

Jossey-Bass Publishers

San Francisco · Washington · London · 1977

Improving Therapeutic Communication
A Guide for Developing Effective Techniques
      by D. Corydon Hammond, Dean H. Hepworth, and Veon G. Smith

Library of Congress Catalogue Card Number LC 76-50704

International Standard Book Number ISBN 0-87589-308-2

Manufactured in the United States of America

JACKET DESIGN BY WILLI BAUM

FIRST EDITION

Code 7707

The Jossey-Bass
   Behavioral Science Series

Preface

The impetus for this book came from the enthusiastic responses of graduate students and practitioners to learning materials we had developed to help others master vital helping skills. Both students and practitioners in the helping professions have long expressed an interest in learning experiences that provide opportunities to master the skills required in clinical practice. However, traditional education has emphasized theories of counseling, casework, or psychotherapy at the expense of practical skills. Moreover, the clinical performance of trainees and professionals has generally lagged behind knowledge about the helping process. This book aims to close that gap.

Only a decade ago, the knowledge available to teachers and learners in the helping professions was largely theoretical. Students and practitioners who requested instruction in skill development were reminded that "skill cannot be taught." The conventional wisdom argued that only principles could be taught and that skill development was an internal process beyond the province of the classroom educator. Since then, marked advances in empirical knowledge of the helping process have made the old wisdom obsolete. That knowledge makes possible training methods that both teach competencies to students and provide the means of assessing objectively whether students have learned the skills they need to practice effectively. Such training is not only possible; it is also necessary. Published research studies demonstrate that skill development must be an integral part of education in the helping professions.

This book is the culmination of the authors' lengthy and extensive efforts to combine theory and skill development in a single volume. We believe the book to be of value to student and practitioner alike. For the student, the book will provide a solid foundation in both the theory of interpersonal skills and their mastery. For the practitioner, the book will be an excellent resource for updating knowledge, assessing current levels of skill, and enhancing professional competence.

Chapter One introduces the reader to the vital ingredients of the helping process and concisely reviews the empirical research linking these vital ingredients to therapeutic outcomes. In Chapter Two, the major phases of the helping process are identified, and the role of each vital ingredient during the major phases of the helping process is discussed. Chapter Three identifies the common counterproductive patterns of communication.

Chapters Four through Ten represent the heart of the book, presenting theory and exercises for developing skills in vital dimensions of therapy: the perception of feelings, reciprocal empathy, additive empathy, respect (nonpossessive warmth), authenticity and relational immediacy, and confrontation. The basic format of each chapter consists of theoretical discussion, introduction to research scales that operationalize the vital ingredient under consideration, examples of counselor response to client messages that illustrate various levels of the ingredient, exercises in discriminating these levels and in formulating responses to actual client messages, and modeled high-level responses.

This format provides learning experiences that progress from relatively simple to increasingly complex tasks, with feedback given on the exercises to enable the reader to assess his understanding. This format lends itself to self-instruction for the novice and skill enhancement for the practitioner.

The authors regard themselves as eclectic educators and practitioners and believe that the contents of the book will have relevance for practitioners from virtually all theoretical persuasions. The authors' combined practice experience of over fifty-five years has involved clinical work with individuals, couples, families, and groups as well as supervision, consultation, and administration in a wide variety of settings: public welfare, child guidance, mental health, marriage and family counseling, drug and alcohol abuse, youth detention, state prison, university academic and vocational counseling, and private practice. The large majority of exercises are taken from actual interviews by the authors in all of these clinical situations. In addition, our various educational and professional backgrounds have enabled us to draw on the skills, theories, and literatures of clinical psychology, social work, counseling psychology, and psychiatry.

In the book the terms *therapist, counselor, caseworker,* and *helping professional* are used interchangeably. Even though the meanings of these terms may change with the nature of the client's problems, the competence of the practitioner, and the nature of the setting, the same interpersonal skills pervade helping relationships in all contexts and thus justify our interchangeable use of the terms. For the same reason, we have used the terms *client* and *patient* interchangeably.

The efforts and cooperation of many people combined to bring this book into the light of day. To our colleagues Dr. Edwin G. Brown, Dr. Jo Ann Larsen, Dr. Gary Q. Jorgensen, and Kay Stanfield, we express our appreciation for their helpful ideas and support. Many willing and gracious people helped in typing the manuscripts, and to them we extend our gratitude. Especially we thank Pat Clark, Diane Florez, Barbara Kollmar, Janet Boyakin, Neva Nielsen, and Doris Mortensen. The greatest debt of gratitude is owed to our spouses, Gloria, Pat, and Clyda, for their patience, constant encouragement, and sacrifices. To them this book is affectionately dedicated.

Salt Lake City   D. Corydon Hammond
February 1977   Dean H. Hepworth
                                           Veon G. Smith

Contents

The Authors

D. CORYDON HAMMOND is a clinical psychologist and the co-ordinator of training and research at the Alcohol and Drug Abuse Clinic, University of Utah College of Medicine. He is also a clinical instructor in the Educational Psychology Department and in the College of Medicine (Division of Physical Medicine and Rehabilitation) and is an associate instructor in the Graduate School of Social Work at the University of Utah. He has served for a number of years on the faculty of the University of Utah Summer School on Alcohol Studies and Other Drug Dependencies.

Hammond is a licensed psychologist and marriage and family counselor. His part-time private practice includes clinical work, consultation, and workshops in counselor communication skills, differential treatment, alcoholism and drug-abuse counseling, and marriage and family counseling. His clinical work over the years has included individual, group, and marital therapy with a variety of populations, including alcoholics and drug abusers, university staff and students, physically disabled individuals, and American Indians. For several years, Hammond has conducted saturation marathon group therapy with inmates and their wives or women friends at the Utah state prison. He is a psychological consultant to the Marriage and Family Counseling Bureau at the University of Utah, the Salt Lake County Court Services program, the Division of Physical Medicine and Rehabilitation, and the Cancer Rehabilitation Project in the University of Utah Medical Center.

Cory Hammond earned his doctorate in counseling psychology at the University of Utah, where he was elected to Phi Kappa Phi. He is a member of the American Psychological Association and a clinical member of the American Association of Marriage and Family Counselors. He has made presentations at several national conventions and has recently co-authored a multimodal assessment and planning form and the accompanying counselor's guide. He is married, has two sons, and resides in Salt Lake City.

DEAN H. HEPWORTH is associate dean and professor of the Graduate School of Social Work, University of Utah, and he maintains a part-time private practice in marriage and family counseling, general psychotherapy, and consultation. A frequent contributor to professional journals, he has also made presentations to national conferences in social-work education and in marriage and family counseling.

Hepworth earned an M.S.W. in 1958 and a Ph.D. in educational psychology in 1968 at the University of Utah, where he was elected to the scholastic honor society Phi Kappa Phi. He began social work practice in 1952 as a caseworker with the Utah State Department of Public Welfare, later becoming a casework supervisor and instructor in staff development with that agency. In 1959 he affiliated with a private psychiatrist in Provo, Utah, to practice psychotherapy, also providing services part-time in the Utah County Child Guidance Clinic. In 1963 he entered marriage and family counseling practice, joining the Marriage and Family Counseling Bureau, University of Utah. The following year, he was appointed to the faculty of the Graduate School of Social Work, University of Utah, retaining his clinical position in marriage and family counseling. He also served as a part-time staff member of a traveling mental health clinic serving the needs of a rural population until 1973. He was honored as the outstanding faculty member of the Graduate School of Social Work in 1967 and 1968.

Hepworth is best known as a clinician, educator, and researcher in casework and psychotherapy. He has given many guest lectures in different regions of the country and has conducted numerous workshops on communication and human relations. He is a certified social worker, licensed marriage counselor, member of the Council on Social Work Education, and a clinical member of the American Association of Marriage and Family Counselors.

Hepworth resides with his wife, Patricia, an accomplished artist, in Salt Lake City. They have two married sons and two grandchildren.

VEON G. SMITH is a professor in the Graduate School of Social Work and the director of the Marriage and Family Counseling Bureau, University of Utah. His experience includes teaching, instruction of professionals, supervision, administration, and extensive clinical practice. He has had fifteen years part-time experience in a mental health clinic outside the university and thirty years of part-time private practice. Before joining the university faculty, he did psychiatric social work in the military and with the Veterans Administration.

Smith received his bachelor's degree in English and education with high honors from Brigham Young University. He received an M.S. in Social Administration from Western Reserve University in 1948 and did additional graduate work in sociology and educational psychology at Brigham Young and the University of Utah.

He has contributed to the professional literature, done extensive consultation for agencies and programs, conducted workshops on marriage and family counseling, and presented conference papers. For twenty years, he has been an active member of the American Association of Marriage and Family Counselors (AAMFC), and currently he is a clinical member, a fellow, and a designated supervisor in that organization. He is serving as a member of the AAMFC accreditation committee, which reviews training programs in marriage and family counseling. A licensed marriage and family counselor and a certified social worker, he has served as chairman of the Utah State Licensing Committee for marriage and family counseling.

Smith has been married thirty-seven years and has six children and nine grandchildren.

Improving Therapeutic Communication

A Guide for Developing Effective Techniques

Chapter 1

꠹꠹꠹꠹꠹꠹꠹꠹꠹꠹꠹ ꠹꠹꠹꠹꠹꠹꠹꠹꠹

Effective Elements
in Counseling
and Psychotherapy

It has been argued that the foremost requirement for the ethical practice of any profession is competence. The logic behind this assertion is compelling, for when the services of professional practitioners are required, financial security, health, and even life are often at stake. Prudence dictates that people beset by serious medical or legal problems should make demonstrated competence the primary criterion for choosing a doctor or lawyer. Few would argue that the same logic obtains when mental health and well-being are at stake. People troubled by depression, interpersonal conflicts, feelings of inadequacy, marital conflict, drug or alcohol problems, adjustment to drastic changes in life style, or any other difficulty in living need and deserve competent service, be it from therapists, counselors, or caseworkers. Competence is of importance not only to those seeking professional help, but also to professionals themselves. Mindful of their sometimes awesome responsibilities in helping others make crucial choices and changes in their lives, therapists seek to identify and master the knowledge and skills they need to practice competently.

1

At the heart of the concerns of both client and practitioner is a basic question: "What are the elements of competent counseling and the qualities of competent practitioners?" Fortunately, empirical research in recent years has partially answered this question with documented evidence. This book addresses itself to the question of competence and to the quest for that competence by students and practitioners.

To become more aware of what you already know intuitively about the nature of helpful relationships, assume for a moment that you yourself are going to consult a counselor. Your goal in counseling will be to explore yourself in depth, learning more about yourself and in the process revealing deep personal information. Ponder for a few moments what qualities you desire in a person to whom you are going to reveal private and intimate material. You are encouraged to write down the characteristics you identify so that you can compare them later with the characteristics discussed in this book.

The authors have tried this exercise in many workshops and classes and have found a striking similarity in the desirable qualities the participants ascribe to a hypothetical counselor. These characteristics are in fact the subject of this study.

The authors work from the conviction that counseling, and all interpersonal relationships, may be either therapeutic and growth-enhancing or psychonoxious and destructive. We also believe firmly that skills in responding helpfully to others, whether those others be clients, spouses, children, employees, or friends, can be acquired through learning, modeling, and extended practice. Thus this book provides principles, practical guidelines, and exercises whose aim is to instill and enhance skill in responding to others helpfully. This chapter lays the groundwork for the rest, by identifying the therapeutic ingredients and reviewing the research that relates desirable counselor qualities to positive therapeutic outcomes.

Empathic Communication

The most fundamental, vital, and complex therapeutic skill is the ability to convey accurate empathy to the client. The first dimension of empathy involves the counselor's ability to perceive and recognize the private, inner feelings and experiences of the client as the client experiences them. Empathic communication requires a willingness to walk in another person's shoes, seeking to grasp the meaning of his* experience, rather than imposing meaning on that experience from the outside. Thus empathy is an understanding *with* the client, rather than a diagnostic or evaluative understanding *of* the client. External, or counselor-centered, knowledge is not the same as empathic knowledge. Being empathic means going beyond the role of a technician, who rigidly applies mechanical skills and techniques, to becoming deeply and personally involved. Focusing intensely on "being with" another person, rather than relating to the other as an object for analysis or manipulation, entails a personal struggle. The empathic counselor must see beyond conventional facades, refrain from imposing personal interpretations and judgments, and be willing to risk understanding another person's private logic and feelings, which in superficial daily contacts the counselor might view as weak, foolish, or undesirable.

Empathic responsiveness requires the ability to go beyond factual knowledge and detail, and to become involved in the other person's affective world, but always with the "as if" quality of taking another's role without personally experiencing what that other person experiences. To experience the identical emotions of the client would be to be overinvolved. Sympathetic responding involves the expression of care and the compassion to comfort another person. Empathic responding, by contrast, does not involve the direct expression of one's own feelings but rather focuses exclusively on the feelings expressed by another, conveying thereby an understanding of them.

Being empathically attuned to a client also requires much more than merely identifying the flow of his apparent feelings. It also includes "sensing meanings of which he/she is scarcely aware, but not trying to uncover feelings of which the person is totally unaware, since this would be too threatening" (Rogers, 1975, p. 4). Thus deeply empathic responses go well beyond merely reflecting

*The traditional use of the pronouns *he* and *his* has not yet been superseded by convenient, generally accepted pronouns that mean either *he* or *she* and *his* or *her*. Therefore, the authors will continue to use the masculine but hereby acknowledge the inherent inequity in doing so.

or parroting the client's surface feelings and labeling underlying or hinted feelings. In actuality, then, empathic interventions are mild to moderate interpretations (Rogers, 1966; Truax and Carkhuff, 1964; Bergin, 1966). Additionally, however, the empathic counselor must grasp the dynamic meaning, personal significance, and purposiveness of experiences as well as the affective state. Thus the counselor must achieve a moment-to-moment awareness of the affective, perceptual, and cognitive worlds of the client. The counselor must also observe such subtle cues as facial expressions, tone of voice, tempo of speech, and posture and gesture that amplify or perhaps contradict verbal meanings or that hint at underlying feelings or meanings.

Despite the enormous concentration and effort such a task requires, empathic *recognition* is only the first dimension of this creative process. One must also be able to accurately convey his understanding to the client. Life really enters therapeutic relationships when the counselor is able to reach out and "touch" the client through perceiving accurately and then conveying sensitively what he has understood. Understanding alone is not enough; we must also communicate that understanding accurately.

Occasionally, neophyte counselors hesitate to elicit and acknowledge such powerful, underlying, negative client feelings as despair, inadequacy, or rage, for fear that exploration and discussion of such feelings will be destructive and will only intensify the feelings. However, our experience suggests that such uneasiness is more often related to the counselor's difficulty or discomfort in responding emotionally than to any real hazard for the client. In fact, empathically identifying such strong, implicit feelings generally benefits the client in that he sees in the person of the counselor someone unterrified by the prospect of exploring threatening feelings and experiences. Gendlin explains his view in these words: "We should never avoid what an individual *implicitly* feels because we fear he cannot take it. He is already taking it! The question is: 'Will you enable him to live it with you or only alone?'" (1970, p. 91).

Empathy has a number of therapeutic benefits. Empathic communication is one of the primary vehicles for establishing a relationship with the client. An individual who feels empathically understood is likely to risk sharing deep and personal feelings. The client's perception of our genuine effort and commitment to understand and his experience of being "empathically received" creates a low-threat environment that obviates self-defense and self-protection. Thus client self-exploration, a prerequisite for self-understanding and subsequent behavior change, is facilitated. Empathic acknowledgment clarifies feelings for the client, elucidating reasons behind previously puzzling behavior patterns. Ginott (1965, p. 40) artistically describes the function of empathic responding with children:

> How can we help a child to know his feelings? We can do so by serving as a mirror to his emotions. A child learns about his physical likeness by seeing his image in a mirror. He learns about his emotional likeness by hearing his feelings reflected by us.
>
> The function of a mirror is to reflect an image as it is, without adding flattery or faults. We do not want a mirror to tell us, "You look terrible. Your eyes are bloodshot and your face is puffy. Altogether you are a mess. You'd better do something about yourself." After a few exposures to such a magic mirror, we would avoid it like the plague. From a mirror we want an image, not a sermon. We may not like the image we see; still, we would rather decide for ourselves our next cosmetic move.
>
> The function of an emotional mirror is to reflect feelings as they are, without distortion.

Respect

Respect refers to a nonpossessive caring for and affirmation of another's personhood as a separate individual. This quality involves a warmly receptive attitude that prizes and preserves the client's feelings, opinions, individuality, and uniqueness. By not arguing, threatening, disapproving, ridiculing, rejecting, belittling, or condescending, the counselor maintains a nonevaluative, nonjudgmental posture. The respectful counselor conveys a commitment to understand the client's feelings and opinions sensitively, and he endeavors to accept the client. Martin Buber refers to the process of acceptance wherein an individual, even "with all his desire to influence the other, nevertheless unreservedly accepts and confirms him in his being this man and in his being made in this particular way" (1966, p. 112). He further elaborates:

Genuine conversation, and therefore every actual fulfillment of relation between men, means acceptance of otherness. The strictness and depth of human individuation, the elemental otherness of the other, is then not merely noted as the necessary starting point, but is affirmed from the one being to the other. The desire to influence the other then does not mean the effort to change the other, to inject one's own "rightness" into him; but it means the effort to let that which is recognized as right, as just, as true . . . through one's influence take seed and grow in the form suited to individuation.

Buber also explains respectful acceptance by saying, "In a genuine dialogue each of the partners, even when he stands in opposition to the other, heeds, affirms, and confirms his opponent as an existing other" (p. 122). This means that even client defenses and resistance are met with respectful patience and a striving to understand their purpose. Ideally, then, the counselor should not be offended by the client's provocation, censure, or hostility, but should attempt to accept such feelings and encourage their open expression so that they might be understood. Respect is an attitude of seeking never to unnecessarily damage or hurt a client's self-esteem or self-image under the guise of trying to be helpful.

The counselor who conveys respect accepts the individual's right to make his own decisions and believes in and trusts the client's ability to do so responsibly. Therefore, a counseling relationship with respect has the flavor of a cooperative partnership in which there is equality, mutuality, and shared thinking about problems. This relationship is drastically opposed to a type of counseling wherein the counselor establishes himself as an authoritative adviser and then proceeds to dictate and manipulate. A manipulative counselor controls the flow of conversation, dominates, selects topics, attempts to override, persuade, and influence without understanding and appreciating, and he evaluates rather than listening responsively and accepting. Implicit in such a counselor's manner is a distrust for the client, as opposed to a belief in and affirmation of the client's capacity and right to make his own decisions wisely. The condescending, authoritative, or manipulative counselor presumptuously believes that his superior knowledge qualifies him to know what is best for another human being. Thus such a counselor is reluctant to respect the client's self-autonomy and right to self-determination.

However, respect does not require the counselor to be namby-pamby or to accept destructive client behavior. When the relationship is well-established and the problem-solving process is well under way, the counselor can convey respect by challenging the other person to act on his capacity to achieve his goals and to take full responsibility for himself. Thus the sharing of expectations and personal reactions such as disappointment, irritation, encouragement, and praise may convey respect when expressed in the context of good will, caring, and helpful intent. Respect permits the honest questioning of the client's behavior, not out of a need to control, dominate, or force conformity upon the client, but rather out of a concern about the damage worked by certain behaviors on himself and those dear to him. Such concern emanates from respect and caring, not from value conflicts. In fact, genuine caring, positive regard, warmth, and interest are important aspects of this dimension, as contrasted with a cool or aloof "professional" attitude. When client behavior appears self-defeating, a good counselor should care enough to be candid and open. But, equally important, the respectful counselor displays a commitment to understand, conveyed through attentiveness and empathic recognition of the client's views, however inappropriate or neurotic they may seem (Strupp, 1973, p. 282). Remembering what the client has said, demonstrating sensitivity and courtesy, and showing respect for the client's feelings and beliefs even when genuinely sharing one's own views constitute respect.

Authenticity

A primary characteristic of the effective counselor's relationship with the client is his authenticity. Authenticity refers to a sharing of self by behaving in a natural, sincere, spontaneous, real, open, and nondefensive manner. An authentic individual relates to others personally, so that expressions do not seem rehearsed or contrived and verbalizations are congruent with actual feelings and thoughts. When appropriate, the authentic counselor can express his feelings as something belonging to him and separate from the other person, without imposing his feelings on that other. For example,

when the counselor is angry and deems it appropriate to express
his feelings, he will express them as something within himself, rather
than blaming or otherwise placing responsibility on the client for
his own feelings. The genuine helper is able to be himself, and he
is human enough to admit his own errors to the client. He realizes
that if he is asking a client to lower his defenses and become real,
he too must be real, provide a model of humanness and openness,
and avoid hiding behind a polite facade of professionalism. The
more authentic the counselor, the more he can trust himself, be
sensitively aware and accepting of his own feelings, and escape a
preoccupation with technique at the expense of the relationship
itself (May, 1958, p. 85).

Authenticity and genuineness require the counselor to do
with his own inner experiencing what he tries to help the client do—
that is, be aware of it, and claim it as his own. Gendlin clarifies this
further (1970, p. 92):

> We must not just blurt out: "You bore me," or "Why
> do you never say anything important?" Instead, we must
> ourselves carry forward our own experiencing for a few
> moments in a chain of content mutation and explica-
> tion. For example, "I am bored. . . . This isn't helping
> him. . . . I wish I could help. . . . I'd like to hear some-
> thing more personal. . . . I really would welcome him. . . .
> I have more welcome on my hands for him than he lets
> me use. . . . but I don't want to push away what he does
> express. . . ." The resulting therapist expression now
> will make a personal interaction, even if the client says
> nothing in return. The therapist will say something like:
> "You know, I've been thinking the last few minutes, I
> wish I'd hear more from you, more of how you really
> feel inside. I know you might not want to say, but when-
> ever you can or want, I would like it."

Even after one has explored and differentiated the meaning
of his own feelings, the therapeutic value of sharing them must
guide the determination of whether they should be expressed to
the client. We must not merely share our feelings and impressions
with the client indiscriminately; the client has probably engaged
in such exchange with other people without facilitative effect. In

fact, authentic expression may at times be destructive. Yalom and Lieberman (1971), in a study of encounter-group casualties, document that attack or rejection by the leader or the members of the group produces many psychological casualties, whether the attack or rejection is genuine or not. Carkhuff and Berenson advocate that when the counselor's only genuine reactions to the client are negative, the counselor should use his expressions constructively as a basis "for further inquiry for the therapist, the client, and their relationship" (1967, p. 29).

Authenticity constrains the counselor from acting contrary to his feelings, but it does not require a constant and total disclosure of those feelings. Rather, such disclosures as are made should be genuine. Truax and Carkhuff (1964) discovered that beyond a certain level, genuineness does not increase facilitation for the client. What seems most critical is that the client does not perceive the counselor as defensive, phony, or merely responding according to a role. Carkhuff and Berenson (1967), therefore, conclude that the therapist must avoid confusing genuineness with free license to do what he will, especially with respect to expressing hostility. Counselor interventions should be in response to client needs and interests and should not shift the central focus to the counselor. Yalom (1975) explains that counselor behavior appropriate at one phase of therapy may be quite inappropriate at another stage. Authenticity must not be construed as an end in itself. The primary role of the helper, whether in groups or in individual therapy, is to facilitate the client's growth, not to demonstrate his own honesty or authenticity.

Confrontation

Confrontation is one of the most controversial concepts and processes in counseling. There is no widely accepted definition of confrontation. Definitions from the dictionary are undoubtedly the source of some of the conceptual confusion. One such definition of confrontation is, "the act of facing in hostility or defiance." Some counselors, unfortunately, use confrontation in just such a negative manner, venting aggressive feelings or frustrations or seeking to set the client straight. Used in this manner, confrontation is punitive, destructive, and out of place in the helping process.

Consider a second dictionary definition, which is, "the act of bringing close together for comparison or examination." This definition better identifies the kind of confrontation employed constructively in therapy. Confrontation, indeed, is the therapist's bringing together of growth-defeating discrepancies in the client's perceptions, feelings, behavior, values, attitudes, and communication to compare and examine them. Confrontation thus involves bringing the client face to face with some aspect of his problem or behavior that he has failed either to recognize or to verbalize (Johnson, 1961).

Confrontation helps the client view his behavior in a different light, activate strengths previously underestimated or unrealized, come to terms with discrepancies between stated goals and actual behavior, and unmask distortions, rationalizations, and evasions. Implied in these functions are the major purposes of confrontation—to expand client awareness of internal obstacles to growth and change and to prompt the client to act toward more effective functioning and increased fulfillment.

Therapist-initiated confrontation involves certain risks because the client usually feels threatened when the therapist in effect challenges some aspect of his usual thinking or behavior. This challenge usually causes the client some temporary disorganization or disequilibrium (Egan, 1975). In an established relationship where the client senses the therapist's good will, such disorganization may serve a constructive purpose by opening the client to influence and change. Even skillful confrontations, however, may elicit defensive reactions. Poorly executed confrontations, however, invariably engender defensiveness (covertly if not overtly), resentment, and perhaps alienation.

Confrontation is not indispensable, for as Berenson and Mitchell (1974) agree, its purposes can be accomplished by other means if time is available. These authors do not regard confrontation as a major vehicle for helping, and they believe it much abused by some practitioners who, because of an inadequate repertoire of clinical skills, use it excessively. They take the position, however, that when time is limited, confrontation may be used appropriately and effectively to accelerate therapy by counselors who have mastered the other facilitative skills.

Egan regards confrontation "at its best" as an extension of advanced accurate empathy, in the sense that the unmasking of the client's distorted understanding of himself is based on the therapist's deep understanding of the client's feelings, experiences, and behavior. He advocates, therefore, that confrontation be done "in the spirit of accurate empathy" (1975, p. 165). Interestingly, Egan's contention is supported by research (Berenson and Mitchell, 1974), which indicates that high-level facilitative therapists employ confrontation differently, both qualitatively and quantitatively, from low-level facilitative therapists.

As we will discuss later, confrontation takes many forms, but the potency of this dimension for helpfulness or destructiveness is so great that the use of any form of confrontation requires finesse and expert timing. Chapter Ten examines this matter in more detail.

The Theoretical Base of the Facilitative Conditions

For many years, experts in the helping professions have been greatly concerned with identifying the essentials of effective therapy. Many publications on this topic have appeared in the literature, but two prominent works deserve particular mention.

In 1950, Fiedler reported the elements of an "ideal therapeutic relationship," as identified most often by therapists from divergent theoretical backgrounds. It is of interest that from a pool of 119 statements describing patient-therapist relationships, therapists of different theoretical schools consistently chose 14 items as the ones most characteristic of an ideal therapeutic relationship. Virtually all of the 14 items, which include "an empathic relationship," "a tolerant atmosphere exists," "the therapist leaves patient free to make his own choices," and "the therapist really tries to understand the patient's feelings," are embodied in the three facilitative conditions: empathic communication, respect, and authenticity.

The second prominent publication, which appeared a few years later in the social work literature, is Biestek's *Casework Relationship* (1957). This book rapidly gained widespread acceptance and is still used extensively as a reference. Biestek identifies the following seven "principles," or elements, of the casework relationship:

individualization of the client, purposeful expression of feelings, controlled emotional involvement, acceptance, nonjudgmental attitude, client self-determination, and confidentiality. Although Biestek's terms are not identical to Fiedler's, their meanings are very close. Moreover, Biestek's seven elements can also be subsumed, for the most part, under the three facilitative conditions. Thus not only do therapists from divergent schools of psychotherapy agree on the essentials of effective therapy, but there is a consensus even among the different helping professions. Truax and Carkhuff write (1967, p. 25):

> Despite the bewildering array of divergent theories and the difficulty in translating concepts from the language of one theory to that of another, several common threads weave their way through almost every major theory of psychotherapy and counseling. . . . In one way or another, all have emphasized the importance of the therapist's ability to be integrated, mature, genuine, authentic, or congruent in his relationship to the patient. They have all stressed also the importance of the therapist's ability to provide a nonthreatening, trusting, safe, or secure atmosphere by his acceptance, nonpossessive warmth, unconditional positive regard, or love. Finally, virtually all theories of psychotherapy emphasize that for the therapist to be helpful he must be accurately empathic, be "with the client," be understanding, or grasp the patient's meaning.

The Empirical Base

It is important to note that the qualities of ideal helping relationships identified by Fiedler and Biestek were based upon practical wisdom—that is, on the opinions and views of experienced counselors, therapists, and caseworkers. At the time there was no persuasive experimental evidence documenting relationships between these qualities and successful therapeutic outcomes. Indeed practitioners complacently accepted this theoretical knowledge as valid, and no compelling reason existed to undertake research for purposes of validation.

Eysenck (1952) summarily shattered this complacency and prompted others to look into the empirical relationship between the nature and the outcome of therapy. In his study, Eysenck first established a baseline recovery rate of untreated patients by reviewing an earlier study that reported the percentage of neurotic patients discharged annually as recovered or improved following only custodial care in New York hospitals and a second study of neurotic patients treated only by their physicians with no psychotherapy. He then gathered data from some nineteen published studies of recovery rates of neurotic patients treated by psychotherapy. Eysenck's comparisons of these two bodies of data led him to conclude that patients treated with psychotherapy fared no better, even did worse in some instances, than those who received no treatment at all. Eysenck concluded in fact that the more psychotherapy received, the lower the recovery rate and that improvement following therapy resulted from "spontaneous remission" rather than the therapy itself.

Eysenck's paper set off a giant earthquake whose aftershocks still rock the helping professions. Although by present standards Eysenck's research design included several serious flaws, which we will cite later, and although his analysis of the data contained error and bias (Bergin, 1971), Eysenck's paper was of enormous value in stimulating much-needed research. The impact of his paper, incidentally, was augmented by other research studies (Barron and Leary, 1955; Leavitt, 1957) that also cast doubts on the value of psychotherapy.

The stimulus provided by Eysenck also led to more sophisticated analysis of the complex issues involved in outcome research and particularly to efforts to identify the variables or factors involved in successful outcomes. It was observed, for example, that Eysenck had drawn his conclusions from average outcome rates, which masked the wide range of improvement or recovery rates reported—from 25 percent in one study to 90 percent in another. What would account for variability of such magnitude? Apparently some potent but undefined factors produced improvement rates sometimes well above and sometimes well below those reported in the control groups. Moreover, Bergin (1967, 1971) argued vigorously that attributing improvement in control patients to "spontaneous remission" was unscientific and simply an admission of ignorance about what was really happening. The variables, he maintained, simply had not been identified as yet. After searching for an explanation of why untreated clients showed about the same rate of improvement on the average as treated clients, Bergin presented persuasive evidence from a nationwide survey of mental health in the United States (Gurin, Veroff, and Feld, 1960) that those who did not seek out professional therapists probably received help from nonprofessionals such as friends, teachers, physicians, clergymen, and others. Indeed, the survey revealed that the majority of Americans with mental health problems sought help from a clergyman or family doctor, whereas only 31 percent had consulted professionals identified as mental health practitioners. Moreover, of those seen by a clergyman or doctor, 65 percent said they were helped or helped a lot, as contrasted to 46, 39, and 25 percent who had seen psychiatrists, other psychological counselors, or marriage counselors respectively.

The findings of this survey cast an entirely new light on the processes that ameliorate psychological suffering. Perhaps, Bergin (1967) speculated, not only is there nothing special about psychotherapy, but persons selected from the natural social environment provide better conditions for helping with psychological problems than do trained mental health experts. Lay therapists, he conjectured, may be chosen because of their known and proven ability to provide help through natural therapy based on a capacity to form therapeutic relationships and to convey wise counsel, whereas professionals are chosen because of academic and professional credentials. The natural consequence of Bergin's line of thinking was to raise questions about the "better" conditions provided by the attributes of these proven helpers, who were subsequently labeled "inherently helpful persons" (Truax and Mitchell, 1971).

It was the same line of thinking that earlier had prompted Rogers (1957), in an article now regarded as a classic, to postulate six therapist and client conditions, which, if met, would assure constructive personality change. Three of these conditions—empathy, unconditional positive regard, and congruence—applied to the therapist. Rogers's formulations proved to be seminal, leading to the development of research scales (Truax and Carkhuff, 1967; Carkhuff, 1969) that operationalized the three therapist ingredients in slightly modified form as accurate empathy, nonpossessive warmth, and genuineness (which here become empathic communication, respect, and authenticity). Following these scales came a plethora of research studies, the majority of which documented a relationship between high levels of the ingredients, or facilitative conditions, and successful counseling outcomes (Rogers and others, 1967; Truax and Carkhuff, 1967; Carkhuff, 1969; Truax and Mitchell, 1971; these references summarize literally dozens of studies relating outcomes to the facilitative conditions).

In addition to the powerful effects of the facilitative conditions on outcomes, similar potent results on specific client behavior have been documented in other studies. For example, the degree of client self-exploration in individual interviews, high levels of which are known to be associated with positive outcomes (Truax and Carkhuff, 1967), has been shown to be a function of the level of facilitative conditions (Carkhuff and Truax, 1965; Holder, Carkhuff, and Berenson, 1967; Piaget, Berenson, and Carkhuff, 1967).

It should be noted that a few outcome studies (Bergin and Jasper, 1969; Beutler, Johnson, Neville, and Workman, 1972; and Kurtz and Grummon, 1972) have failed to replicate the findings of positive relationships between facilitative conditions and outcomes. These studies, however, number many fewer than those which have found such a relationship. Moreover, these studies suffer from methodological weaknesses (Hammond, Hepworth, and Smith, 1975), including the use of unsophisticated raters, low interrater reliabilities, and the failure to compare counselors whose ability to communicate empathy ranged from very low to very high levels.

The potency of the facilitative conditions in determining outcomes has been further documented by disturbing findings that the clients of therapists who relate with low degrees of the facilitative conditions tend to deteriorate—that is, they get worse. Deterioration has been reported in numerous studies which are summarized by Truax and Mitchell (1971) and Bergin (1971, 1975). Deterioration resulting from encounter groups has been documented by Lieberman, Yalom, and Miles (1973), who report a 12 percent "casualty rate." Gottshalk and Pattison (1969) report an even more alarming statistic from a six-month follow-up study of T-group participants. They found that the group experience produced serious disturbance in 19 percent of the participants. Much of the deterioration in encounter groups was attributed to "psychonoxious" group leaders—that is, damaging leaders who used an excessively intrusive, aggressive approach, severely challenging and confronting members of the group without respect for their feelings and individuality. Instead of relating with high levels of the facilitative conditions, these group leaders tended to be impatient and authoritarian, usually pressuring group members into immediate self-disclosure, emotional expression, and attitude changes. These disturbing findings prompted one writer (Anderson, 1975) to emphasize the need for group leaders to be better trained in interpersonal skills, particularly in empathic communication. Similar concerns apparently prompted Bergin to write "When Shrinks Hurt: Psychotherapy Can Be Dangerous" (*Psychology Today*, 1975) to alert the lay public to the potential damage that may be inflicted on unwary clients. There Bergin cites evidence from a dozen well-designed and carefully controlled outcome studies which indicates that the average rate of deterioration for patients in psychotherapy is 10 percent, a rate double that of patients in untreated control groups. Truly, psychotherapy is "for better or for worse."

In a more optimistic vein, however, Bergin presents data from rigorous, well-designed studies that refute Eysenck's original conclusion about psychotherapy's conspicuous lack of success. These data indicate that the average rate of improvement for treated patients is about 65 percent as contrasted to only 40 percent for those who receive no treatment. Subotnik (1972) presents evidence that the rate of "spontaneous" recovery—that is, without therapy—is much lower than 40 percent, suggesting that spontaneous remission may be an artifact.

To this point, our discussion has centered upon empirical evidence of the relationship between levels of the facilitative conditions and outcomes of the helping effort. Mounting evidence, however, indicates as well that the facilitative conditions affect outcomes even in behavior therapy. Unfortunately, many behaviorists, who persist in clinging to the outmoded belief that changes in behavior therapy result exclusively from the technology involved in desensitization, environmental manipulation, and other conditioning techniques, have ignored or belittled these findings. Commenting about the tendency of many behaviorists to limit their interventions to the application of the favored technologies, one internationally prominent behaviorist (Lazarus, 1968) asserts that a clinician who so limits himself evades his duties and that nothing in modern learning theory precludes the behavior therapist from offering human understanding, empathy, support, and other factors that foster hope and mobilize an expectation of help.

Research studies underscore even further the importance of the facilitative conditions in behavior therapy. Vitalo (1970) investigated the effects of empathy, respect, and genuineness in a verbal-conditioning paradigm and found that high-facilitative experimenters had a more significant impact on the subjects than those who related at low levels of empathy, respect, and genuineness. Mickelson and Stevic (1971) report findings that efforts to increase the information-seeking behavior of clients by using verbal reinforcement procedures are significantly enhanced when counselors relate with high levels of the facilitative conditions. Other researchers (E. L. Phillips and others, 1973; Morris and Suckerman, 1974a, 1974b; and Ryan and Gizynski, 1971) have demonstrated that facilitative therapist qualities, especially warmth, contribute significantly to the outcomes of behavior therapy. At this point the extent of that contribution has not been determined definitively, but present knowledge appears sufficient to justify Carkhuff's conclusion that "high levels of interpersonal functioning are prerequisite to obtaining maximum benefits from any behavior modification program" (1971, p. 8).

How Facilitative Conditions Affect Other Relationships

Evidence has been accumulating that the potency of the facilitative conditions extends beyond counseling and psychotherapy into virtually all human relationships. With respect to teacher-student interaction, for example, Truax and Tatum (1966) report that the degree of warmth and empathy communicated by preschool teachers was significantly related to positive changes in children's preschool performance and adjustment to school, teachers, and peers. Aspy and Hadlock (1967) found that the students of grammar-school teachers with high levels of the facilitative conditions achieved as much as two and one-half years of intellectual growth in one school year, while students taught by low-facilitative teachers showed only six months of growth over the same time span. Moreover, truancy rates among students of low-facilitative teachers were double those of the high-level instructors. Other studies by Griffin and Banks (1969) with inner-city students and Hefele (1971) with deaf students report similar findings.

Stoffer (1970) reports significant relationships between the levels of empathic understanding and unconditional positive regard of teacher-counselors and the indices of elementary school achievement and classroom behavior. The relationships between learning and adjustment also seem to hold in college. Wagner and Mitchell (1969) found that the final examination scores of freshmen taking college algebra were related to their perceptions of the empathy, warmth, and genuineness of their instructors. Interestingly, Hollenbeck (1965) also found a positive relationship between the adjustments of students to college and their perceptions of their parents' facilitative dimensions.

A growing body of knowledge also indicates a relationship between levels of the facilitative conditions offered by parents and the adjustment levels of children. Truax and Carkhuff (1967) review numerous studies that substantiate this relationship.

It should also be noted that three of the most prominent books (Ginott, 1965, 1969; Gordon, 1970) written to assist parents in communicating effectively and beneficially with children and teenagers focus heavily on skills embodied in the facilitative conditions. Not surprisingly, the importance of the facilitative conditions is also reflected in major programs developed to help couples learn how to communicate effectively. The skills taught in the Minnesota Couples Communication Program (Miller, Nunnally, and Wackman, 1972) are virtually identical to the facilitative conditions. The same identity holds true for the concepts and skills taught in conjugal therapy (Ely, Guerney, and Stover, 1973). Interestingly, modest evidence also indicates a relationship between the degree of facilitative communication couples achieve in marriage counseling and the outcomes of that counseling (Gurman, 1975).

Some evidence also indicates that the facilitative conditions have a powerful impact on racial and ethnic differences between helper and client. Banks (1971), Cimbolic (1972), and Santa Cruz and Hepworth (1975) all report research findings which indicate that clients are affected more by the counselor's facilitative conditions than by his race or ethnic origin. These authors conclude that high levels of facilitative communication can surmount racial and ethnic barriers, and they have recommended that training programs for counselors be planned accordingly.

Implications for Training Programs

From this great mass of evidence, one cannot escape the far-reaching conclusion that practicing and prospective counselors and therapists have an ethical responsibility to develop to the greatest possible extent the interpersonal skills subsumed under the facilitative conditions. However, disquieting evidence from a survey of the levels of facilitative functioning among counselors and psychotherapists (Carkhuff, 1968) indicate that most function at low levels. These findings are consistent with those of Strupp and his co-workers (1960), who rated the responses given by 126 psychiatrists to standardized sound films of patient-therapist interactions. Of the 2,474 responses analyzed, over 95 percent either were neutral or communicated coldness and rejection. On the measure of therapeutic attitude toward patients, fewer than one third of the psychiatrists were rated as positive or warm. Later comparisons involving a sample of 237 psychiatric social workers, psychologists, psychiatrists, and psychoanalysts yielded similar findings.

The educational implications of these findings clearly indicate the need for training programs that assist future practitioners in the helping professions to develop skills in the facilitative conditions. Unfortunately, however, traditional training programs retain a largely theoretic focus, and the academic degree still provides little or no assurance of the graduate's skill. The neglect of training in skill development in traditional graduate programs in clinical psychology has been documented by Bergin and Solomon (1970), Carkhuff, Kratochvil, and Friel (1968), and Carkhuff, Piaget, and Pierce (1968), all of whom report that doctoral trainees near or at the completion of training functioned substantially below a minimally facilitative level of empathic communication.

Although similar research in social work has not been reported, there is reason to believe that the findings would be no different. Although the practicum component of social-work curricula provides opportunities for skill development, practicum instruction, as characterized by Wells and Miller (1973), is unsystematic, and the richness of experience and the quality of instruction differ widely from setting to setting. Moreover, the vast majority of field instructors have not themselves been systematically trained in the facilitative conditions. This situation also obtains for instruction offered in practicum and internship experiences in clinical and counseling psychology. Field or practicum instructors cannot and do not advance students beyond the levels of skill they themselves possess (Pierce, 1966; Payne and Gralinski, 1968; and Pierce and Schauble, 1970).

To fill the gap left by traditional academic programs, researchers have experimented with instructional methods that provide trainees with opportunities to practice such skills under the direction of highly skilled trainers. The results are impressive. Carkhuff and Truax (1965), for example, found that with 100 hours of didactic and experiential learning, lay persons and clinical psychology trainees could function at a level roughly equal to highly experienced and prominent professionals. Moreover, these trained aides had a significant impact as group therapists, a fact that demonstrated not only the potency of the instructional methods but of the facilitative conditions. Poser (1966) provides additional experimental evidence that with similar systematic training lay therapists can equal and in some instances surpass professionals in level of functioning. Encouraged by these and other similar findings, Truax and Carkhuff (1967) published a description of the training methods, which Carkhuff (1969) further refined and detailed.

Despite the proven success of Carkhuff's instructional format, graduate schools have been slow to incorporate the methods into their curricula. As knowledge of the facilitative conditions has become more widespread, however, a few graduate schools have experimented with workshops or laboratories offered to limited numbers of students (Oxley, 1973; Wells and Miller, 1973; Canfield, Eley, Rollman, and Schur, 1975). Favorable results, manifested in student enthusiasm and increased skill development, have been reported, but the results were not measured systematically. Empirical validation of the efficacy of systematic skill training in schools of social work, however, has been provided by Wells (1975) and by Larsen and Hepworth (1975). In the latter study, the ninety-four students of a first-year graduate social work class were randomly assigned to experimental groups, which received systematic training in the facilitative conditions over one academic quarter, or to control groups, which received traditional didactic instruction. Pre- and post-test measures indicated that experimental groups significantly outperformed the control groups. The former groups achieved mean skill levels equivalent to those regarded as minimally facilitative (Anthony, 1971) in approximately ten hours of actual training, whereas the control groups were still functioning at substantially lower levels. Many of the training materials employed in conducting the experimental groups are presented later in this book. The materials, which were developed by the authors for self-instruction, employ aspects of the proven Carkhuff format and thus have a strong empirical base.

Another empirically-based feature of the format employed in this book is the provision of modeled responses for the communication exercises. Perry (1975) has documented the effectiveness of modeling in learning empathic communication. The materials presented here, which combine didactic instruction with systematic practice of the skills, can be readily adapted to group learning experiences like the experimental skills-development course just described.

Empirical and Theoretical Bases of Confrontation

Whereas empirical evidence abounds to support the relationship between the facilitative conditions and therapeutic outcomes, few studies have been made of confrontation, and these few have been inadequate to ascertain the effects of confrontation on therapy. The authors could locate only one outcome study of confrontation (loosely defined), and this study concerned encounter groups. Lieberman, Yalom, and Miles (1973) studied a dimension of group-leader behavior they identified as "emotional stimulation," which includes behavior that "emphasizes revealing feelings, challenging, confrontation, revelation of personal values, attitudes, beliefs, frequent participation as a member in the group, exhortation, and drawing attention to self" (p. 235). Their concept appears to fuse confrontation with authenticity. They reported that a moderate level of this dimension was closely related to productive outcomes. If the degree of this leader dimension was low—that is, if the group leader challenged and stimulated little—the group's participants improved only modestly, even if other critical dimensions were high. By contrast, if the leader provided too much emotional stimulation, the risk factor increased, and psychological casualties were more frequent.

Other research on confrontation consists of comparative or process-type studies not directly related to counseling outcomes. Mitchell and Namenek (1972), for example, investigated the effects of therapist-initiated confrontation on the depth of client self-exploration during initial interviews, a factor associated with counseling outcomes. They concluded that confrontation had little impact on the absolute level of self-exploration during initial interviews. However, this finding revealed little about the results of the *effective* use of confrontation, because confrontation during the early phase of the helping process is premature, often destructive, and therefore generally contraindicated. We will look at this matter in more detail in Chapter Ten.

In a study of the level of client self-exploration, Kaul, Kaul, and Bednar (1973) contrasted confrontive therapists with speculative therapists and found no differences between the two groups. The findings of this comparative study, while informative, unfortunately do not yield information about the specific effects of the confrontive and speculative styles, making interpretation difficult.

Thus the empirical evidence of the effectiveness of confrontation in promoting client self-exploration is inconclusive despite assertions that confrontation is related to client self-understanding and action (Carkhuff, 1969). Unfortunately, studies of the effects of confrontation during later stages of counseling, when it is most appropriate, have not been reported. Before the effects of confrontation can be definitely determined, such studies must be completed.

Additional process studies indicate marked differences in the use of confrontation between therapists whose helping relationships are characterized by high levels of the facilitative conditions and those whose levels are low. Based on a study in which the initial interviews of fifty-six different practitioners were rated on various helping dimensions, Berenson and Mitchell (1974) report that "high-functioning" (on the facilitative dimensions) helpers initiated significantly more confrontations than did "low-functioning" helpers. The clients of high-functioning therapists, as expected, engaged in self-exploration more extensively than did clients of low-functioning therapists. Moreover, the frequency of different types of confrontation differed sharply between high- and low-functioning helpers. The latter group rarely used confrontations aimed at identifying and mobilizing latent client strengths. The low-functioning helpers, on the other hand, used frequent "weakness confrontations," which were rarely employed by high-functioning helpers. Commenting about this disparity, Berenson and Mitchell observed that the low-functioning helpers appeared to be searching for client vulnerabilities rather than strengths. They write, "Strength and, particularly, weakness confrontations are very likely specific helper behaviors which lead directly to helpee improvement or deterioration" (p. 78).

Berenson and Mitchell also observed marked differences in the frequency of experiential confrontations by high- and low-functioning helpers (p. 51). Experiential confrontations focus on "any discrepancy between the helpee and helper's experiencing of the . . . relationship or [on] any discrepancy between the helpee's overt statement about himself and the helpee's inner covert experience of himself or [on] any discrepancy between the helpee and the helper's subjective experience of either the helper or helpee." This low frequency of experiential confrontations by low-functioning helpers ". . . suggests the lows are really not in tune with the helpee's experiences" (p. 51).

Apparently, the constructive use of confrontation and high-level functioning on the facilitative conditions are intertwined. Taking an even stronger stand, Berenson and Mitchell maintain that only those helpers who relate with high levels of the facilitative conditions are "entitled to confront" (pp. 89–93).

Although the research on confrontation is scanty, the technique is hardly new to therapy, and in recent years it has received increasing theoretical attention. Douds and others (1967) assert that "facilitative conditions, techniques, and insight are not enough for effective therapy" (p. 179). Confrontation, they maintain, is essential to positive outcomes. Grinker and his associates (1961) argue further that with clients who lack motivation to change, the therapist who prolongs nurturing transactions beyond the point at which rapport, trust, and positive regard are firmly established instead of helping the client become more aware of the nature of his own responses and behavior may perpetuate dysfunctional behavior. Berne (1964) similarly maintains that at a certain point in the therapeutic relationship, the therapist may deliberately "cross transactions" to stimulate the client to become more aware of the nature of his own responses. "Crossing transactions," as used by Berne, means moving from a complementary "nurturing parent-to-child relationship" to a more reality-oriented, confrontive situation.

Numerous types of confrontation are identified and suggestions made for their use by Egan (1970), Berenson and Mitchell (1974), and Shulman (1971). Kelly (1975) gives guidelines for the effective confrontation, and Hawkins (1976) discusses the use of confrontation in marriage and family counseling. Hawkins also explicates further the relationship between confrontation and self-disclosure and provides a rich discussion on determining when the client is ready for confrontation. These topics will be discussed at length in Chapter Ten.

The Research Scales

We have referred above to research scales that operationalize the dimensions of therapy and specify levels of those dimensions along a continuum ranging from low to high. Here we will introduce the scales briefly. In subsequent chapters devoted to the facilitative conditions, each scale will be delineated in greater detail, and the reader will be provided with exercises that provide practice in recognizing the various levels.

Each scale has levels ranging from 1 (the lowest) to 5 (the highest). One exception is the Empathic Communication Scale, which also includes half-levels (for example, 1.5, 2.5) for purposes of finer discrimination. Level 3.0, the intermediate level, on each scale represents the level believed to be minimally facilitative—that is, the minimal level at which the therapist's response is helpful or therapeutic. A therapist whose mean level of functioning on one of the scales is below 3.0 is regarded as low functioning or low-facilitative on that scale as contrasted to a high-facilitative therapist, whose mean level is higher than 3.0.

THE EMPATHIC COMMUNICATION SCALE

On this scale (presented at length in Chapter Five), the crucial variable is the extent to which the therapist conveys understanding of the feelings the client manifests. On the intermediate level (3.0), the therapist conveys understanding at the same level as the client's expression of feelings; hence, the term *reciprocal empathy* designates this level. Responses that fail to capture the explicit feelings manifested by the client are termed *subtractive* and are rated below level 3.0, depending on how much they subtract from the expressed feelings (verbal or nonverbal). By contrast, other responses may be *additive* (levels 3.5–5.0), in that they add to expressed feelings by identifying implicit or underlying feelings or meanings not verbalized or not recognized by the client.

In abbreviated form, the meanings of the various levels are as follows: 1.0, highly subtractive; 1.5, markedly subtractive; 2.0, moderately subtractive; 2.5, slightly subtractive; 3.0, reciprocal (neither additive nor subtractive); 3.5, slightly additive; 4.0, moderately additive; 4.5, markedly additive; 5.0, highly additive.

THE RESPECT SCALE

At level 3.0 on this scale (detailed in Chapter Seven), the therapist communicates positive concern and respect for the client's feelings and his ability to act constructively on his own problems. The therapist suspends judgment of the client and demonstrates openness and a willingness to enter into a relationship. Level 4.0 involves deep respect for the client manifested in affirming the client's feelings and his capacity to act constructively on his problem. A high level of respect for the client's worth is also demonstrated. At the highest level, 5.0, the deepest respect for the client's worth and potential as a self-determining individual is conveyed. Moreover, after the relationship is well established, the therapist holds the client to the expectations that he achieve his goals and assume responsibility for himself.

Level 1.0 on this scale indicates that the therapist communicates overt disrespect by actively criticizing, dominating the conversation, attempting to impose values or beliefs, or depreciating the client's worth in some other manner. Level 2.0 responses manifest moderate disrespect by according little significance to the feelings, potentials, or experiences of the client. The therapist may ignore the client's expressions or respond in a casual, uninvolved, or passive manner that conveys a lack of interest or concern.

THE AUTHENTICITY SCALE

At level 3.0 on this scale (presented in Chapter Eight), the therapist's responses are not incongruent, defensive, or phony. However, the therapist is not truly open nor does he reveal personal feelings and reactions to the client. Level 2.0 responses are moderately low in authenticity. At this level, the therapist responds in a sterile, "professional" manner. The therapist may also hedge or make statements that are incongruent with his actual feelings and thoughts. At the lowest level, or 1.0, the therapist responds negatively by being defensive or retaliatory when challenged by the client. Striking incongruities and phoniness also characterize level 1.0 responses.

Level 4.0 responses are moderately high in authenticity. The therapist is congruent but may be hesitant or uncomfortable in expressing personal thoughts and feelings. He communicates negative feelings selectively and nondestructively if they serve to strengthen the relationship. The highest level of authenticity, level 5.0, is manifested when the therapist is openly and freely himself in the relationship. All types of feelings are openly shared when they are relevant to the client's needs and situation and when the sharing will facilitate constructive exploration in the helping relationship.

THE CONFRONTATION SCALE

On this scale, level 3.0 represents the minimally facilitative level (presented later in Chapter Ten). At this level the therapist's responses draw attention to or raise questions about inconsistencies and discrepancies in the client's behavior. Level 3.0 responses may also be those formulated to facilitate self-confrontation. Responses rated as moderately low (2.0) on this scale include confrontations that are premature and otherwise poorly timed. Other level 2.0 responses are characterized by the therapist's failure to identify discrepancies and inconsistencies in the client's behavior explicitly. Thus, although the therapist is aware of the inconsistencies, he fails to deal with them directly and reponds instead by mirroring the client's reactions to the problem behavior. At the lowest level, 1.0, the therapist ignores, overlooks, or passively accepts inconsistencies, or he employs confrontations that are abrasive or blaming or otherwise demean the client.

Confrontive responses moderately high (4.0) on the scale focus on and explicitly identify inconsistencies and dysfunctional behavior. The timing is appropriate, and the dignity and self-esteem of the client are protected. At the highest level (5.0), the therapist employs a keen sense of timing in directly confronting inconsistencies. Confrontations entail a high level of respect for the client's growth potential and convey the therapist's caring and helpful intent.

Chapter 2

ＸＯＸＯＸＯＸＯＸＯ ＸＯＸＯＸＯＸＯＸＯＸＯＸＯ

Processes and Phases in Counseling and Psychotherapy

In this chapter, we will discuss the facilitative conditions and techniques aimed at inducing therapeutic change in the context of the major phases of counseling. It is important to keep it in mind that although each of these interpersonal skills and processes plays a role throughout the counseling process, the significance and function of each one varies markedly with the phase of counseling. Consequently, one must understand the varying applications of these skills and processes in order to use them effectively.

We do not intend to elaborately analyze all the various stages constituting the major phases of counseling. That task lies well beyond the scope of this book. Instead, we will show how the interpersonal skills and therapeutic processes introduced in Chapter One are applied differentially throughout the phases of counseling.

Individualization and Systematization in Counseling

To some extent, it is artificial and misleading to divide the counseling process into discrete phases and stages characterized

28

by specific objectives, processes, and behaviors. Counseling, indeed, should not be described as a standardized and unitary process, for such a description reduces it to a rigid, mechanistic, and dehumanizing affair lacking the very characteristics that foster human growth. Rather, counseling is best seen as a highly individual process shaped by the personality and style of the counselor, tailored to the personality, problems, and motivation of the client, and varied according to its setting. Thus each counseling venture, indeed each interview, differs from every other.

Despite its highly individual nature, however, effective counseling contains many systematic elements, and research (Fiedler, 1950; Strupp, 1955) shows that many common threads draw the divergent schools of counseling and psychotherapy together. The novice counselor should bear this unity in mind, seeking diligently to master the fundamentals of effective counseling identified in Chapter One. No one should take the individual nature of counseling as giving license "to do his own thing" and to disregard the empirical knowledge and clinical wisdom that has evolved over many years. Nor should the student seek to become a carbon copy of his mentors, supervisors, or other models. The "use of self" is a powerful tool in counseling, and individual counseling styles are therefore desirable.

In final analysis, then, each budding counselor confronts the challenge of developing an inner core of knowledge and skill and adapting that core to his own personality. But the challenge is difficult, for knowledge and personality are not static. Knowledge has a persistent habit of becoming obsolete. The counselor's knowledge must be open to new input, or the counselor, like his knowledge, is doomed to obsolescence. Furthermore, healthy personalities are always "becoming," and the counselor's style, therefore, should incorporate changes that flow from emerging knowledge, accumulated clinical wisdom, and the personal growth that accrues from maturation and from the richness of human experience from working closely with many people.

Thus the counselor should cultivate the essential qualities of openness and flexibility. Competent practice—the foremost ethical responsibility of a helping professional—requires these qualities, for competence is relative to the knowledge and technical skill extant in the profession. A counselor may be competent at one point, yet slide into incompetence a few years later by failing to keep abreast of advances in knowledge and skill and to modify his practice accordingly. One caution, however, deserves mention. The counselor is urged to be wary of accepting new theories and techniques that have not been rigorously tested in practice or research. Theoretical fads in counseling and psychotherapy come and go fairly frequently, and the authors have observed numerous practitioners over the years, many lacking fundamental counseling skills, who have eagerly jumped from one bandwagon to another, only to be disenchanted as each new approach fails to produce the miracles its proponents tout (Thorne, 1968). Openness does not mean gullibility. Openness, indeed, should be tempered with skepticism.

The Major Phases of the Therapeutic Process

We divide the processes of counseling or psychotherapy into three major phases: (1) the initial, or early, phase; (2) the middle, or change-oriented, phase; and (3) the terminal phase. Although each phase has distinct objectives and involves different processes, the phases are not sharply demarcated, and the processes applied in the therapy differ more in frequency and intensity than in quality. Empathic communication, for example, is important throughout the course of counseling, but it plays a critical role during the early phase and a relatively minor role in later stages of the change-oriented phase.

In the following discussion, we will discuss each of the facilitative conditions and change-oriented processes in relationship to each of the major phases.

THE EARLY PHASE

The early phase of counseling is crucial, for unless the counselor succeeds in engaging the client during this phase, the client is likely to stop seeing the counselor. Moreover, the patterns of interaction established during the early phase tend to persist during subsequent phases of counseling. Engaging the client successfully means that the counselor must develop rapport as well as adequate levels of trust and confidence in the client. At the point of intake, clients vary widely in their motivation to use counseling, but the degree of motivation to continue counseling after the first interview is determined largely by the degree of rapport achieved during that initial interview. Any client's motivation to continue depends on the client's experience in looking the counselor over during the initial interview. A negative experience may keep a highly motivated client from coming back, while a positive experience may well induce a poorly motivated client to return.

Empathic communication during the early phase. Rapport, a primary objective of the early phase of counseling, is fostered by the counselor's use of empathic communication. For rapport to develop, the client must feel that he is understood and accepted as a person. Empathic communication contributes to understanding and acceptance with messages that, in effect, say, "I am with you; I hear and understand what you are telling me and what you are experiencing." In all interviews, but particularly in initial ones, the counselor must be keenly attuned not only to the client's verbal messages but to nonverbal signals as well. Many clients are intensely uncomfortable in sitting down face-to-face with a stranger in whom they must confide personal and sometimes painful information, emotions, and experiences in order to solve their problems. Understandably, many clients find it difficult to begin, and struggle in their search for words to express themselves. For some clients, the struggle is further compounded by strong distrust or by a fear that the counselor will condemn, ridicule, or reject them.

Empathic responses to nonverbal cues indicating intense discomfort, anxiety, or fear may break the ice and help the client reveal his reasons for coming. Responding to the client's quivering lips, tight facial muscles, or uneasy shifting about in the chair with a warm expression of concern such as, "It was difficult for you to come," or "I can sense how hard it is for you to get started," often elicits a knowing and appreciative acknowledgement. Beginning where the client is by responding empathically serves to reduce the client's anxiety and, even more importantly, fosters an initial impression of the counselor as a sensitive, concerned, and understanding person. Sowing the seeds of rapport in such a fashion is the first step toward the goal of creating a safe climate wherein the client can risk revealing more of his problems, feelings, needs, thoughts, and behavior.

It takes much more than an empathic opening response, however, to achieve this goal. As the client begins to test the climate by sending up trial balloons in the form of verbal expressions, the counselor must continue to demonstrate understanding and acceptance through additional empathic responses, which will include both verbal reflections of client feelings and nonverbal facilitative responses, such as attentive listening and understanding nods of the head, which convey the message, "I am following you; please continue."

It is important to note that feedback that accurately reflects the feelings the client expresses best conveys empathic understanding. For example, the response, "I gather you're feeling very discouraged and overwhelmed by your son's truancy and rebelliousness," conveys far more understanding of the client's emotional state than the words, "I understand how you feel." The latter response, in fact, often indicates that the counselor has not explored the client's feelings sufficiently to genuinely understand them.

Continued empathic responses by the counselor tend to reduce threat and lower the defenses, permitting more thorough exploration of the client's problems and expectations. When the client's tensions and fears have been supplanted by trust and confidence in the competence and humanness of the counselor, a primary goal of the early phase—to build a sound working relationship—has been accomplished.

The length of the early phase of counseling varies widely from client to client according to the individual's level of interpersonal functioning. Clients with high levels usually require only short periods of testing and may plunge into exploring their problems in depth after only a few minutes of looking the counselor over. Other clients, however, particularly those who characteristically maintain considerable distance in interpersonal relationships as a result of long-standing fears and distrust of themselves and others, may test and probe for weeks or even months before they can bear the risk of opening themselves to another. With such clients, a great deal of patience and persistence is required of the counselor. Pushing for client self-disclosure before a working relationship is established may alienate the client, needlessly prolong the period of testing, or if the pressure is strong, actually produce psychological casualties (Lieberman, Yalom, and Miles, 1973).

Empathic communication is a potent force in overcoming the fears and distrust plaguing alienated persons (Anderson, 1975).

Anderson also maintains that empathic relationships foster the capacity to give love as well. Empathy for another involves understanding, which in turn flows from a desire to understand. It is this desire to understand that conveys our concern, our caring for another, and that, in final analysis, is what the client is testing during this early phase of the encounter. Only as he experiences this caring, will the alienated person venture from his self-imposed protective shell.

Empathic communication also is crucial in working with involuntary or captive clients and with those who have been pressured, often by an ultimatum, into seeing a professional. Such situations typically include counseling in mental-health or correctional institutions, probation and parole work, protective-service work in child-welfare settings, and work with adolescents or adults who have been ordered or coerced to seek help by the courts, parents, or marital partners. During initial contacts, such clients generally lack positive motivation to use professional help, and they feel angry, resentful, and perhaps bitter about having to see the helping professional. These reactions often are manifested in overt hostility, sullen and uncooperative behavior, or obsequious compliance.

Establishing a working relationship with an involuntary client is difficult at best, but empathic communication again is an indispensable tool. Before the client can acknowledge that a problem exists and explore it, he must first release and work through negative feelings about seeing the counselor in opposition to his own wishes. Beginning where the client is by conveying empathy with and acceptance of the client's negative feelings helps the client ventilate those feelings. As the client releases his hostility and resentment toward those who precipitated his referral and toward the counselor, he frees himself from their grasp and becomes amenable to exploring his difficulties. This will occur, however, only if the counselor is empathic and avoids both trying to persuade the client that he needs help and confronting the client prematurely with the reality of his part in the problems.

Empathic responsiveness helps defuse or neutralize hostility. Empathic responses such as, "I can see how you'd be mad as blazes about having to come here under threat," convey understanding of the client's reaction and foster a positive image of the counselor opposed to the preconceived punitive and authoritarian image the

client brings to the initial interview. However, empathizing with
and accepting the client's feelings should not be confused with
agreeing with or condoning the client's views. The counselor must
express empathic understanding from a neutral standpoint, avoiding the appearance of siding with either the client or with those
toward whom his antagonism is directed. The use of empathy and
acceptance with involuntary and inadequately motivated clients is
extensively discussed and illustrated by Wolberg (1967, pp. 528–
545). Resistance will be more extensively discussed in Chapters
Eight and Nine.

Empathic communication in the early phase of counseling
serves the vital purposes of facilitating the development of a working relationship and fostering the climate of understanding necessary to communication and self-disclosure, thereby setting the stage
for deeper exploration of feelings during subsequent phases. These
purposes are best accomplished by using a reciprocal level of empathy—that is, responding to the client's feelings on basically the
same level. Thus the counselor neither subtracts nor adds appre-
ciably to the feelings or meaning the client manifests. On the scale
of empathic communication, empathic responses should fall in the
intermediate range from 3.0 to 3.5. Responses in this range capture
feelings experienced by the client at the conscious level or slightly
beyond. The goal of responding at the reciprocal level is to convey
understanding and interest at a level that does not threaten the
client. Reciprocal empathy and the Empathic Communication
Scale will be discussed in Chapter Five.

Additive empathic responses, those ranging from 3.5 to 5.0
on the Empathic Communication Scale, exceed the level of feelings
and meanings expressed by the client. Such responses serve to
expand the client's awareness of underlying feelings, meanings, and
goals of behavior. Pursuing these objectives during the early phase
of counseling is counterproductive. Any attempt to uncover feelings
beyond the client's awareness before a working relationship is firmly
established tends to mobilize resistance and may precipitate premature termination (Hollis, 1968).

Respect during the early phase. The facilitative condition of respect also plays a vital role in fostering rapport during the early
phase of counseling. Many clients, as noted earlier, enter counseling
with feelings of guilt and shame and failure, discouragement with

self, and fears that the counselor will perceive them as weak, inadequate, immoral, stupid, or worthless. Obviously, to create a climate of trust wherein the client can risk revealing the very aspects of his personality, feelings, and behavior he fears to reveal, the counselor must consistently respond in a warm, accepting, and nonjudgmental manner that conveys respect, no matter what the client's problem and his past or present behavior. In essence, respect requires the counselor to communicate good will toward the client. An extensive discussion of the ingredients of respect, the Respect Scale, and training exercises will be found in Chapter Seven.

During the early phase of counseling, the counselor does best to exhibit respect for the client at level 3 of the Respect Scale (see Chapter Seven). At this level, the counselor conveys a positive and understanding attitude toward the client, suspending all negative feelings, attitudes, or judgments. In Rogers's (1957) words, we extend "unconditional positive regard" to the client. Respect does not prevent the counselor from having opinions about the rightness or wrongness and advisability or inadvisability of the client's actions, nor does it rule out positive or negative reactions toward different clients. The counselor is a human being with feelings, values, preferences, and attitudes. The important point about respect is that these human qualities must be disciplined in the helping process so that negative reactions are suspended in the interest of forming a working relationship. Relating to clients with respect also fosters the development of self-respect, a quality essential to sound mental health and deficient in many clients.

Exploring problems. Once rapport is established, the second major objective of counseling arises: exploring the problem thoroughly with the client and deciding with him whether counseling can produce the outcome he wants. Accomplishing this goal involves weighing the client's problem, expectations, level of functioning, and motivational level against the competencies of the counselor and the type of services sanctioned by the agency. These professional factors are critical, of course. If the problem calls for skills beyond the counselor's or services outside the agency's function, like prescribing medication or providing intensive psychotherapy, referral to another professional or another agency will likely be indicated.

Empathic communication is vital to exploration both for the

reasons cited earlier and because it paves the way into the client's emotions. How the client feels about the problem affects the problem greatly, and in many instances the emotions themselves are the central problem, a point we will discuss further in Chapter Four. Empathic communication facilitates the "drawing out" of the client's feelings, fostering self-disclosure and self-exploration. As the counselor elicits and explores emotions and the client expresses and experiences them, both are better able to discern the part the emotions play in the client's problem.

Eliciting and following the client's feelings, of course, are not the only skills involved in the exploration process. Relating exclusively to the client's feelings can result in aimless wandering in an emotional quagmire. Feelings, by their very nature, are highly subjective, and an assessment based solely on the client's subjective views and feelings can be highly distorted. Discerning the client's subjective world of experience is crucial to understanding his problem, but an adequate assessment of that problem and the client's level of functioning requires additional information, often very concrete in nature.

Even to understand the client's emotions, the counselor must elicit specific relevant information. It is important to keep in mind that clients tend to speak in generalities, particularly during the initial interviews, and that generalities can be very misleading. A client of one of the authors sought marriage counseling because she was certain her husband did not love her and she felt depressed and lonely as a result. Aware that the feelings the woman expressed involved a conclusion or interpretation, the counselor, after reflecting her feelings of hurt and rejection, probed for the details of the marital interaction on which she based her feelings. Asked for recent examples that indicated her husband's lack of love, the woman informed the counselor that her husband never wanted to take her anyplace. Again, realizing that this elaboration lacked specificity, the counselor, after reflecting the woman's hurt and frustration, requested specific examples of her husband's refusals. The client then explained that her husband refused to take her to a movie the previous Tuesday evening. Further requests for specific interactional details, expressed as a desire to understand better exactly what had happened, yielded the explanation that her husband was willing to take her out but could not because the only theater in the small rural town they lived in was closed on Tuesdays. Additional exploration along similar lines soon made it apparent that this client had a serious thought disorder, projecting feelings of worthlessness onto her husband, who in fact appeared to care for her and had tried hard but unsuccessfully to please her. In this situation, both the client's subjective feelings of hurt and rejection elicited by empathic communication and specific factual information yielded by probing responses were essential to a balanced understanding of the client's problem. This type of communication, termed specificity of response or concreteness, is discussed further in Chapter Five.

Additional interviewing skills, including open-ended responses ("Tell me more about that") and pointed questions ("How many children do you have?"), are needed to elicit factual information essential to understanding the client's problems. The counselor's role goes beyond eliciting this kind of information, however; it should facilitate expression and self-disclosure by the client, a task accomplished most effectively by responsive communication, especially empathic communication. This fact is perhaps best expressed by the principle that the richness of information and self-disclosure the client provides is inversely proportional to the number of questions the counselor asks. The weaknesses and limitations of gaining information by excessive questioning are discussed in the next chapter, which deals with counterproductive patterns of communication.

Goals and expectations. The client's goals and expectations must be explored during the early phase to determine whether they are appropriate and can be achieved, to help the client modify any unrealistic expectations, and to clarify counselor and client roles. Many clients, especially those who are naive about counseling and psychotherapy, bring to the initial interview misconceptions about the helping process that must be discussed and skillfully handled if the client is to be constructively engaged. It is not uncommon for the client to impute to the counselor unlimited wisdom and power that can somehow be dispensed magically to solve his difficulties immediately. Parents of a wayward and rebellious adolescent, for example, may expect the counselor to make the child "shape up" in predefined ways without exploring or modifying their own behavior. Marital partners often have similar expectations, requesting the marital therapist to influence the other partner to be more responsible, less violent, more loving, or less critical. Other clients may present themselves in a childlike, dependent manner, pledging cooperation if the counselor will only tell them what to do. Thus various clients may anticipate and perceive the counselor as a parent, a stooge, a threat, a possession, an absolver of guilt, an idol, an authority, a stabilizer, or a friend.

Clients also come with varied expectations about what they will concentrate on in counseling: symptoms, oneself, the past, others, sex, and so forth. These expectations vary with the client's social class, and the counselor must be careful not to impose his perceptual set or problem-solving style on the client. Research findings reported by Aronson and Overall (1966) indicate that clients from lower socioeconomic levels generally expect more action, direction, and support from helping professionals than do middle-class clients. These authors also report that middle-class clients, in general, are more sophisticated about the therapeutic process, recognizing that "much of the initiation and direction in a dynamic interview must come from the patient" (p. 40). When the expectations of client and therapist differ, they must be acknowledged and discussed, or else the client, according to Aronson and Overall, will be likely to doubt the therapist's ability and will suffer a counterproductive increase in anxiety. Unacknowledged discrepancies in expectations, these authors believe, may account in part for the well-documented (Baum, 1966) higher rate of premature discontinuance of lower-class clients as compared to middle-class clients. *What the counselor does must make sense to the client.* Observance of this cardinal principle will bridge the gap of discrepant expectations.

For example, in a study involving research interviews with clients who were dissatisfied with service given them for interpersonal problems, Mayer and Timms (1969) found that when some clients tried to make sense of the counselor's behavior, they reasoned that the counselor's passivity and failure to give concrete advice stemmed from a lack of interest and desire to help. Other clients concluded that the counselors did not understand their difficulties and consequently failed to offer effective and realistic help. The reasons clients attributed to the counselor's failure to act in ways they thought appropriate led Mayer and Timms to conclude that the clients, most of whom were working class, were almost totally unaware that the counselor's approach to problem solving differed fundamentally from their own. Interestingly, many of the dissatisfied clients had not clearly indicated their expectations to the counselor, underscoring further the necessity for counselors to explore carefully this dimension of the client's request for help. Arguing that the high rate of discontinuance by lower-class clients is due to discrepancies in expectations and styles of problem solving, the authors characterize the situation as "two persons ostensibly playing the same game but actually to rules that are private" (p. 37).

Clarifying the helping role. From these and similar research findings several guidelines for dealing with discrepant expectations can be drawn. First, the counselor must be sufficiently flexible to adapt his style to clients whose expectations and problem-solving approaches differ markedly from his own. He must not expect the client to do all the adjusting. The counselor must be able to take a more active and directive role than is typically required in work with middle-class clients.

Second, when the counselor encounters unrealistic expectations, he must skillfully help the client understand that he is not unwilling or uninterested in helping. In fact, the counselor can say that he would like to help the client in the way the client wants, but that it is simply impossible. The counselor may then detail ways in which he can be of help and explain how they may prove helpful in the long run. The counselor's empathy is crucial in "tuning in" keenly to the client's reactions to these clarifications. If the client acts confused or disappointed, the counselor will need to respond to these feelings and attempt further to help the client with them. Otherwise the client will be left to wrestle with them alone, a struggle often culminating in discontinuance.

A third guideline deals with how the counselor can help and how the client can use that help most effectively. Many clients know little about the counseling process and are bewildered by the counselor's behavior, which is alien to their own problem-solving patterns. Taking the time to clarify roles and to explain what the client can expect has been demonstrated to be of considerable value in lowering discontinuance rates of lower-class clients. The research findings of Hoehn-Saric and his colleagues (1964) document that patients prepared for therapy by a "role induction interview" continue at a higher rate and do better than patients in a control group who receive no special preparation.

A fourth guideline taken from the research findings is that the counselor must explore the client's problems and goals thoroughly, taking care that he perceives them as the client does and checking with the client from time to time to make sure that their perceptions continue to coincide. Stark (1959) reports that therapy is frequently discontinued because the counselor, working from his own formulations and not the client's, initiates the problem-solving process prematurely, promoting action and behavior change before the client feels himself ready. Thus it is imperative that the counselor regularly check his perceptions against the client's.

Assessing and enhancing client motivation. Another aspect of the exploratory process involves assessing the client's motivation and goals. Experts agree that the motivational level is probably the single factor most crucial to successful counseling outcomes, an idea supported by research findings (Ripple, 1964).

Prerequisite to adequate motivation is at least a minimal level of discomfort, self-dissatisfaction, anxiety, or—to use Rogers's (1957) original term—incongruence. In other words, the client's usual equilibrium, or steady state, must be disrupted to such an extent that the client perceives that something must be changed to make the discomfort tolerable. The stress producing the discomfort may take many forms, including the need to make a vital and difficult decision, grief stemming from loss of a loved one or of a job, marital conflict, parent-child difficulties, inadequate school or job performance, failure to live up to self-expectations, inability to adjust to changes in one's life situation, depression, interpersonal difficulties, arrest for violation of the law, severe guilt, and any of a host of other common stresses.

Many clients, however, manifest inadequate motivation. Some may see a counselor out of curiosity because a friend has talked about positive experiences in therapy. Others may experience distress and have a desire for change but lack the determination to do something about it. Perlman (1957) characterizes such a situation as the client's having "want" but lacking will. Willingness to assume responsibility for acting on the problem is indispensable to counseling. Wanting without willing is tantamount to wishful thinking and will not generate the energy needed for movement in counseling. The problem, it must be emphasized, is the client's, and the counselor cannot solve it for him. Whenever a client manifests inadequate motivation, it is essential to test whether sufficient motivation can be generated to justify continuing with the client. Efforts to continue counseling with an inadequately motivated client are generally doomed to failure.

When the client fails to acknowledge a problem, as happens with some involuntary clients, Reid and Epstein (1972) recommend negotiating with the client a brief period of "problem search" limited to a maximum of two interviews. During the problem search, the counselor and client explore many aspects of the client's life, and the counselor is alert to areas in which the client may be experiencing some pressure or discomfort. Empathic skills are required to "tune in" to painful emotions and to assist the client in expanding awareness of emotions he may have overlooked or suppressed. If at the end of the problem search, the client still fails to acknowledge any difficulties, counseling is discontinued by previous agreement. To continue without adequate motivation, according to Reid and Epstein, is futile. We heartily agree. Discontinuing therapy, however, does not mean that the counselor agrees with the client's view that there are no problems. The counselor may, in fact, be quite candid in sharing perceptions, making it clear that termination is based on the client's perceptions and that continuing under such circumstances is futile. The client may be invited to return if his perceptions of the situation change. Many clients handled in this way do return later more open and less resistant than before.

Some agencies, however, bear a legal responsibility to provide services to clients whose behavior is offensive or potentially threatening to the public interest. In such agencies, which include various institutional settings as well as probation, parole, and child-welfare departments, the professional staff often do not have the option of discontinuing service if the client is poorly motivated. The interests of society, including the protection of children from parental neglect or abuse, must be safeguarded. In these situations, the impetus for service often derives more from the authority of the law vested in the agency and in the person of the professional worker than from the client's motivation to change. Often the only motivation of clients in such situations is to achieve release from an institution, to avoid incarceration or prosecution, or to avoid losing the custody of children. The professional worker employed in these settings must possess not only the skills we have already discussed but also techniques for "reaching out" and using authority benevolently. Those readers who wish to learn more about the unique aspects of practice in these settings are referred to the writings of Goldberg (1975), Herre (1965), Studt (1959), and Yelaja (1965).

Negotiating a contract. The final objective of the early phase is to reach an explicit understanding with the client about "where we go from here." In some instances, the practitioner will refer the client to other agencies or to other helping professionals. In other instances, the decision may be to discontinue counseling. In still other instances, the client, the counselor, or both may not be sure whether to continue or to stop. In such cases, an extended exploratory or trial period of specified length, usually just a few interviews, may be negotiated. Some clients may need time to think it over before committing themselves to further counseling. The client's wish for time to think should be respected, although the counselor may offer to help the client explore further the various factors involved in his struggle to decide. Attempts to persuade or pressure the client to continue are counterproductive and to be avoided. Often clients who agree to continue in opposition to their own feelings may cancel or fail to keep future appointments, thus expressing indirectly the feelings they could not express verbally.

With those clients who are motivated to continue counseling—and this will be the majority of those who seek help voluntarily—the early phase will conclude with the negotiation of a contract about the goals, the respective roles of the client and the counselor, the frequency of interviews, the number of interviews (when time limits are employed), the nature of the interviews (individual or conjoint—that is, including other family members—or a combination of both), and the financial arrangements for payment of fees. The degree of formality of the contract will vary with the agency's policy and the counselor's preferences. Some agencies use a written contract, signed by the client and the counselor specifying all the conditions of the therapy. Others reach merely a verbal understanding. Regardless of the nature of the contract, the observance of certain guidelines will help enhance client motivation and avoid the hazard of the client's and counselor's working at cross-purposes, which may cause premature termination.

The goals set must be agreed on mutually. If the client has one set of goals in mind and the counselor another, the client is likely to become disillusioned soon, and, for good reason, to terminate counseling. Thus goals should be negotiated openly, and final authority for choosing the goals should rest with the client. This does not mean that the process is unilateral or that the counselor should withhold his impressions. On the contrary, the counselor willingly shares impressions with the client as it is his responsibility to do so. Counselor feedback, of course, is given indirectly through reflective and exploratory responses and directly through the expression of opinions. These responses both sharpen the client's perceptions of his problems and influence his thinking about goals. The counselor may have impressions and suggestions which, if not included in the client's goals, should be presented. If the counselor offers these impressions and the rationales behind them as ideas to consider, the client will be much more receptive than if they are presented as dogmatic assertions.

From this process of mutual negotiation, the participants should emerge with a definite understanding of the direction and focus counseling will take. Excellent discussions of goal selection and contract negotiation will be found in Gottlieb and Stanley (1967), Reid and Epstein (1972), Mahrer (1967), and Thorne (1968). Seabury (1976) discusses the uses, limitations, and abuses of contracts.

Other guidelines in goal-setting relate to the nature of goals. A first and basic principle is that the goals must be achievable. Based on research findings, one prominent social worker (Reid, 1970) concludes that helping professionals in the past overestimated the capacity of people to change and consequently formulated overly ambitious and unachievable goals. Tyler (1960), a prominent theoretician of counseling, takes the same position, advocating a move to "minimum change therapy." These writings make apparent that goals have been formulated idealistically rather than realistically. Perhaps one reason for this is that earlier goal-setting tended to be a counselor-centered process that excluded mutuality and input from the client.

A number of criteria must be considered in setting realistic goals: the personality strengths of the client; the opportunities, resources and constraints provided by the client's environment; the time frame of counseling; and the competence of the counselor relative to the goals sought by the client. Perlman (1957) provides an excellent discussion of these and other factors. In addition, the counselor must consider the range of goals. Some clients present a wide array of problems extending into many facets of their functioning. Effective problem-solving, however, requires sharp and continued focus, and tackling many diffuse problems with a shotgun approach will only dissipate the therapeutic effort. For this reason, after the array of problems has been explored, it is important for client and counselor to determine which problems have highest priority. Generally, two or three major problems are more than enough to consume considerable counseling time and effort. Moreover, if the client makes considerable progress on a few of his difficulties, he may gain the skill and confidence to tackle other problems on his own. This phenomenon has been referred to as the "spread of effect."

Still another guideline in setting goals relates to the specificity with which they are stated. Based on research findings, writers in both social work and psychology have criticized practitioners for stating goals in such general terms that the results cannot be measured, making it impossible to evaluate counseling results effectively (Bandura, 1969). Moreover, when goals are not specific, the lack of a sense of direction sends counseling into an aimless drift or confuses the client (Reid and Epstein, 1972; Schmidt, 1969).

In a broad sense, problem exploration and goal setting are interdependent, and the latter can be no more specific than the former. Problem exploration begins with the eliciting of the client's difficulties, which may range from a single narrowly defined problem at one extreme to a huge heap of general difficulties at the other. At first, clients usually state their problems in general terms (for example, "I have trouble making decisions," or "I don't get along with people"), but subsequent exploration leads to increasing specificity. Only when problems (excesses or deficits) have been pinpointed in such areas as behavior, affect, sensation, imagery, cognition, and the environmental-interpersonal context, can goals be stated in operational or behavioral terms and appropriate treatment interventions selected (Lazarus, 1963; Kanfer and Saslow,

1969). Once goals and treatment are set, the counselor and the client are ready to enter the next major phase of counseling.

Authenticity during the early phase. Before we consider the second major phase of counseling, we should clarify the functions of authenticity, relational immediacy (managing therapeutically the client's reactions to the therapist), counselor self-disclosures, and confrontation during the early phase. Each of these dimensions has a low-key role during the early phase, playing a major part during the middle (change-oriented) phase of counseling.

Authenticity during the early phase is demonstrated more by the absence of phoniness and inauthenticity than by fully authentic counselor behavior. The counselor also demonstrates his authenticity in being open and unevasive to feedback from the client. Counselor self-disclosure—that is, revealing personal feelings, reactions, and experiences—however, is kept to a minimum until trust is well established. Otherwise, the client may misinterpret the counselor's motives or be threatened by what he perceives as a move toward possessive closeness by the counselor. Thus the client's need to keep a safe distance is respected until a working relationship has evolved. The level of authenticity manifested by the counselor during the early phase hovers around level 3 on the research scale (see Chapter Eight).

As to relational immediacy, the counseling relationship in the early phase is not strong enough to permit exploration of the client's here-and-now experience and reactions in the counselor-client interaction. The counselor, therefore, avoids exploring or interpreting relational immediacy. One exception to this guideline, however, should be noted. When the client's strong and apparent reactions to the counselor block exploration, the counselor will need to digress and to explore those feelings with the client. If, for example, the client is very uncomfortable and preoccupied with a resemblance between the counselor and another person of significance in his life, exploration will be needed to help the client to discriminate among his perceptions and to divest the feelings that are impairing free interaction in the interview. The exploration should be no longer nor deeper than necessary.

Confrontation during the early phase. A powerful change-oriented technique, confrontation is largely contraindicated during the early phase. The premature use of confrontation may, in fact, undercut the establishment of a working relationship. Until the client is convinced of the counselor's good will, he may distort or misinterpret the counselor's intent. He may take confrontations, therefore, as a reflection of blame, criticism, or rejection from the counselor.

Some high-level functioning clients, however, may demonstrate a readiness for mild confrontations during the early phase by focusing voluntarily on discrepancies or inconsistencies in their behavior. It is critical to note, however, that such instances entail a self-confrontation initiated by the client rather than an actual counselor confrontation. Even in these instances, the mild confrontation is more probing and tentative than direct (level 3).

The hazards of premature confrontations are documented by the research findings cited in Chapter One. In addition, Hollis reports that a major factor in early discontinuance of marriage counseling was "the worker's efforts to promote understanding prematurely in a way that involved anxiety for the clients" (1968, p. 171).

One exception to the general contraindication for confrontation during the early phase involves clients with major character disorders who deliberately attempt to dupe, deceive, or otherwise manipulate the counselor. Permitting such ploys to pass without discussion does not help establish a relationship because the client is not likely to develop confidence in or respect for a person who is easily played for a sucker. Rather, the client will perceive the counselor as ineffectual and gullible. The counselor thus is well advised to be open and authentic in gently but firmly confronting the client and expressing his concern that little or nothing can be accomplished if the client persists with such avoidance behavior. Such confrontations may actually foster the development of a relationship inasmuch as these clients tend to respect a person who sees through their manipulative behavior.

THE MIDDLE (CHANGE-ORIENTED) PHASE

Once the objectives of the early phase have been accomplished, the helping process enters the middle phase. This phase constitutes the heart of counseling, for the therapeutic effort now concentrates on accomplishing the goals earlier agreed upon. These goals aim at relieving the pressures on the client, thereby freeing his energies for satisfying and productive living. Embodied in this overall goal are the primary objectives of expanding the client's awareness of the barriers or dynamics involved in his impasse and of working through and surmounting these barriers, thereby developing new and functional behaviors.

In those instances in which the exploration of the early phase reveals that the client's difficulties appear to result from external forces and can best be solved by interventions aimed at structural changes in the client's environment, the first objective of the middle phase will already have been largely achieved. In such instances, the middle phase will consist largely of planning and implementing changes, and the focus on intrapsychic forces will be minimal. If the client needs certain resources that are unavailable or which for some reason have been denied him, the worker may assume the role of broker, mediator, or advocate. These roles and the "structural change model" are discussed by Middleman and Goldberg (1974), and any further elaboration is beyond the scope of this book. It should be noted, however, that effective structural interventions require mastery of the very interpersonal skills that constitute the focus of the present volume. Furthermore, as the counselor and client engage in externally oriented activities, emotional reactions by the client are common, and their therapeutic management may be indispensable to achieving maximally successful results. For example, exploration may reveal that a client has been denied medical services or employment opportunities as a result of discrimination by a given institution or staff member. The counselor may determine that mediation or advocacy on the client's behalf is the most appropriate course of action. Before proceeding, however, the counselor must obtain the client's consent and participation. In exploring the client's response to the proposed course of action, the counselor will commonly encounter a strong emotional reaction from the client, which poses a barrier to action and must be resolved before action can proceed. Similarly, another client may manifest a physical symptom that requires hospitalization. Effecting hospitalization, however, is not often a simple task, for some clients may have markedly irrational fears, superstitious beliefs, distrust of doctors or other similar emotional reactions that must be explored and resolved before they will consent to hospitalization.

Expanding awareness. The barriers to change vary from client to client and situation to situation. For example, virtual paralysis in deciding on a career may be rooted in many factors. One client's lack of a decision may result from insufficient information about and awareness of various occupations, personal aptitudes, and interests. Another client, however, may possess adequate information, but be torn between following his personal preference and currying parental approval, which may be a powerful force in his life. Still another client may be struggling with forces rooted somewhat more deeply in the personality such as fears of failure masquerading as indecision. These fears, similarly, may be an offshoot of even deeper and more pervasive feelings of inadequacy and massive self-doubt.

Likewise, the impasses clients experience differ markedly in nature. Many clients, for example, are alienated from others and request help in overcoming painful loneliness. The causes of these difficulties may be easily discerned in some instances as, for example, with aged clients who are geographically separated from loved ones and are hampered by poor physical mobility and limited access to transportation. By contrast, other lonely clients are shy, self-conscious, and so socially inhibited that their relationships are unfulfilling. These personality traits may result from social ineptness produced by inadequate socialization opportunities during critical periods of development or may derive from deep-seated feelings of inferiority rooted in early-life deficiencies in parental love and emotional sustenance. Still others may be lonely because their usual behavior, such as biting sarcasm, temper outbursts, unreasonable demands, clinging dependency, excessive aggressiveness, or ingratiating behavior, is abrasive or offensive.

Whatever the nature of the client's difficulties, the objective of this first major aspect of the middle phase is to help the client expand his awareness of the forces behind the impasse. This goal is very important. People too little aware of the basic nature of their difficulties waste time and energy fighting phantoms—working on the wrong problems—using avoidance patterns that only perpetuate or exacerbate the difficulties, or becoming discouraged, overwhelmed, and sometimes depressed.

As both the client and the counselor gain additional and more precise understanding of the client's difficulties through progressively deeper exploration, the original formulations of the nature of these difficulties may be revised considerably. Deeper exploration of the client's world of experience often brings to light newly discovered feelings, interpersonal themes, patterns of behavior, and factual information that may lead both the counselor and client to view the difficulties from a perspective far different from the original. If the assessment of difficulties thus changes, the goals will be modified accordingly. A female client, for example, who originally expressed resentment and indignation toward men for exploiting her sexually, may, as a result of thorough exploration, gain awareness into how she yields sexually to men to avoid the pain involved in displeasing them by resisting their sexual overtures. Such insights make it possible for people to free themselves from immobilizing patterns of thought, feeling, and behavior. Without insight a person is at the mercy of unknown forces.

It is important to recognize that insight is not the basic goal of counseling or psychotherapy. Rather, insight is a means to the end of change, whether in the environment, in the client, or in both. Obviously one can ask whether insight is necessary to change and, if it is, how much insight is needed. As to the necessity of insight, various positions have been taken by theorists from divergent schools of thought. On one extreme, the psychoanalytic point of view is that changes without insight are superficial or symptomatic at best, tantamount to taking aspirin for chronic headaches. Thus, unless the basic causes of the problems are discovered and resolved, the symptoms may be expected to recur, perhaps in somewhat modified form. The goal of psychoanalysis is, therefore, to explore, analyze, and work through the nuclear causes of conflicts, enabling the patient to replace dysfunctional patterns rooted in the past with functional patterns based in the present.

At the other extreme is the position of the behavior therapists, who minimize the role of insight, considering it informative but not necessarily remedial. Behavior therapists concern themselves with analyzing problem behaviors and deficiencies in behavioral repertoires and with developing shaping programs that extinguish problem behaviors and strengthen or develop functional behaviors. Insight into the historical roots of problems is irrelevant. Of basic importance in behavior modification is an analysis and specification of current reinforcers that sustain dysfunctional behaviors and of available reinforcers that can be used to promote functional behaviors. Thus it is behavior that is important, not deep-seated causes. Enduring changes in behavior can be effected without modifying psychic structure. Indeed, beneficial cognitive and emotional changes may occur, according to exponents of this theory, as a byproduct of behavior changes. In other words, action changes feeling and thought, and not—as the psychoanalysts would have it—the other way around.

Many schools of thought occupy a position between the psychoanalysts and the behavior therapists. The authors take such an intermediate position, maintaining that there is partial validity to both points of view and that practitioners should be sufficiently knowledgeable and flexible to incorporate both methods, applying them in a creative, highly individual manner as circumstances and the needs of the client require. Insight, in our view, paves the way for change by helping the client realize that his difficulties can be understood as a product of the interplay of identifiable factors that can be changed, freeing the client from believing that he is at the mercy of mysterious forces beyond his control. Furthermore, awareness enables an individual to take corrective action and to keep similar difficulties from recurring in the future. However, insight is clearly not enough, and must be followed with techniques that foster behavioral change.

As to how much insight is required, the law of parsimony has particular application. In other words, insight should be pursued only as far as it is essential to removing the barriers to change. The counselor's ethical responsibility is to assist clients as rapidly as possible, and in some instances little insight is required before the client can undertake corrective actions. For example, considering the alternatives available for solving a problem may identify courses of action that have not occurred to the client before, and this new awareness may be all the client needs. In other instances, as a client initiates a potentially remedial course of action, he may encounter formidable new barriers to change in the forms of anxiety, fear, or even panic. These emotional reactions may so immobilize the client that new insights are required before further action is possible.

At this point, the authors' assertion that the various phases of counseling are neither discrete nor mutually exclusive should be obvious to the reader. Action, as we just noted, often precipitates emotions that necessitate further exploration and resolution. Change-oriented actions may be initiated even during the early phase in some cases, and even though relationship-building particularly characterizes the early phase, efforts to sustain the working relationship continue through the remainder of counseling. Our point is that despite its essentially systematic nature, counseling is implemented in a highly fluid manner. Guidelines must be adapted to the nuances of each client, each problem, and to the constantly changing dynamics of each individual interview.

An important aspect of expanding awareness or gaining insight is identifying themes, or patterns of thought, feeling, and behavior. As the client begins to work toward the goals negotiated during the early phase, the counselor assists in exploring all of the facets of the client's experiences that pertain to his difficulties. Empathic communication, relational immediacy, confrontation, and authentic feedback play vital roles in expanding the client's awareness. (Levels of these facilitative dimensions during the middle phase are discussed later in this chapter.)

As the experiencing of the client is examined in detail over the span of several interviews, a redundancy (Watzlawick, Beavin, and Jackson, 1967) of certain feelings, thoughts, and behaviors will become apparent to the trained observer. Some clients, in fact, become spontaneously aware of recurring dysfunctional thoughts, feelings, and behaviors experienced in separate but similar situations. This insight often has a dramatic "Eureka!" impact, precipitating energetic efforts by the client to liberate himself from the dysfunctional patterns. The client may express such insight as, "Aha! Now I see what I've been doing. So that's been the problem all along!"

Spontaneous awareness of patterns or themes is highly desirable, but the counselor will need to take the lead in helping the client tie together similar thoughts and feelings through empathic interventions and through the crucially important process of meaning attribution (Lieberman, Yalom, and Miles, 1973). It appears that many clients, and particularly those who lack psychological sophistication, cannot discern themes or patterns in their own behavior because their own presence in their perceptions obscures those perceptions. Therefore, counselors need to assist clients in attaching meaning to behavior and experiences.

Interestingly, establishing themes and patterns runs against concreteness, or specificity, of response. To gain specificity, the counselor responds to messages from the client couched in general terms, such as views and conclusions, by eliciting details that clarify the client's sense. Meaning attribution, on the other hand, extracts general themes from those specifics, themes the client must be aware of before remedial action can begin. Specificity is believed to be most critical in the early phase of counseling for gaining understanding and in the later phase for planning concrete behavioral changes. In the middle phase, generalization is helpful for enhancing insights into patterns.

Awareness facilitates change but does not assure it. When the client is sufficiently aware of the essential elements of his difficulties, he must then undertake the second major objective: translating the awareness into effective remedial action. This is much easier said than done, for the process of change is often complex, difficult, and painful. Dysfunctional behavior, to be sure, causes suffering, but at least the suffering is familiar to the client. Despite the pain, some clients cling tenaciously to their dysfunctional patterns rather than risk new and unfamiliar ones. A few very discouraged people, indeed, choose to spend their entire lives emotionally incapacitated rather than confront the risks of traversing what they perceive as unknown and potentially horrifying regions of human experience. Fortunately, however, the majority of clients, partially as a result of warm and empathic encouragement from their counselors, attempt, and sometimes relish, experimenting with new patterns of behavior.

Efforts to change are also frequently impeded when powerful and distressing emotions that contributed to the original development of the dysfunctional pattern emerge into conscious awareness. For example, when the young woman mentioned earlier, who had problems in being sexually exploited by men, experimented with asserting her right to decline sexual overtures, she experienced intense anxiety and virtual panic, despite some insight into the source of her fears of rejection, humiliation, and retaliation. These fears required further working-through before she could master them sufficiently.

Some counselors work under the assumption that once feelings have been explored and insight gained, the client should be able to cope effectively with the problematic situation thereafter. Nothing could be further from the truth! Emotional patterns become deeply ingrained over many years and are mastered only with persistent determination. This does not mean that professional help need extend over a lengthy period, for some clients can master dysfunctional patterns on their own once they have gained sufficient awareness of their problems and of the needed remedies. However, the working-through process is seldom smooth and rapid. To prevent discouragement and consequent premature termination, the rigors and the erratic course of change should be discussed with the client during the later portion of the early phase or the beginning of the change-oriented phase. Role-induction interviews have the advantage of preparing the client for the vicissitudes of therapy by explaining that progress usually involves ups and downs and telling the client to expect periods of both enthusiasm and of discouragement. The client is advised that when discouragement sets in, he should not discontinue therapy but instead discuss his feelings with the therapist. Growth and mastery are attained through incremental changes, and the client is counseled not to expect magically sudden and smooth progress. Counseling, like life, "is hard by the yard but by the inch is a cinch."

Task accomplishment. As the client demonstrates readiness to engage in change-oriented actions, it is important that such actions be determined mutually rather than by the counselor alone. The client's commitment to implement the actions or tasks deepens when he has been a willing and active partner in planning them. The counselor should weigh the client's chances of success at the tasks under consideration and discourage the client from biting off more than he can chew. Failures are not necessarily disastrous, and they are to be expected occasionally. In fact, they can sometimes be used to therapeutic advantage in facilitating further exploration of barriers and resistance to change. More commonplace failures, however, can devastate the client's morale. If a client persists in pursuing an impossible task, the counselor may cushion the destructive impact of failure by authentically expressing his own misgivings about the validity of the task. This may later help the client attribute failure to the unrealistic nature of the task rather than to personal inadequacy or ineffective therapy.

The success of change-oriented tasks also increases when the counselor helps the client prepare for carrying them out. Reid (1975) has developed some helpful guidelines called the task implementation sequence, or TIS. The sequence, whose effectiveness has been empirically validated, consists of the following steps: (1) encouraging the client and enhancing his commitment by considering with him the potential benefits of carrying out the task; (2) further specifying the task and developing plans for implementing it; (3) mutually considering obstacles that may be encountered and ways of handling them; (4) modeling, rehearsal, and guided practice preparatory to carrying out the task; and (5) summarizing the task and the plan of implementation.

Even when the counselor uses a systematic approach such as the TIS, the success of change-oriented actions is not assured. Change, at best, is difficult to achieve. If this were not the case, people could work through their difficulties without turning to professional help. Laymen can often readily see what change the troubled person must make, but seeing is not enough. Indeed, the hallmark of the professional therapist is his ability to make the client aware of the barriers that impede change and to help the client hurdle those barriers. The professional also facilitates change by encouraging the client and by believing in his capacity to change (Nikelly and Dinkmeyer, 1971). Encouragement is vital in maintaining the client's hope, an indispensable prerequisite to change. Believing in the client is equally essential, for many clients have grave doubts about their ability to change and they derive courage and strength from the counselor's convictions until they begin to succeed and become more self-confident.

There are numerous change-oriented tactics to choose from, including assertiveness training (Alberti and Emmons, 1970; Rose, 1975), behavioral rehearsal (Rose and others, 1970), use of paradoxes (Watzlawick, Weakland, and Fisch, 1974), talking to the empty chair (Perls, 1969; Fagan and Shepherd, 1970), reframing or reformulating problems (Watzlawick, Weakland, and Fisch, 1974), desensitization (Wolpe, 1969), modeling (Schwartz and Goldiamond, 1975, Bandura, 1969), contingency contracting (Alexander and Parsons, 1973; DeRisi and Butz, 1974), aversive therapy (Rachman and Teasdale, 1969), flooding (Morganstern, 1973), fixed-role therapy (Kelly, 1955), homework assignments (Shelton and Ackerman, 1974), behavioral self-control techniques (Bandura, 1969; Mahoney and Thoresen, 1974; Thoresen and

Mahoney, 1974) and many others (Kanfer and Goldstein, 1975; Thorne, 1968). Each of these techniques works well when employed judiciously, but may fail dismally when applied indiscriminately. None is an adequate substitute for interpersonal skills. The potentials for success, as noted in Chapter One, are significantly enhanced when the techniques are employed in a helping relationship characterized by high levels of the facilitative conditions.

The facilitative conditions and the change-oriented processes of confrontation and relational immediacy are the workhorses of most nonbehaviorist therapists for expanding the client's awareness, surmounting barriers to change, and effecting essential changes in behavior. The remainder of this chapter, therefore, will look closely at these basic objectives of the change-oriented phase of counseling.

Empathic communication during the middle phase. Empathic communication is critical in helping the client gain the awareness needed for effective action. Once the working relationship is established and goals are negotiated, empathic communication primarily helps the client understand himself and his difficulties better and better. Trusting in the counselor's good will, the client is ready to engage in self-exploration with much less risk of misperceiving the counselor's intent as the client's emotions, deeper motivations, and patterns of behavior are probed.

For the client to understand himself better, the therapist must go beyond the reciprocal level of empathy to additive levels—that is, 3.5 to 5.0. Additive empathic responses exceed the client's own awareness, helping illuminate feelings and meanings that he perceives only dimly. The therapist helps the client experience vague feelings more sharply, become aware of feelings that have been suppressed or experienced physically (for example, tightness in the throat or chest, nervous perspiring, and so forth), take note of themes or patterns, and discover motives and meanings underlying behavior that have been unknown or misunderstood.

The depth of self-exploration required, of course, will vary with the nature of the problem and the client's goals. Some clients want "depth-oriented" therapy, and others, even though they could benefit from it, are not so inclined. One guideline, however, is crucial. The counselor should avoid any consideration of alternative actions before the essential facets of the problem are understood. To move on to action without understanding is tantamount to embarking on a trip without a map or an itinerary.

Premature action may prolong rather than accelerate counseling, for many false starts and detours can delay effective action or cause the client to terminate early. Deep understanding of a problem, by contrast, yields a sense of direction. What needs to be changed and how to change it gradually become clear to both counselor and client. This does not mean that effective counseling need always be lengthy. The nature and sources of difficulties can often be rapidly discerned, making early planning and implementation of remedial actions possible. This will be particularly true when problems are of recent origin and not located in deep layers of the personality and when the client's usual level of functioning has been high.

Empathic responding at additive levels also serves a vital function in facilitating the translation of awareness or insight into action. Level 5 empathic responses embody the basic feelings and themes in the client's difficulties and in addition contain goal-oriented messages that direct the client's motivation toward making essential changes in himself or acting upon the environment. Thus, at this highest level, empathy relates to the client's thrust toward growth and change, highlighting the available alternatives and actions that have been mutually discovered by deep exploration. As Carkhuff aptly states, "The highest and ultimate form of empathic understanding is action" (1969, p. 85).

Deep empathic understanding and communication are also vital to the change-oriented processes of confrontation and authentic responding. As the counselor employs confrontations or responds to experiences in the immediacy of the helping relationships, he must be keenly attuned to client reactions. Because these therapeutic activities involve working with emotions and patterns at the edge of the client's awareness and even beyond, unfavorable reactions are always possible. It is imperative, therefore, that when such untoward reactions occur, the therapist shift the focus of the interview to the immediacy of the client's experiencing. This tactic allows negative reactions such as hurt or resentment to be discussed, explored, and resolved, thus averting resistance and safeguarding the working relationship.

The additive levels of empathy are the subject of Chapter Six.

Respect in the middle phase. As the client increasingly discloses himself, the counselor experiences more fully various facets of the client's personality and gains additional insights into "what makes him tick." This expanded experiencing provides a basis for genuine positive feelings and higher levels of respect, which augment the good will and nonjudgmental attitude of the intermediate level (level 3) manifested during the early phase of counseling. In turn, these positive feelings make it possible for the counselor to share authentic feelings in the immediacy of the relationship, as will be discussed briefly later in this chapter and extensively in Chapter Nine. The point is that the counselor's authentic respect for the client often serves a vital therapeutic purpose in increasing the client's self-respect.

Although increased understanding of the forces behind the client's dysfunctional behavior usually results in greater tolerance, acceptance, and respect on the counselor's part, negative feelings toward the client may occasionally arise. If such feelings persist, the counselor will not be able to offer the conditions that facilitate growth and change, and he in fact may deleteriously affect the client. In such instances, the counselor has an ethical responsibility to attempt to resolve his negative feelings by introspection or consultation with another professional and, if these measures fail, refer the client to another person. If a counselor experiences negative feelings toward more than just an occasional client, he may have a problem that should be resolved before subjecting additional clients to potentially damaging experiences. Some such counselors, of course, may be well advised to consider changing occupations in the interests of themselves, potential clients, and the helping professions.

In the middle stage, the counselor shows respect in the highest level (level 5) by emphasizing the client's potentials for effecting changes and for achieving maximal autonomy and responsibility for self. The best therapists, according to existentialists, are those who perceive the client not as he "is" but as he "might become." Relating to the client's potentials, encouraging their activation, and holding the client accountable for their development characterize the counselor's respect in the middle phase. In a sense, then, this level of respect entails some conditionality. The counselor does not accept feeble excuses or approve halfhearted efforts to carry out the tasks agreed on. Certainly the counselor does not reprimand, belittle, or reject the client, but he does unmask resistances for what they are and expect the client to assume responsibility for carrying out as best he can the actions to which he has committed himself.

Respect is discussed extensively in Chapter Seven.

Authenticity and relational immediacy during the middle phase. It will be recalled that during the early phase of counseling, authenticity consists largely of an absence of phoniness or defensiveness. The objectives of the early phase require the counselor to be responsive, and they provide no basis for more than minimal self-disclosure by the counselor. During the change-oriented stage of the middle phase, however, higher levels of authenticity (levels 4–5) not only are appropriate but may contribute to the objectives of enhancing awareness and fostering change-oriented actions. In contrast to the responsive posture of the early phase, authentic responding becomes a natural part of the middle phase and may be used to initiate growth-oriented counseling activities. The counselor's ever-expanding experiencing of many aspects of the client's feelings, thoughts, behavioral patterns, and various idiosyncrasies provides a rich fund of information from which the counselor can provide valuable feedback for the client. Appropriate self-disclosure by the counselor thus is a major aspect of authenticity in the change-oriented stage.

Most of the client's interpersonal patterns will gradually become apparent within the helping relationship, and the counselor who is alert to these patterns and to personal reactions to them will be able to use them to expand the client's self-awareness. For example, a client of one of the authors, Mrs. W., complained that her husband seldom let her know how he felt about various aspects of their lives. The counselor, after several interviews, became aware that trying to communicate with the woman left him frustrated because she frequently interrupted, seldom listened for long, and persisted in complaining about her husband's passivity. Realizing that she probably behaved with him much as she did with her husband, the counselor shared his own feelings of frustration in not being listened to and wondered whether similar feelings might account in part for her husband's reluctance to express himself more openly. Mrs. W. was somewhat taken aback, as such a possibility had never occurred to her before. She subsequently was able to apply this newly gained insight to both the marital and counseling relationships, improving her progress in both.

In this example, it should be noted that the counselor shared his immediate experiencing to foster the client's self-awareness and further her self-exploration. This is the primary and fundamental reason for self-disclosure by the counselor. Indiscriminate self-disclosure can be destructive. Negative feelings such as anger, irritation or disappointment are best restrained; they should be expressed only after the counselor has himself explored the dynamics of such feelings and is certain that disclosure of the negative feelings will encourage profitable explorations of the helping relationship. Though increased authenticity often plays a role in the change-oriented stage, the purpose of counseling remains unchanged—to help the client, not to use him to gratify the counselor's needs or to work out his frustrations.

Authentic sharing may also help foster insight in numerous other instances. The earlier discussion of respect, for example, pointed out that positive feelings toward the client may be shared to foster the client's self-respect. Disclosure can also help with clients who make the counselor uncomfortable and with those defensive, supersensitive patients who have to be handled with kid gloves lest their feelings be hurt. The counselor should remember that the client probably behaves the same way toward people outside the helping relationship and that awareness of the behavior may help the client modify his interpersonal patterns. Such disclosure, though, must convey the counselor's helpful intent. Even then, disclosures of this type often cause the client pain, simply because they conflict with the client's self-perceptions. Human beings readily see weaknesses and imperfections in others but overlook the same flaws in themselves.

During the change-oriented phase, the authentic being of the counselor may also be increasingly disclosed by spontaneity and humor. Both of these desirable qualities evidence further the counselor's humanness and invite the client to relate too with openness and spontaneity. If the counselor cannot himself be spontaneously open, how can he justifiably expect the client to be open? If openness and humor do not belong in helping relationships, where, indeed, do they belong? The counseling relationship is most helpful in the long run when it has positive transferability to other relationships and when it provides a model. Openness, spontaneity, and humor have such transferability.

One final word about authenticity relates to the counselor's self-awareness and integration. To help others gain self-awareness, the counselor must be in touch with various aspects of his own being and integrate these various aspects in a healthy fashion. The counselor who lacks self-awareness will have difficulty distinguishing between the feelings and reactions that derive from self and those that derive from the client. With the rapid changes in our society that often embody value-laden issues, including abortion, pornography, open marriage, and changing sexual roles, the counselor is confronted with clients representing an array of values, beliefs, and life styles. To help such clients, the counselor must first come to terms with his own feelings about such controversial issues. This does not mean that the counselor need espouse any given position or reveal that position to the client, but it does mean that the counselor who has not addressed these issues and examined his personal feelings may let his covert feelings influence perception and interactions, all the while unaware that he is doing so. This danger in the feminist movement is cogently discussed by Sherman (1976).

Confrontation during the middle phase. A powerful means of facilitating change, confrontation assumes major importance during the middle phase in assisting the client both to expand self-awareness and to implement change-oriented actions. Employed only sparingly and at low levels during the early phase, effective confrontations advance to high levels (4–5) during the middle phase. Confrontation is used with additive levels of empathy, which often facilitate self-confrontation—that is, discovery by the client of inconsistencies, discrepancies, and resistance to change in his behavior. Self-confrontation is preferable to therapist-directed confrontation because the client is more likely to accept the validity of awareness gained from the former than from the latter. Nevertheless, confrontations by the therapist are vital in making the client aware of feelings, behaviors, and patterns he remains unaware of. The therapist must remember that the portion of the self in the client's awareness is but the tip of the iceberg of the total personality. It is the therapist's task to bring to awareness those aspects of the client's undiscovered self that have posed barriers to the changes the client seeks.

Confrontations are needed to unmask the meanings of many aspects of the client's behavior, particularly those which impede progress and otherwise perpetuate dysfunctional behavior. Because counseling tends to be painful and because change seldom occurs without a difficult struggle, the counselor commonly encounters resistances, which if not recognized and resolved, may prolong or even undermine counseling. Resistances are commonly directed toward counseling or the counselor and may take a variety of forms: failing; canceling; changing appointments or arriving late; a flight into feigned health by denying or minimizing problems; avoiding the discussion of problems or attempting to divert the discussion from painful areas; failing to pay fees; attempting to dilute the helping relationship by conventional social conversation, shifting the focus to the counselor, seductiveness, flattery, or ingratiation.

Such resistances must be explored and worked through; otherwise the client is left to sort out the underlying feelings independently. Should that occur, the client's solution often is to terminate counseling. The handling of resistances of this sort is discussed in Chapter Nine, which deals with relational immediacy, and in Wolberg's (1967) important book.

Confrontation also is vital in identifying and working through the universal resistance to change. The client commonly manifests resistance to change by bringing up topics unrelated to current tasks, dissociating counseling from daily life by facing problems only in the counseling office, procrastinating in carrying out the actions agreed upon, intellectualizing about the dynamics of difficulties with no attempt to translate insight into action, adopting a position of weakness or helplessness, rationalizing inaction, questioning the validity of chosen actions, and many of the behaviors listed above. Obviously, such discrepancies and inconsistencies between behavior and avowed goals must be confronted if the client is to succeed in making essential changes.

Working through the resistances, however, involves much more than merely pointing them out to the client. The emotions underlying the resistances must frequently be explored and resolved before the client can muster the courage for further change-oriented actions. Again, high-level empathic communication is called into service to illuminate the underlying feelings. Later, the therapist may use strength confrontations—that is, reminding the client of the strengths he has already demonstrated, thereby encouraging and urging the client to mobilize those strengths. Conveying a belief in the client's capacity to change and an expectation that he mobilize that capacity involves the highest level of respect.

It sometimes happens that the client chooses not to carry out actions which he himself has helped plan. Respect dictates that we honor the client's right to make that choice. It also dictates, however, that we confront the client with the possible negative consequences of that choice. Moreover, other clients must be confronted with the reality that inaction and procrastination also often involve choice by default, whether the choice is favored or not.

Obviously, confrontation affords the means by which we help a client face his moment of truth about his part in the difficulties. Confrontation may open the door to new possibilities for growth and change, and when used skillfully in a context of good will, it is a most important tool in the counselor's armamentarium. When used poorly, however, confrontation can be very destructive (Lieberman, Yalom, and Miles, 1973; Berenson and Mitchell, 1974). Poor timing, excessive use, vigor and dogmatism, overtones of criticism or belittling, insensitivity to the client's reactions following confrontation—these and other errors may produce alienation rather than insight. The reader is advised to study carefully Chapter Ten, which discusses confrontation extensively.

THE TERMINAL PHASE

The terminal phase varies in length and significance with the type of counseling. In planned short-term counseling, termination actually begins during the initial period of contract negotiation, when the total number of interviews or the terminal date is specified. Termination, thus, is anticipated well in advance and the process occurs in a relatively straightforward manner. In other types of open-ended counseling—no time limit is specified—deciding when to terminate is a matter of major concern, involving careful assessment and skillful handling. When goals have been formulated in observable and measurable terms, however, the decision to terminate is much simplified for both counselor and client. If, for example, the goals are for the client to approach others, initiate and maintain conversations, and ask for dates, it will be relatively simple to ascertain when the goals have been achieved.

In instances when goals are less specific, guidelines about termination are likewise less specific. If the goals, for example, have been to overcome certain guilt feelings or to alleviate depression, the criteria for goal accomplishment are somewhat nebulous, for "overcoming" or "alleviating" cover many degrees of relief. The degree of freedom from the troubling feelings that the client desires is the most appropriate criterion, but this varies from client to client and often cannot be accurately predicted by either the client or the counselor. Evidence from numerous research studies, summarized by Reid and Epstein (1972, Chapter Four), indicates, however, that most problems are alleviated rapidly, indicating that in the majority of cases, a point of diminishing return is probably reached by the sixth interview. A review of studies of continuance in therapy (Garfield, 1971) indicates that in ten representative psychiatric clinics the average number of interviews per patient was five. Moreover, in the majority of instances therapy ended not by mutual planning but because the patient failed to return for scheduled appointments.

Unilateral termination by the client has been traditionally regarded as "premature" because of the assumption that change takes a long while, and, therefore, that the client has discontinued treatment before much has been accomplished. Reid and Epstein, however, ascribe the high rate of supposedly premature terminations, to the client's lack of motivation to continue because his discomfort has been alleviated within a few interviews (1972, p. 84). This view, which many have accepted, is the theoretical cornerstone of time-limited therapies.

The point of this discussion is not to present a case for planned short-term therapy—although a strong case does exist—but to emphasize that unilateral client terminations suggest that therapists either frequently fail to explore the client's feelings about progress in counseling or to perceive manifestations of enhanced client functioning. In either event, unilateral termination rules out the beneficial counseling experiences that occur in well-conducted, planned terminations. For this reason, we strongly recommend that counselors be constantly alert to indications that the client feels ready to terminate. Such indications include reports of diminished anxiety, more relaxed demeanor, improvements in mood and out-look, relative absence of pressure accompanied by a lack of things to talk about, missed or forgotten appointments, reduced inter-personal conflicts, increasing and more satisfying involvements with others, reports of improved feelings about self, and greater self-confidence. Some of these indications may manifest resistance, but there is no reason to assume categorically that such is the case. A rule of thumb is to explore the client's feelings to determine the meaning behind the change in behavior. If the client is satisfied with his progress and is entertaining thoughts of termination, mu-tual planning can be initiated.

A skillfully planned termination can benefit the client. The client's gains can be augmented by, for example, reviewing with him the sources of his basic difficulties and the process by which they were ameliorated. This process may expand the client's aware-ness, better preparing him to cope effectively with similar problems in the future. Elements of the problem-solving process may also be reviewed, including identifying the nature and source of the prob-lem, considering other persons and factors involved, identifying and weighing various alternatives and their consequences, select-ing the most promising alternative, anticipating possible obstacles, developing strategies for surmounting them, and implementing the chosen course of action.

This process of anticipating possible problems in the future and considering the remedies has been termed "anticipatory guid-ance" by theorists of crisis intervention. A client helped through this process, which need not take long, is not only better prepared for future coping, but also leaves counseling with greater confidence. Moreover, the counselor will be able to emphasize the client's strengths and successes and thereby reinforce his self-esteem and self-confidence for meeting difficulties in the future.

In addition, the therapist can challenge the client to apply the learning gained during counseling to future daily living. Life presents opportunities for continuous growth, and the client can be encouraged to pursue growth-oriented activities after termination, applying insights and principles learned in formal counseling. One of the authors once received a Christmas card from a former client approximately eighteen months following termination. In the card the client wrote, "I want to thank you again for helping me. You may not know it, but you are still helping me. I often think about our interviews, and I have applied what we discussed on numerous occasions."

Another benefit of planned termination is the opportunity to invite the client to return for help, should overwhelming difficulties occur in the future. The counselor can express continued interest in the client, leaving the door open for future service. By contrast, a client who has terminated unilaterally may find it difficult to return, fearing criticism or blame.

Termination is often difficult for both parties. The client frequently experiences ambivalent feelings about termination, particularly when counseling has lasted a long while. On one hand, the client may feel a sense of accomplishment and exhilaration at being ready to try his wings without the counselor. On the other hand, he commonly suffers from apprehension and uncertainty about facing the future on his own. A certain amount of dependency is inherent in the helping process, and the client may experience termination as the end of a relationship with a person who has become precious to him. The sense of loss, however, is not limited to the client, for if the counselor has really permitted himself to become meaningfully involved with the client, termination also means relinquishing a valued relationship. Obviously, however, the loss will be less for the counselor than for the client.

It should be apparent to the reader that each of the vital dimensions of the helping process is employed at moderate and high levels during the terminal phase of counseling. High levels of empathic communication are essential in eliciting and exploring the client's feelings about readiness to terminate. Empathic communication and high levels of respect are also vital in discerning and responding to possible painful feelings of separation. High levels of respect are also involved in emphasizing client strengths and accomplishments and in challenging the client to continue tapping these strengths as he continues to pursue personal growth. High levels of authenticity and empathic communication play a role in responding to and sharing the deep and personal feelings engendered by the pending termination of the relationship. The mutual expression and shared appreciation of these feelings appropriately brings an appropriate closure to a deeply significant and positive human encounter.

Chapter 3

๖๏๖๏๖๏๖๏๖๏๖๏ ๖๏๖๏๖๏๖๏๖๏๖๏๖๏๖๏

Barriers to Effective Communication

To develop therapeutic communication skills, the practitioner must first understand counterproductive communication patterns. Such an understanding enables the therapist to recognize and avoid pitfalls in communication that may produce such undesired consequences as eliciting defensiveness, causing the client to terminate prematurely, forming relationships with clients inimical to growth and problem solving, and, in some instances, causing deterioration in the client's functioning. As noted in Chapter One, research indicates that counseling may affect the client adversely. These detrimental effects are most likely associated with the use of destructive patterns of communication. In this chapter, dysfunctional or destructive communication patterns will be identified and discussed.

Passivity

Ongoing dialogue between the counselor and the client is essential to the helping process for several important reasons. The exploration of problems, feelings, and motivation and the capacity to work on the problems require extensive self-disclosure by the client. The counselor's encouragement of the client by listening attentively and by nonverbal gestures that convey interest and concern tends to facilitate self-disclosure, but verbal activity in varying degrees is also vital. If the counselor merely remains silent, his response is ambiguous and thus subject to misinterpretation. Many clients, and particularly those who are insecure, dependent, or prone to interpersonal perceptual distortions, may interpret silence as indicating the counselor's lack of interest, criticism, or rejection. Silence, likewise, may raise the anxiety level of some clients. Though increased anxiety is desirable in some instances (Sifneos, 1967), it may virtually immobilize those clients whose anxiety levels are already high. The findings of one study (Heller, Davis, and Myers, 1966) reveal that when counselors are active rather than passive and silent, clients, too, are more verbally active, and they are more likely to continue in counseling and to perceive their counselors as friendly.

The degree of verbal activity required of the counselor will vary from client to client and from interview to interview involving a given client. Some clients possess verbal facility and reveal rich information and emotion with minimal activity on the counselor's part. Other clients lack verbal skills, are guarded, or find it difficult to reveal much about themselves. In such instances, the counselor will need to actively maintain the client's verbalization. Empathic responses and other verbal and nonverbal facilitative responses are indispensable in maintaining adequate verbal exchange. These skills are discussed extensively in subsequent chapters.

The timing of the counselor's silence, verbalization, and intervention is important. The counselor should remain actively involved but place the responsibility for the progress of the interview on the client. There are times when the counselor should be relatively quiet in order, for example, to reduce the pace or intensity of the interview, to place pressure on the client to talk and to accept responsibility in the interview, or to allow the client time to think.

No therapist should expect constant verbal interchange. Pauses occur naturally when the client or the counselor needs a moment to reflect on an idea or when the client attempts to remember details of a relevant event. Strong emotions may also emerge, temporarily interrupting the flow of the client's verbalization, as a result of the discussion of painful material, recall of emotionally laden events, or sudden insights. Such natural pauses normally last only a short while and usually do not warrant interruption. Frequent or prolonged pauses, however, generally indicate client resistance or ineffective counseling. Therapeutic handling of silence involving the client's feelings toward the counselor is discussed in Chapter Nine, which deals with "relational immediacy." An excellent discussion of techniques for managing silence associated with resistance may also be found in Wolberg's *Technique of Psychotherapy* (1967).

Counselor Dominance

Domineering counselor activity contrasts markedly with passivity, and it may take several different forms. Some helping persons, by dominating the interview, fail to elicit from the client sufficient information, feelings, and views. Instead of entering the client's world of experience and thinking with him about possible remedies, such counselors prematurely and often erroneously jump to conclusions about the causes of and the solutions to the client's problems. They may readily offer advice and move prematurely to action approaches without first understanding the situation adequately. Operating largely from an external frame of reference, the domineering counselor is prone to act all-knowing, omnipotent, and infallible and to advance his own prestige by pushing the client to improve. These modes of behavior meet the therapist's needs, not the client's.

Domineering counselor behavior is characterized by frequent interruptions, impatience, changes of the subject, vigorous persuasive efforts, arguments, and lectures. Although some clients, especially those who are excessively dependent, may welcome the counselor's dominance, the majority take offense and may resist. Resistance may well be, as Masserman (1965) has aptly put it, a healthy response to poor counseling in the same sense that resistance is a healthy response to rape. Even those clients who welcome counselor dominance are more often hindered than helped. Inappropriate solutions proffered by the counselor may exacerbate rather than alleviate problems. Moreover, the client who becomes more dependent as a result of what should be a helping relationship has been rendered an unfortunate disservice.

Dominating counselor behavior conveys disrespect for the client's capacity to solve his own problems. The importance of respect to therapy is discussed at greater length in Chapter Seven.

Inappropriate Self-Disclosure

Another ineffective pattern of communication is self-disclosure that focuses inappropriately on the counselor instead of the client. Some counselors dwell at great length on their educational achievements, professional reputations, hobbies, families, or "valiant struggles" in achieving success despite difficult obstacles. Clients often are understandably bewildered about how these "ego trips" relate to their own problems. Obviously, it is not the client's needs that are met by such attempts to demonstrate the counselor's importance, prominence, brilliance, or success.

Some counselors subscribe to the philosophy of "letting it all hang out"—that is, freely revealing any or all of their feelings whether appropriate or not. Although there is merit to authenticity in counseling, a topic to be discussed in Chapter Eight, indiscriminate self-disclosure serves the needs of the wrong person. Consider, for example, how a client might be affected by a counselor's revealing his own marital problems, sexual indiscretions, or feelings of repulsion toward a physical attribute or trait of the client. This last disclosure would likely leave the client feeling hurt and rejected. Revealing information about the counselor's marriage troubles or affairs would probably reduce the client's confidence in the counselor and perhaps lead him to wonder whether the counselor needs help more than the client does. The cherished definition of counseling as "two persons working together on the problems of one—hopefully the client's" should be kept in mind for its relevance and wisdom as well as its humor.

Self-disclosures by the counselor may at times serve valid therapeutic purposes, but they should be used prudently and sparingly. The appropriate use of self-disclosure is discussed more extensively in Chapter Eight.

Interrogation or Grilling

The excessive use of questions is counterproductive because it limits client verbalization and self-disclosure. Questions tend to structure or to circumscribe the client's responses and hence elicit information or feelings less revealing than those which emanate more from the client. For example, a counselor seeking to elicit information about the adjustment of children in a family may ask, "Are your children getting along OK?" and get little more than "Yeah" or "Not really" for an answer. Additional questioning or probing is needed to gain more specific information. By contrast, an open-ended counselor message such as, "I'd like to know more about your children; please tell me about them and how they're getting along," will elicit an expanded and richer expression because the client is free to respond from a much broader domain. Thus the response will reveal more of his views and feelings.

Relying largely on questions to elicit information and feelings is counterproductive also because the counselor largely determines the relevant information or emotion. This limits the client's participation and may establish a pattern of interaction that is difficult to change. If early in counseling, the counselor takes a strongly directive role characterized by excessive questioning, the client may consider this situation the expected pattern and assume a passive role. Such a pattern, of course, tends to inhibit rather than foster client autonomy and growth, both of which are fundamental goals of the helping process.

Questions, of course, must be used frequently to elicit essential information. Skilled interviewers, however, are able to elicit much of the information essential to adequate assessment by using open-ended, empathic, and other forms of facilitative response rather than grilling the client with question after question. Facilitative response is discussed extensively in subsequent chapters.

Distancing Patterns

Other patterns of communication are ineffective because they keep the client at a distance, thus blocking the development of trust, openness, spontaneity, and genuine caring, all of which characterize an effective helping relationship. There are many types of such distancing patterns, but all serve the common purpose of protecting the counselor from anxieties, discomfort, or fears associated with deep involvement in the client's emotional experience.

TABOOS AGAINST CRYING

An extreme measure to protect the counselor from discomfort in the presence of strong emotion is simply to explicitly or implicitly prohibit crying by the client. This drastic measure, of course, indicates that the counselor has unresolved problems associated with crying and that the prohibition, therefore, meets the needs of the wrong person. The meaning the client is likely to attribute to such a prohibition is that weeping is wrong or indicative of weakness. As a result, he or she may avoid discussing problems that are emotionally laden, perhaps those which are most troubling. Ironically, many people's problems stem from keeping emotions so tightly bottled up that either they are converted into physiological symptoms or they erupt violently when pressures mount out of control. Moreover, individuals experience a beneficial release of tension when troubling feelings are ventilated. Thus, not only is inhibiting the expression of painful emotions counterproductive in most instances, but it may also reinforce the client's dysfunctional patterns of managing emotions. One exception involves clients who emote excessively and for whom this emotionality is itself defensive and dysfunctional. Such clients may emote dramatically and profusely using this as a pattern to manipulate others. The therapeutic goal is to help such clients to learn more effective patterns of coping and to bridle their emotions.

FOSTERING SOCIAL INTERACTION

Another way to maintain distance is to communicate with the client only about safe topics that are unlikely to elicit emotion or to foster increasing self-disclosure. Thus, channeling the discussion to matters typifying conventional social intercourse avoids the risk of becoming involved in painful, highly personal, or emotional subjects. Discussions of the weather, sports, news, mutual acquaintances, hobbies, common interests, or other topics extraneous to the client's problems tend to foster a social rather than a therapeutic relationship. Although the client may need friends and although therapeutic relationships frequently do develop emotional ties akin to friendship, clients need much more than friendship to solve their problems effectively. Indeed, research indicates that counseling relationships are most sharply differentiated from friendships by their concreteness, otherwise designated as specificity of the counselor's response (Martin, Carkhuff, and Berenson, 1964). In other words, communication in counseling relationships is characterized by sharp focus and specificity as contrasted to the lighter and more diffuse communication typical in social relationships.

Two qualifications to this general rule against social banter should be noted. During the "getting acquainted" period of initial interviews or during early portions of subsequent interviews, a brief discussion of conventional topics may be appropriate and helpful in reducing the client's tension before moving to an exploration of potentially painful areas. A second qualification pertains to work with children and adolescents, many of whom are threatened by the unknowns of counseling and are afraid of the counselor, whom they tend to perceive as a figure of authority intending to punish or to control them in some as yet undefined manner (Markowitz, 1954). Discussing safe topics and consciously cultivating a quasi-friend role often help lower defenses and promote a less threatening climate wherein the child or adolescent can gradually risk increasing openness with the counselor.

SKIRTING UNCOMFORTABLE ISSUES

Another distancing pattern is often harder to detect, because the counselor, although emotionally engaged in many of the client's problems and feelings, consistently avoids confronting facets of the client's behavior that may elicit discomfort, hostility, defensiveness, or resistance. In essence, the counselor keeps a safe distance by playing the "nice guy" and thereby avoids the riskier but deeper involvement that occurs when the client is confronted with his part in the problems. The client needs more than warm support from an empathic counselor. As Bettelheim (1950) says, "Love is not enough." The client needs a corrective emotional experience, and such techniques as confrontation are usually critical elements of the helping process.

Skill in confrontation is one of the many tools required of the effective counselor. Those who lack this skill may establish good working relationships but be unable to move beyond the "honey-moon period" of counseling. Ultimately, the client must be helped to assume responsibility for modifying problematic aspects of his or her behavior. Skillful confrontation, which requires much finesse, is discussed extensively in Chapter Ten of this book.

FALSE REASSURANCE

Reassuring the client prematurely or without justification is another distancing pattern that enables the counselor to avoid exploring the client's feelings of despair, anger, helplessness, or hopelessness. Statements such as, "Don't worry; it'll be ok," "Everyone has problems," "When I was your age, I guess I was just like you," or "Things will work out, you'll see," fail to provide the reassurance they intend. Instead, the client, whose feelings oppose such exhortations, is convinced that the counselor fails to understand. Conveying hope when indeed there is hope may provide the client much-needed emotional support. Instead of fostering hope, however, the hollow ring of glib reassurance has the opposite effect. Grim situations are often encountered in counseling, and the counselor is better advised to elicit and to explore the client's feelings and to acknowledge painful realities than to avoid discomfort for both parties by conveying the attitude of a phony Pollyanna.

Reassurance should be used selectively and only when a genuine basis for it exists. With anxious, insecure, or depressed clients, reassurance may be used to good advantage if employed judiciously. Used indiscriminately, reassurance may promote dependency, engender doubt about the counselor's authenticity, reinforce inappropriate behavior, or unwittingly reduce the anxiety and conflict that may be essential motivators to effective therapeutic work by the client.

EMOTIONAL DETACHMENT

Distancing may take the form of aloofness or detachment. Detachment may be manifested by passivity, as noted earlier, or by taking the role of technical expert engaged in a sterile, detached analysis and dissection of the client's problems and experiences. The detached counselor who acts as if he is merely a reflective mirror rarely relates authentically, with the effect that the client's communication becomes increasingly guarded. As noted earlier in Chapter Two, authenticity is basic to effective helping relationships. The reader who would like more extensive exposure to the clinical significance of the counselor's authenticity or "transparency" is referred to Jourard's (1971) and Colm's (1966) important writings on this subject.

INTELLECTUALIZATION

Closely related to detachment is the practice of intellectualizing about the etiology or psychodynamic significance of the client's problems to stave off involvement in the client's here-and-now world of experience. Theorizing about the early roots of problems and dysfunctional behavior may be intriguing and indeed occasionally helpful. Unfortunately, however, insight into etiology tends to be more informative than remedial. Insights gained experientially through counseling are much more potent in producing change because they are more relevant and more readily transferable from the interview to the client's current life situation than are intellectual discussions of emotions conjured up from the remote past.

Cognitive conceptualization and analysis of the various forces involved in the client's problems, of course, may be essential and therapeutic when preceded by careful and adequate exploration of the relevant feelings and information. Intellectualization, as an habitual pattern of communication, however, is inimical to effective counseling. Certain responses by the counselor invite intellectualization and are, therefore, generally counterproductive. Questions such as, "Why do you suppose it is so important for you to please others?" or "What is your theory about the origin of your fear?" foster sterile excursions into the realm of intellectual speculation.

The counselor may not be the only one guilty of intellectualizing. Some clients use intellectualization as a defense or distancing mechanism to avoid contact with their own painful and often deeply buried emotions or to escape the risk of possible hurt and rejection in allowing themselves to move emotionally closer to the counselor. With such clients, the counselor should avoid responding in kind. Otherwise the encounter becomes sterile, the communication abstract, and the results unsuccessful.

Using Crude Language

In sharp contrast to intellectualization is the counselor's use of four-letter words, often of the gutter variety, and his insistence that the client do the same. This pattern, which is often referred to as "coming on straight," is based on the rationale that the use of sophisticated terms such as *having intercourse* or *making love* tends to foster discussion devoid of the emotional intensity the client attaches to the experience he is dealing with. Although there may be a modicum of validity to this argument, many "sophisticated" clients need not resort to language generally regarded as crude or vulgar to express emotions openly. Moreover, skillful counselors are alert to patterns of intellectualization or to cues of hidden emotions, and they employ techniques other than obscenity to expand the client's expressions of those feelings.

Although some clients, especially those for whom crude language is a natural pattern of expression, do not object to and in fact may welcome the use of such language by the counselor, it offends many others so much that some clients simply fail to return for additional interviews. In our judgment, the counselor can best establish rapport by skillful interviewing without resorting to crude language. Indeed, if such language is not a natural part of the counselor's verbal repertoire, the client will probably perceive it as phony, and the crudity will therefore be counterproductive. In other instances, rapport and respect may be fostered by avoiding crude language even when the client uses it. Many individuals who use profanity and vulgarity freely do not condone the use of such language by themselves or by others. Rather, they may respect those who have not adopted such habits of speech.

Using Jargon

Professional jargon means little to most clients and often confuses or bewilders them. A rule of thumb for good counseling is to use language no more complex than the client can understand readily. Such terms as *narcissistic, psychotic, ego-structure, transference, repression, schizoid, Oedipus complex, fixation,* and a host of others may be commonplace to the counselor but alien to the client. Counselors who employ such terms in interviews often need to dazzle clients with their knowledge. Certainly such ostentatious displays of knowledge will impress the client, but the impression gained is likely to be one of pomposity rather than helpfulness. The client will probably resent, not admire, the counselor.

Moralizing or Admonishing

Another type of communication for counselors to avoid is moralizing, sermonizing, admonishing, or otherwise passing judgment on the client or his behavior. The client, like anyone else, tends to respond defensively, inwardly if not overtly, to criticism or judgment by others. Consequently, a client is not open to examining the self or to considering alternative frames of reference when he feels evaluated or criticized. Even though the helping person may intend to be helpful, the other person rarely perceives moral judgments in that light. Messages such as, "You shouldn't have done that," "That wasn't a very honest thing to do," "You should respect your parents," "Why don't you grow up?" or "You ought to pay your bills," leave the client resentful and alienated. Moralizing behavior stands in opposition to the facilitative condition of respect, which is discussed at length in Chapter Seven.

Patronizing or Condescending Behavior

Another pattern of communication, also ineffective because it lacks respect and authenticity, is patronizing or condescending behavior. Most people feel demeaned by patronizing behavior because it places them in a position inferior to the other person. Although the counselor may have the best of intentions, the client rarely perceives patronizing favorably and is more likely to be resentful than grateful.

Common forms of patronizing behavior are flattery, unearned or feigned praise, effusive sympathy, catering to win favor, giving advice, or insisting on doing things for clients that they can do for themselves. The first three forms lack sincerity, and the client will perceive them as phony. As such, they are low in the facilitative condition of authenticity, which is discussed at length in Chapter Eight. The others lack respect because the counselor's advice or insistence on doing things for the client minimizes or ignores the client's strengths and potentials. Underestimating the client's capacity to assume responsibilities, including the responsibility to reveal and to explore problems in counseling, tends to be demeaning, and clients may be expected to respond with inner resentment.

Inept Confrontation

Although, as noted earlier, confrontation is indispensable to effective counseling, premature or excessive use of this technique causes many terminations and failures. Counselors who employ confrontations excessively often base their action on the spurious premise that people are best helped by facing the realities underlying their dysfunctional behavior as rapidly as possible. Under the guise of "reality therapy," some counselors confront clients prematurely, failing to observe Glasser's (1965) emphasis that preconditions for confrontation include emotional involvement and the development of a relationship. When clients fail to return for additional interviews, such counselors usually attribute the termination to inadequate motivation or resistance on the client's part.

Confrontation always involves a certain amount of risk to the helping relationship because of the ever-present danger that the client will misinterpret the counselor's motives. Until a working relationship is firmly established and the client is certain of the counselor's good will, the client feels highly vulnerable and may misinterpret confrontations as criticisms, "put-downs," blame, or rejection. The degree of risk involved in a confrontation, therefore, depends upon the counselor's sense of timing and his or her finesse. Effective confrontations generally require delicate handling, and they must occur in the context of empathic understanding. Skills in the use of this vital technique are discussed extensively in Chapter Ten.

ARGUING

Arguing is not to be confused with confrontation. Abrasive, ineffective, and often destructive to the helping relationship, arguing in any guise is to be avoided. In arguing, the counselor ignores the client's feelings and views, seeking instead to prove the rightness of his own views. The ensuing contest, in which the client feels at a loss because of the counselor's greater expertise, often engenders feelings of resentment, alienation, passive resistance, or overt hostility. Rarely does arguing produce benefical results.

It is often appropriate and helpful for the counselor to disagree. Disagreement, however, will not evolve into competitive interaction as long as the context is one of good will and helpful intent and as long as the client does not feel that he or she must accept the counselor's views as necessarily right.

DOGMATIC INTERPRETATION

Interpretations presented by the counselor as dogmatic assertions are another form of inept confrontation. Interpretations of the dynamics of the meaning of behavior, as explained in Chapter Six, may be helpful, but not when offered in a rigid or authoritarian manner. The authoritarian counselor or therapist may be meeting his or her own need to demonstrate perceptiveness or erudition. The client's impression, however, is more likely to be that the counselor is imperceptive and arrogant.

Pressure Tactics

During the action-oriented or working-through phase of counseling, some helping professionals make the serious error of attempting to pressure the client into accelerating the rate of progress. Pressure tactics include unilaterally assigning "homework" tasks that the client cannot or will not carry out, prodding the client to make changes deemed desirable by the counselor but not necessarily by the client, browbeating or belittling the client for not making changes, predicting dire consequences if changes are not made, discrediting the client's sense of responsibility, or questioning the sincerity of his motivation to change if the client does not meet the counselor's expectations. Each of these tactics ignores the feelings or other factors involved in the client's failure to achieve what the counselor calls success. Rather, the tactics involve imposing assignments on the client and responding punitively when the client fails to accomplish the assigned changes.

Pressure tactics generally elicit untoward responses, among them fear of the therapist, feelings of inadequacy or failure, apology and acquiescent behavior aimed at regaining the therapist's favor, activation of negative transference feelings associated with authoritarian parental relationships, or strong feelings of resentment toward the therapist. When the client is resentful, he may bring counseling to an end by simply failing to return for additional interviews. In other instances, the client may respond to pressure tactics with deterioration in functioning. The destructive results of pressure tactics have been documented by Lieberman, Yalom, and Miles (1973), whose research reveals that psychological casualties are associated with pressure tactics employed by leaders in encounter groups. Moreover, the use of pressure to produce change places the responsibility for providing the impetus to change with the therapist rather than with the client. The therapist who assumes this responsibility is not only setting himself up for failure, but also for taking the blame, perhaps appropriately, for that failure.

Therapists who employ pressure tactics often fail to understand how difficult and painful it is for people to change deeply entrenched patterns of behavior. Resorting to pressure tactics may also reflect the counselor's insufficient grasp of the principles and psychodynamics involved in helping people overcome the inevitable obstacles encountered in change. Some therapists are impatient. Others lack awareness of their own motivations for employing pressure tactics. Some such therapists appear to need to dominate others, to validate their competency as therapists, or to meet their own needs vicariously through their clients. An example that came to the attention of one of the authors involved a therapist who encouraged his young, attractive, married female client to engage in extramarital sexual relations because she was sexually unfulfilled in her marriage. He made this recommendation even though it was incompatible with his client's moral values. Wisely, she changed therapists instead of sexual partners.

In this chapter, counterproductive communicational patterns have been identified and discussed. The reader is urged to become thoroughly familiar with these patterns so that he can recognize them and eliminate those which are included in his repertoire of responses. In subsequent chapters, effective styles of communication will be introduced and exercises provided to facilitate their mastery.

Chapter 4

⁂⁂⁂⁂⁂⁂⁂⁂⁂⁂⁂⁂⁂⁂⁂⁂⁂⁂⁂⁂⁂

Developing
Perceptiveness
to Feelings

The Significance of Feelings

Feelings or emotions are a vital, universal, and major part of human experience, exerting powerful influences on behavior. The eminent psychologist and philosopher William James wrote, "Reason is but a fleck on the sea of emotion." Certain emotional states may govern human behavior for short periods. Terms like *crime of passion* and *blind rage* evidence the belief that emotions may be so intense as to be ungoverned by reason. But emotions also invest life with zest and meaning. Joy, elation, ecstasy, pride in accomplishment, bliss, passionate love—these and other strong positive states of feeling are associated with those events and experiences most prized in human existence. These emotional states may override cognitive processes, as is signified by such phrases as *beside oneself with joy*.

Emotions also play a vital role in interpersonal relationships. Emotional reactions to others determine in large measure the quality of feelings experienced in relationships with them, such as whether they attract or repel us. We tend to cultivate relationships with people who are congenial, easy-going and even-tempered and to shun those who are grouchy, irritable, or morose. Whether we seek a deep relationship with another person depends largely on whether we generally feel good in the other's presence. Moreover, the extent and quality of feelings shared in relationships often determine the degree of satisfaction experienced.

Strong emotions or states of feeling invariably play a central role in the problems of people who seek help. The powerful role of emotions is readily apparent in some problems, as, for example, with persons who are emotionally volatile and get into difficulties because they have a "short fuse" and discharge their anger through violent outbursts of temper. Such individuals are governed excessively by their emotions, and we refer to them as emotionally unstable or immature. Other individuals may be stable emotionally under ordinary circumstances but may become temporarily distraught and immobilized by depressive states resulting from acute stresses such as the death of a loved one, a divorce, or an overwhelming sense of failure in some effort deemed vital.

Many people who see counselors are pulled in different directions by opposing feelings and seek help to resolve their emotional dilemmas. A person may, for example, be torn by love and hate toward the same person. Similarly, someone facing a difficult marital situation may be in conflict over whether to remain in a highly frustrating situation or face the agony of a divorce. In such instances, the helping professional may render a valuable service by assisting the client to become aware of and to sort out feelings involved. When this is accomplished, the client may be able to see and choose the most appropriate course of action.

Human beings vary widely in the range of emotions they experience. Some people, for example, fluctuate markedly from elation to depression, as in manic-depressive reactions. Others change but little, seldom experiencing strong emotions and rarely, if ever, losing control of themselves. Some, in fact, are overly controlled, as will be discussed later. The stability of emotions is likewise variable. Flightiness, or emotional ability, characterizes some people, who may react strongly even to mild provocations. Others have a remarkable tolerance for frustration, demonstrating strong emotions only under the most unusual circumstances. Still others manifest emotional characteristics that typify their personalities and earn them such labels as moody, brooding, petulant, querulous, or tempestuous, to name just a few. By contrast, others are said to be affable, lovable, even-tempered, or incurably optimistic.

Just as people vary in their emotional reactivity, so do they vary in their emotional expressiveness. One person may readily identify and express most of his feelings. Another, however, may be emotionally detached, withholding, and unexpressive. Variance is also common within a given individual. Some people are highly expressive of certain emotions such as anger but restricted in expressing tender feelings. Some individuals cannot express love and sentiment well, a deficiency that often causes marital difficulties because the normal need for emotional sustenance and security in the love of the partner is frustrated. Consider these lines from "The Buried Life" by the celebrated English poet Matthew Arnold:

> Alas, is even Love too weak
> To unlock the heart and let it speak?
> Are even lovers powerless to reveal
> To one another what indeed they feel?
> I knew the mass of men conceal'd
> Their thoughts, for fear that if reveal'd
> They would by other men be met
> With blank indifference, or with blame reproved:
> I knew they lived and moved
> Trick'd in disguises, alien to the rest
> Of men, and alien to themselves—and yet
> There beats one heart in every human breast.

Feelings and the Therapist

Many, if not most, basic problems presented to therapists involve emotional states. Clients may be dominated by irrational fears or by depressive states, for example, and the counselor will need skills in working with these emotions to help effectively. Other clients may experience difficulties because of outbursts of temper or feelings of guilt or personal inadequacy. In other instances, as with those individuals who are overcontrolled emotionally, the role of feelings or emotions is more subtle. Out of touch with their feelings, these individuals may develop physical symptoms caused by tension resulting from the inadequate release of emotions naturally and inevitably associated with daily living. Because they are out of touch with their emotions, such persons may be unaware of the sources of the tension that overstimulates certain systems of the body and often produces or aggravates such physical symptoms as ulcers, colitis, asthma, skin rashes, headaches, muscular aches, and tics. The counselor can help these individuals toward awareness and expression of the emotions that earlier were handled by denial or some other exclusion from conscious awareness. As awareness of emotions develops, the person can be helped to cope with his emotions in a healthier fashion and to integrate his emotionality into the totality of human experiencing. In the final analysis, how one deals with his emotions determines to a great extent his physical and mental health and the nature of his interpersonal relations.

Emotions often are experienced as transitory responses to occurrences in the environment, such as fear or panic in the event of a near accident. The extreme fear and anxiety associated with certain stressful situations may be warded off temporarily by depersonalization—that is, psychological removal of the self from the situation. For example, a late-adolescent female client of one of the authors experienced depersonalization one night while waiting on a carful of young males at a drive-in hamburger stand. The young men were flirting with her and making mild sexual references. The client, who had never adequately integrated her own sexuality, virtually panicked. Suddenly she found herself viewing the situation, including herself, in a detached manner, as though she were looking down on it all from the top of a nearby lightpole. The woman's emotional reaction to the experience was so intense that she sought protection against being overwhelmed by engaging in depersonalization.

In other instances, emotional reactions to traumatic events such as rape may persist and mount for extended periods of time, increasingly impairing functioning until the victim is virtually immobilized. Extreme trauma or seemingly inescapable and intolerable frustration may also produce emotional reactions so severe that the person seeks psychological escape in amnesia, a partial or total loss of memory that at least temporarily blocks awareness of the stressful situation. Somewhat similar are delayed mourning reactions to the loss of loved ones by death or divorce. Essentially, the person represses feelings of bereavement as a psychological protection against depression, appearing to take the loss in stride. Months or even years later, however, the person experiences the full impact of the loss, and the effects may be devastating, producing a profound depression.

The potentially damaging impact of stressful events may be diminished if the therapist helps the person ventilate his emotions. Ventilation of pent-up emotions facilitates emotional healing much as lancing a boil to drain the pus helps heal the sore. Fostering ventilation and expanding awareness of feelings require that the therapist be skilled in accurately identifying and responding to the client's feelings, both apparent and underlying. Therapists who are uncomfortable in relating to strong emotions or who lack skill in eliciting and empathizing with them will be ineffective with a substantial proportion of clients.

Certain states of feeling exist as enduring inner patterns. Of profound importance, these enduring states tend to be deeply ingrained and are associated with personality patterns that govern interpersonal transactions in large measure. Such states usually involve feelings about the self or others, including inferiority, worthlessness, helplessness, aloneness in the world, and self-contempt. These feelings often derive from experiences in early life, but they persist long after because they remain unresolved as "unfinished business." Such states of feeling may be the motivating force behind the development of such dysfunctional patterns as social isolation, aggressiveness, passivity, and excessive dependence. Individuals victimized by these patterns often seek professional help because they are unhappy. Frequently unaware of the feelings underlying their dysfunctional patterns, they can be helped to expand their awareness and to master these patterns, thereby enriching their satisfaction in living.

Because human problems invariably involve emotions and feelings, effective counseling requires that the counselor be highly perceptive to the complex emotions and states of feeling the client manifests. This statement does not exclude cognition from therapy. Feelings, indeed, do not exist independent of thoughts, a point discussed more extensively in Chapter Ten. Even cognitive therapists acknowledge the significance of emotions. Although cognitive theorists (Ellis, 1962, 1973a; Raimy, 1975) make erroneous assumptions and misconceptions the primary determinants of behavior, they nevertheless acknowledge the power of emotions. They acknowledge further that emotions are the surface manifestations of underlying misconceptions and thus are significant even in cognitive therapy. Emotions and feelings are of pivotal significance in the theories of virtually all schools of counseling and psychotherapy.

Effective therapists must be able to elicit, respond to, and understand the role of emotions in the many and varied problems clients present. Moreover, skills in perceiving the feelings of others are prerequisite to the mastery of empathic communication, which involves sensing or "tuning in" to the feelings of another and conveying to that other that one has accurately perceived his feelings.

The Vocabulary of Feelings

Helping professionals encounter a broad spectrum of emotions and feeling states in their daily work. Conveying an accurate understanding of these emotions and feelings to the client requires full awareness of the diversity of human emotion. Accurate perceptiveness, moreover, requires a high degree of sensitivity to the intensity of feelings the client experiences. Anger, for example, may be experienced in the mildest degree as mere annoyance or in the most intense degree as violent rage or fury. Similar ranges of intensity characterize other emotions and feelings.

To achieve high levels of empathic communication, the helping professional must not only be attuned accurately to both the quality and the intensity of the client's feelings, but also must be able to communicate back to the client the exact feeling he perceives. This latter skill requires a rich vocabulary of words and expressions of emotion the helping person can use to reflect each feeling in its proper intensity. Even experienced therapists have deficient vocabularies of feeling. In a critical vein, May observes, "When the therapists do respond on the level of feelings, the range of affects picked up and dealt with is definitely limited" (1969, p. 438). In identifying feelings for empathic communication, the therapist must also be able to go beyond single words to phrases and metaphorical expressions that vividly portray and add to the feeling and experiencing of the client. Too often, as May says, "the therapist reflects the words of

THE VOCABULARY OF FEELINGS

Levels of Intensity	Happy	Caring	Depressed	Inadequate	Fearful	Confused	Hurt	Angry	Lonely	Guilt-Shame
Strong	thrilled	tenderness toward	desolate	worthless	terrified	bewildered	crushed	furious	isolated	sick at heart
	on cloud nine	affection for	dejected	good for nothing	frightened	puzzled	destroyed	enraged	abandoned	unforgivable
	ecstatic	captivated by	hopeless	washed up	intimidated	baffled	ruined	seething	all alone	humiliated
	overjoyed	attached to	alienated	powerless	horrified	perplexed	degraded	outraged	forsaken	disgraced
	excited	devoted to	depressed	helpless	desperate	trapped	pain(ed)	infuriated	cut off	degraded
	elated	adoration	gloomy	impotent	panicky	confounded	wounded	burned up		horrible
	sensational	loving	dismal	crippled	terror-stricken	in a dilemma	devastated	pissed off		mortified
	exhilarated	infatuated	bleak	inferior	stage fright	befuddled	tortured	fighting mad		exposed
	fantastic	enamored	in despair	emasculated	dread	in a quandary	disgraced	nauseated		
	terrific	cherish	empty	useless	vulnerable	full of questions	humiliated	violent		
	on top of the world	idolize	barren	finished	paralyzed	confused	anguished	indignant		
	turned on	worship	grieved	like a failure			at the mercy of	hatred		
	euphoric		grief				cast off	bitter		
	enthusiastic		despair				forsaken	galled		
	delighted		grim				rejected	vengeful		
	marvelous						discarded	hateful		
	great							vicious		
Moderate	cheerful	caring	distressed	inadequate	afraid	mixed-up	hurt	resentful	lonely	ashamed
	light-hearted	fond of	upset	whipped	scared	disorganized	belittled	irritated	alienated	guilty
	happy	regard	downcast	defeated	fearful	foggy	shot down	hostile	estranged	remorseful
	serene	respectful	sorrowful	incompetent	apprehensive	troubled	overlooked	annoyed	remote	crummy
	wonderful	admiration	demoralized	inept	jumpy	adrift	abused	upset with	alone	to blame
	up	concern for	discouraged	overwhelmed	shaky	lost	depreciated	agitated	apart from others	lost face
	aglow	hold dear	miserable	ineffective	threatened	at loose ends	criticized	mad	insulated from others	demeaned
	glowing	prize	pessimistic	lacking	distrustful	going around in circles	defamed	aggravated		
	in high spirits	taken with	tearful	deficient	risky	disconcerted	censured	offended		
	jovial	turned on	weepy	unable	alarmed	frustrated	discredited	antagonistic		
	riding high	trust	rotten	incapable	butterflies	flustered	disparaged	exasperated		
		close	awful	small	awkward	in a bind	laughed at	belligerent		
			horrible	insignificant	defensive		maligned	mean		

elevated neat	warm toward friendly like positive toward	terrible blue lost melancholy	like Casper Milquetoast unfit unimportant incomplete no good immobilized		ambivalent disturbed helpless embroiled	mistreated ridiculed devalued scorned mocked scoffed at used exploited debased slammed slandered impugned cheapened	vexed spiteful vindictive	left out excluded lonesome distant aloof	regretful wrong embarrassed at fault in error responsible for blew it goofed lament

Mild

glad	unhappy	lacking	nervous	uncertain	put down	uptight
good	down	confidence	anxious	unsure	neglected	disgusted
contented	low	unsure of	unsure	bothered	overlooked	bugged
satisfied	bad	yourself	hesitant	uncomfortable	minimized	turned off
gratified	blah	uncertain	timid	undecided	let down	put out
pleasant	disappointed	weak	shy		unappreciated	miffed
pleased	sad	inefficient	worried		taken for	irked
fine	glum		uneasy		granted	perturbed
			bashful			ticked off
			embarrassed			teed off
			ill at ease			chagrined
			doubtful			cross
			jittery			dismayed
			on edge			impatient
			uncomfortable			
			self-conscious			

the patient, not his feelings; words *about* rather than the experiences themselves" (p. 437).

A rich vocabulary of feeling is essential also to communicating with high levels of authenticity and relational immediacy, both qualities which often involve the counselor's sharing emotions he experiences in the context of the helping relationship. These two important aspects of communication are discussed in greater detail in Chapters Eight and Nine.

It has been our experience that beginning counselors lack an adequate repertoire of feeling words and tend to employ excessively those few words they do know. Vague feeling words such as *upset* and *frustrated,* which may embrace somewhat diverse feelings, often are overused because the counselor is unaccustomed to more precise words like *bewildered* or *perplexed.*

To help you expand your vocabulary, the Vocabulary of Feelings has been compiled as a resource. Although the list is by no means exhaustive, it does include the emotions and feelings most commonly encountered in helping relationships. The emotions and feelings are subsumed under ten categories, which appear at the top of each list of feeling words in the category. The feeling words are further classified by the intensity each denotes.

You are encouraged to use the Vocabulary of Feelings in formulating responses to the exercises in this and subsequent chapters. At first, you should draw from your own vocabulary. As you compose your response, keep in mind that emotions are complex and that messages often involve more than one feeling. After formulating a response, review the Vocabulary of Feelings to determine whether another word would make your response more accurate. Also scan the categories of feelings to determine whether the client's message involves feelings in addition to those you identified. By using the Vocabulary of Feelings, you will find that your own vocabulary will gradually expand and that you will increasingly employ words that you rarely, if ever, used before. As you broaden your vocabulary, you will have less occasion to refer to the Vocabulary of Feelings.

Improving your ability to perceive emotions and feelings accurately and to convey your perceptions skillfully will help your client expand his own awareness of his inner experiencing. Often the client has difficulty communicating his feelings to others because he cannot identify or label his emotions. A perceptive and skillful helping person will be able to draw out the client's feelings and thereby help to label them so that both the helping person and the client will understand the troubling emotions and patterns of feelings that play a role in the client's problems.

Skill-Development Exercises in Perceiving Feelings

To assist you in increasing your perceptiveness to feelings, exercises involving client messages taken from actual interviews have been provided. Read each message carefully, and then write down the feeling word that you believe captures the essence of the emotion the client experiences. Keep in mind that clients often do not use feeling words and that feelings may be only implied. It is the responsibility of the helping person to "tune in" to feelings even though they may be expressed indirectly. You may find it helpful to ask yourself the questions, "What would the person have to feel or experience to send such a message?" and "What would I be feeling in the same situation?" With the second question, however, you must be careful not to project your feelings onto the client. It takes a high degree of self-awareness to avoid the common error of assuming that others feel as you would in a given situation. Nevertheless, although each person is unique, human beings are much more alike than different, and your personal experiences may help you perceive the experiencing of others.

The exercises are divided into two parts. The first group of fifteen messages provides practice in identifying feelings in typical client statements. Exercises 16 through 23 involve sharper discriminations between readily apparent feelings and probable deeper feelings—that is, emotions that may be somewhat removed from the client's immediate awareness. For example, when probable deeper feelings are involved, it is not unusual for a person to experience a surface emotion of anger, which in actuality derives from feelings of hurt. Friction or antagonism between two persons may be resolved if feelings of hurt are disclosed, whereas expressions of anger may produce defensiveness and alienation, thus perpetuating and perhaps exacerbating the problem. In other instances the dynamics may be reversed. A person who believes that anger is bad may experience hurt when the more appropriate feeling of anger is suppressed. The significance of apparent and probable deeper feelings and the importance of the ability to discern both levels will be elaborated in Chapters Five and Six.

Read each message and write the feelings involved in the space provided. If possible, use the Vocabulary of Feelings to improve your response. As you complete each exercise, check the feelings you identified with those given by the authors. In the authors' answers, similar feeling words are grouped under labels a, b, and so forth. If you have identified words not on the list but very close in meaning, consider yourself as accurate. If you were unsuccessful in identifying the feelings correctly, study the message further to see whether you can discover the cues you missed.

In subsequent chapters, particularly Chapter Five, you will have much more extensive practice in identifying feelings and in formulating responses.

EXERCISES IN THE PERCEPTION OF FEELINGS

1. "Life just doesn't seem worth struggling with anymore. I just don't think I can make it. I just can't go on anymore."
    Feelings Involved:

2. "I wrote Fred a special tune for his birthday, and he never said anything about it—whether he appreciated it or didn't like it. I felt really bad."
    Feelings Involved:

3. "I think this is just a complete waste of time! I never wanted to come. I wouldn't be here if my husband didn't make me. I don't know why *I* should be here! He has more problems than me!"
    Feelings Involved:

4. "I don't shower after gym. I'm embarrassed about my body, about being overweight."
    Feelings Involved:

5. "It's my turn to give a five-minute talk in speech class Tuesday. Every time I think about it I get goosebumps."
    Feelings Involved:

6. "My husband loves his job as a bus driver, but I wish he'd consider working at something else. When he's gone for five days on a trip, the house seems so big and empty I can hardly stand it."
   Feelings Involved:

7. "I've been feeling good about how things are going. My husband has been trying harder and he's been opening up more. But I'm even more pleased with myself. I've handled my emotions better, and I've felt for the first time that I'm an intelligent human being."
   Feelings Involved:

8. "My girlfriend is pressing me for a decision as to whether or not I'm going to get a divorce. My wife says I have to give up the girlfriend or get out. I'm not ready to decide what I want and I don't know which way to turn."
   Feelings Involved:

9. "I wonder if I do too much for my husband. He doesn't do much for me or for any woman. I knocked myself out painting the house and he didn't lift a finger to help me."
   Feelings Involved:

10. (Fourteen-year-old boy:) "I don't feel I'm ever considered at all. Everybody tells me to do this, do that. All I am is a thing."
    Feelings Involved:

11. "No one ever takes me seriously. I can tell people something serious, and they think I'm just joking around."
    Feelings Involved:

12. "You have no idea how warmly I feel toward you. No one else has ever cared enough to listen or understand."
    Feelings Involved:

13. (Woman:) "The house is just constantly in turmoil. I never seem to have any peace or a minute for myself. I just sit down and the kids are either fighting, or they want me to wait on

them, or something happens. I can't ever sit down to rest and enjoy a TV show or read a magazine."
Feelings Involved:

14. "I know that the statistics say that ninety-five percent of the males masturbate, but somehow that doesn't make me feel any better."
Feelings Involved:

15. (Fifteen-year-old boy:) "I finally got up enough courage to ask a girl out for a date. After we went to the show, she asked me if I wanted to 'make out.' I didn't know what she meant and had to ask her. I felt really stupid when she told me."
Feelings Involved:

EXERCISES IN APPARENT AND PROBABLE DEEPER FEELINGS

16. "I know my children are busy, but wouldn't you think they could find time to at least call their mother on the telephone to see if she is dead or alive?"
Apparent Feelings:
Probable Deeper Feelings:

17. (Girl:) "I'm going to leave home. No matter what I do I'm always wrong. My mother keeps telling me my dresses are too short, that I'm going to get in trouble with boys. I can't stand it any longer. I'm going to run away."
Apparent Feelings:
Probable Deeper Feelings:

18. "My husband has started kissing me every time he leaves. I can't stand that; I've never been demonstrative. I don't like people 'kissing on me!' I can't stand at times to have people touch me. I've never let people smother me with affection."
Apparent Feelings:
Probable Deeper Feelings:

19. "I really got into a battle with my wife last night. I was an hour late for dinner because I had to go to a union meeting. She got

on my back because I didn't call to tell her I'd be late. I don't feel like I should have to check in with her like I'm one of the kids."
Apparent Feelings:
Probable Deeper Feelings:

20. "I decided to go to the dance after the football game, but it was a real drag. I didn't dance a single dance. I've had it with the boys in our school. They're a bunch of creeps."
Apparent Feelings:
Probable Deeper Feelings:

21. "I know we talked last time I saw you about my not losing my temper with the kids. But what do you do when they don't seem to learn. Just before I left home today my four-year-old ran out in the street twice after I'd warned him. It made me so mad I lost my cool and whalloped the hell out of him."
Apparent Feelings:
Probable Deeper Feelings:

22. "I can't tolerate my husband's flirting. Last night at a party you can't believe how attentive he was to that divorced floozie from work. I'd swear he talked more to her last night than to me. When I told him that afterwards, he got uptight and told me it was all in my head."
Apparent Feelings:
Probable Deeper Feelings:

23. "This was the fourth time in the last two weeks that Henry forgot to pick me up. And he can't understand why I didn't melt in his arms when he made affectionate overtures later that evening."
Apparent Feelings:
Probable Deeper Feelings: a.
                          b.

ANSWERS TO EXERCISES

Client Statement 1: (a) depressed, despondent, in despair, demoralized

                    (b) overwhelmed, helpless, defeated, like giving up

Client Statement 2: (a) hurt, rejected, rebuffed, unappreciated, disappointed, crushed

                    (b) resentful, offended, angry

Client Statement 3: (a) angry, resentful, bitter, indignant, antagonistic

                    (b) controlled, dominated, unjustly coerced, put upon, unfairly blamed

Client Statement 4: (a) embarrassed, ashamed, self-conscious, humiliated, horrible, afraid of ridicule or criticism

                    (b) inadequate, inferior, deficient, exposed

Client Statement 5: (a) apprehensive, scared, anxious, dread, fearful, afraid of failing

                    (b) unsure of yourself, lacking confidence

Client Statement 6: (a) lonely, isolated, all alone, lonesome

                    (b) downcast, blue, unhappy, sad

                    (c) dissatisfied, discontented, displeased, neglected

Client Statement 7: (a) happy, pleased, encouraged, delighted, just great, good about yourself

Client Statement 8: (a) confused, bewildered, perplexed, trapped, in a quandary, troubled, frustrated, in a bind, overwhelmed, torn up

                    (b) distressed, pressured

Client Statement 9: (a) confused, perplexed, frustrated, disconcerted

                    (b) irritated, resentful, used, aggravated

Client Statement 10: (a) hurt, overlooked, depreciated, devalued, ignored, unappreciated, rejected

                    (b) dominated, bossed, controlled

                    (c) resentment, anger

Client Statement 11: (a) discredited, taken lightly, misunderstood, unappreciated
(b) resentful, offended, put out, uptight

Client Statement 12: (a) close, caring, warm
(b) appreciated, respected, valued, gratified
(c) have been feeling alone, cut off, excluded, estranged

Client Statement 13: (a) burdened, pressured, overwhelmed, exhausted, frustration, in turmoil
(b) unfulfilled, deprived, powerless, immobilized
(c) aggravated, annoyed, irritated, agitated

Client Statement 14: (a) guilty, crummy, horrible, bad

Client Statement 15: (a) embarrassed, humiliated, exposed, ridiculous, mortified, like an idiot, like a klutz

Client Statement 16—*Apparent Feelings:* neglected, unappreciated, lonesome, hurt, let down
Probable Deeper Feelings: indignant, bitter, resentful, angry

Client Statement 17—*Apparent Feelings:* angry, offended, put upon, resentful, antagonistic, unjustly accused, unfairly criticized, fed up, never understood, picked on
Probable Deeper Feelings: hurt, degraded, belittled, hopeless, alienated, rejected

Client Statement 18—*Apparent Feelings:* repulsed by, uncomfortable, irritated, annoyed, turned off, smothered, distasteful, anxious
Probable Deeper Feelings: afraid (of letting someone that close or of not having control), fearful (of tender feelings), guilt

Client Statement 19—*Apparent Feelings:* resentful, angry, aggravated, mad, burned up

Probable Deeper Feelings: afraid (of being dominated), fear (of being controlled)

Client Statement 20—*Apparent Feelings:* disappointed, disgusted, fed up, mad, ticked off
Probable Deeper Feelings: left out, rejected, hurt, lonely, inadequate, lacking, unimportant

Client Statement 21—*Apparent Feelings:* frustrated, angry, exasperated, out of patience
Probable Deeper Feelings: concern, afraid, worried, protective

Client Statement 22—*Apparent Feelings:* jealous, angry, aggravated, indignant, irked, chagrined
Probable Deeper Feelings: insecure, hurt, afraid (fear of rejection or abandonment)

Client Statement 23—*Apparent Feelings:* cool, distant, cross, grouchy, annoyed, irritated
Probable Deeper Feelings: a) angry, resentful, burned up, galled
b) neglected, unimportant, mistreated, unloved, rejected

Chapter 5

⋉⋊⋉⋊⋉⋊⋉⋊⋉⋊⋉⋊⋉⋊⋉⋊⋉⋊⋉⋊⋉⋊⋉⋊

Responding Empathically to the Client's Expressions: Reciprocal Responses

In Chapters One and Two, we explained the critical importance of empathic responding, showing how it stimulates the client's self-experiencing and his exploration of feelings and conflicts, thereby laying the foundation of insightful understanding necessary for behavioral change. Furthermore, the counselor's communication of empathic understanding reduces threat and defensiveness, conveys interest and helpful intent, and facilitates the establishment of a therapeutic relationship wherein the counselor becomes emotionally significant in the client's life. This relationship provides the necessary trust, regard, and encouragement for the client to remain in therapy and to endure the anxiety, fearfulness, and growing pains of deep self-examination and constructive change. The therapeutic relationship also provides the interpersonal context and atmosphere in which the client's conflicts, distortions, and projections may be reexperienced, understood, and resolved.

97

Communicating empathic understanding, however, takes more than merely believing in its vital importance (Bergin and Solomon, 1970). Acquiring the skill requires focused practice and high-level modeling. The purpose of this and the following chapter is to provide abundant materials for practical skill training in empathic responsiveness. Initially the reader will be trained to perceive varying levels of empathic communications through the introduction of a rating scale, examples of varying levels of counselor responses, and exercises to refine perception and discrimination. The reader will then be prepared to undertake exercises in learning how to communicate empathic understanding. Practical guidelines and recommendations for responding empathically are presented, as well as clinical indications and contraindications.

Levels of Empathic Responding

The Empathic Communication Scale is presented below, followed by examples of varying levels of empathic responses by the counselor to messages from the client. The reader is encouraged to memorize the essential characteristics of each level of the scale, and to refer back to it consistently while studying the examples and working the rating exercises.

EMPATHIC COMMUNICATION SCALE*

Level 1.0. The counselor's verbal and behavioral responses are irrelevant, *subtract significantly* in affect and content, and do not attend appropriately to the other's expressions. The counselor communicates no awareness of even the most obvious, expressed surface feelings of the other person. The responses include premature advice-giving, arguing, changing the subject, criticizing, pontificating, and asking questions that shift the focus from the expressions of the client.

Level 1.5. Counselor responses qualify as negligibly accurate, and any of the client's feelings that are not distinctly defined tend to be entirely ignored. Counselor responses may mislead or block off the client. The client does not go to a deeper level of self-exploration.

*Adapted from earlier versions of accurate empathy rating scales (Rogers, Gendlin, Kiesler, and Truax, 1967; Truax and Carkhuff, 1967; Carkhuff, 1969; Gazda, 1973).

Level 2.0. The counselor responds to at least part of the surface feelings of the other person, but the response *noticeably subtracts affect* or *distorts the level of meaning.* Awareness of the client's expressed feelings is only partially communicated. The counselor may respond to his own conceptualizations rather than to what the client expressed. Some responses may have diagnostic or psychodynamic accuracy, but not empathic accuracy.

Level 2.5. The counselor wants to understand and makes the effort, but his responses subtract slightly from the level of feelings the other expresses. Responses that merely parrot expressions of the other person in the same words belong to this level.

Level 3.0. Responses communicate understanding at the level of feeling the client expresses. The counselor's responses are essentially *interchangeable, or reciprocal, in affect* with the surface, explicit expressions of the other individual, or they accurately reflect his state of being. The responses do not add affect or go below the surface feelings, nor do they subtract from the feelings and tone expressed. Factual aspects of the client's message (content), though desirable, are not required; if included, content must be accurate.

When expressed feelings are vague or ill defined, inquiries used to expand the expression of feeling or to explore meaning are appropriate. However, if feelings are stated explicitly or are clearly implied, then inquiries alone, without responsiveness to the feelings, are noticeably subtractive (level 2.0).

Responses at level 3.0 are minimally facilitative and helpful.

Level 3.5. The counselor's responses reflect not only the feelings but also the reasons for the feelings that the other person expresses—in other words, the counselor's responses complement feelings with content.

Level 4.0. The counselor's responses accurately identify implicit, underlying feelings somewhat beyond the expressions of the client *and* complement feelings with content that adds deeper meaning.

Level 4.5. Responses exceed level 4.0 but fall short of level 5.0.

Level 5.0. The counselor's responses *significantly add* to the affect and meaning explicitly expressed by the client. Additionally, the counselor's responses accurately communicate the affect, meaning, and intensity of the other person's deeper feelings by word, voice, and intensity of expression.

Whenever appropriate, responses at this level may empathically identify the client's implicit goals which point the direction for personal growth, paving the way to action. The counselor may relate current feelings and experiences to previously expressed experiences or feelings, or he may accurately identify implicit patterns, themes, or purposes.

LEVELS OF EMPATHIC RESPONDING: EXAMPLES

Client Statement 1:

"At work I've been trying so hard to please my boss. I can't seem to please him and he's really sharp and blunt when I make a mistake. Yesterday I misspelled a word and he glared at me and said he'd like to have a secretary who uses better grammar and spells better than he does."

Level 1.0 response. "Why don't you tell him that no one's perfect and that you're doing your best?"

Explanation. The counselor communicates no awareness of the person's feelings. The advice-giving in this instance is inappropriate and might be expected to inhibit rather than expand expression of the client's feelings.

Level 1.5 response. "I wonder if you've considered changing jobs."

Explanation. The response has some relevance and is not given directly as advice, so it is higher than level 1.0. However, it entirely ignores the client's feelings and will probably block their further expression. Therefore, the level of response is lower than level 2.0.

Level 2.0 response. "Sounds like he's really a tough guy to work for."

Explanation. The counselor refers indirectly to the client's feelings, but the response is noticeably subtractive because it does not clearly identify the feelings. The response is subtractive also because it focuses primarily on the employer rather than on the client's feelings. Since the response is relevant and not markedly inaccurate, it is higher than the 1.5 level.

Level 2.5 response. "You're feeling pretty discouraged about the whole thing."

Explanation. This response is accurate but slightly subtractive because it makes no reference to the client's concern that she is not meeting the boss's expectation. The response thus falls short of being reciprocal.

Level 3.0 response. "You want to please your boss but are discouraged about being unable to. I gather you're concerned after his remark yesterday that he isn't satisfied with your performance."

Explanation. Essentially interchangeable, this response expresses accurately the surface emotions in the client's message. The content of the response is accurate, but deeper feelings and meaning are not added.

Level 4.0 response. "You're feeling overwhelmed and lost as to how to please him. I gather that it's most discouraging and hurtful when he's as blunt and critical as he is and that you're worried right now about keeping your job."

Explanation. This response conveys not only the surface feelings and content, but also is noticeably additive in reflecting the client's deeper feelings of being overwhelmed and lost in not knowing how to cope with the situation. The reference to worry over losing the job is also additive.

Level 5.0 response. "I gather you're just so overwhelmed and distressed with the futility of trying to please your boss that you're feeling it may be hopeless. You're afraid your job may be in jeopardy and are wondering what to do in light of the stress and uncertainty."

Explanation. Significantly additive, this response goes well beyond the surface feelings in reflecting the underlying feelings of distress, futility, and possible hopelessness of the situation. In addition, the latter part of the response includes an action statement that may preface exploration of possible alternatives available to the client.

Client Statement 2:

College-age male: "I'm caught in a dilemma. I would like to stay in town on the weekends to see Paula, but my parents like me to come home to visit them. I don't want to hurt my parents, plus they really make me feel guilty when I don't come home. But at the same time what I'd most like to do is spend my free time with my girl."

Level 1.0 response. "Your parents probably are doing what they feel is in your best interest. They really don't understand how you feel about Paula. I think they really mean well though and you need to try to understand their position."

Explanation. This response ignores the client's feelings and demonstrates no understanding at all of his frame of reference. The focus shifts from the client to his parents, and this response may lead the client to feel that the helper is taking sides with the parents. This irrelevant response would probably shut off self-exploration.

Level 1 response. "How do you think Paula and your parents see the situation?"

Explanation. This question shifts the focus away from the experiencing of the client and communicates no grasp of the client's inner world.

Level 2.0 response. "It seems that you are uncertain what to do. You're at an age where you'd like to break away from those parental apron strings and stand on your own, but you still have some conflicts over whether you want to be dependent or independent."

Explanation. The initial sentence demonstrates an effort to understand, although it subtracts slightly from the expressed feelings of the other person. However, the second sentence is the counselor's own conceptual formulation, which may be diagnostically accurate, but is not empathically attuned to the client's expression.

Level 3.0 response. "I can see your bind over wanting to be with Paula, yet not knowing how to do it without hurting your parents."

Explanation. This response neither adds to nor takes away from what was expressed. It tunes in on the expressed feelings of confusion and the concern over the impact on the parents, and, in addition, it includes the important content of the message.

Level 3.0 response. "Kind of feeling very confused as to how to satisfy both your parents and yourself."

Explanation. This response reciprocally captures the tone, neither adding nor subtracting affect.

Level 4.0 response. "I hear your bewilderment over how in the devil to see Paula as much as you'd like without leaving your parents feeling neglected. But I think I might hear more too. Could you try changing the word *guilt* into the word *resentment* when you refer to how you feel with your parents, and see if it fits?"

Explanation. This response first communicates the affect and content expressed by the client, then goes on to make an additive inference about what appear to be underlying feelings.

Level 4.5 response. "Seems like you're saying, 'I'm in a real conflict over whether to satisfy my parents or to do what I'd really like and see Paula.' You may be feeling some resentment over their wishes, yet also feeling some caring for them, and you're confused over how to reconcile the feelings."

Explanation. This response meets all of the requirements of a level 3.0 response, and it adds implicit, underlying feelings. It should be emphasized, however, that to achieve this rating, an additive response must be accurate. Therefore, in an actual therapeutic situation, the client's next response would need to confirm the accuracy of the counselor's statement in order to achieve this rating. If an additive response is inaccurate, it is rated level 2.0.

Level 5.0 response. "So you're really in a bind between feeling very fond of Paula and wanting to be with her and not wanting to reject your parents. I also seem to sense some resentment toward your parents for expecting you to be home and a wish that you could help them understand without feeling hurt."

Explanation. This intervention tunes in on both the feelings and content expressed by the client, adds underlying feelings, and contains a goal statement that prepares for future action. Again, in an actual counseling encounter, the accuracy of the additive portion of the response would need to be confirmed by the client to achieve this rating.

Exercises in Assessing Levels of Empathic Communication

These exercises in rating varied counselor responses for the degree of empathy communicated are designed to refine your perception of empathic messages in preparation for practice in communicating empathy. Five client statements are given, followed by several possible counselor responses. Refer back to the Empathic Communication Scale and rate each response in the space provided at the left of the counselor response. The discrepancy score will be explained below, after you have finished the exercise.

CLIENT STATEMENT 1

"It was scary when life seemed so empty and black—I was very discouraged and almost decided to put my child on the bus and send him to my sister's place, then just disappear."

Your Rating	*Responses:*	*Discrepancy Score*
_____	1. "You were eager to be by yourself so you seriously considered sending your child to your sister's place."	_____
_____	2. "You felt discouraged—like you had to have some time to yourself away from your child."	_____
_____	3. "Your feelings of despair and hopelessness were so intense that you felt desperate enough to make up plans for disappearing."	_____
_____	4. "You really must cheer up, and I should think having your child with you would help you keep from getting discouraged."	_____
_____	5. "You were frightened when you realized how discouraged you were, especially when you actually wanted to send your child to your sister's for safekeeping."	_____
_____	6. "I gather you were very discouraged, and it was scary when you thought of sending your child to your sister's."	_____
_____	7. "You feel depressed and frightened that your thoughts would go so far as to make plans for your child and then think of disappearing."	_____
_____	8. "It seems to me you need to get hold of yourself and realize you have a child to think about as well as yourself."	_____
_____	9. "You were very frightened when you realized you were so depressed that you were ready to initiate plans to care for your child and then vanish. But your coming for help tells me you are hoping there can be another solution."	_____
_____	10. "Your world seems to be completely desolate, and you felt so demoralized	_____

and totally helpless that you just wanted to send your child away and get away from it all."

Sum: _____

Average Discrepancy Score: _____

Check your ratings with those provided on page 109. Figure the difference, disregarding whether it is positive or negative, between each of your ratings and the authors' ratings, and enter the differences in the blanks to the right of the responses. Then add the differences between your ratings and the ratings provided for the ten responses. Divide this sum by 10 (the number of counselor responses) to get your average discrepancy score, which provides a guide to your ability to discriminate the levels of empathic responses accurately. The goal is to achieve an average discrepancy score of 0.5 or less by the end of these exercises. After each exercise, study the responses for which your ratings differ from the authors', refer to the rating scale, and try to pinpoint the reason why the authors rate it as they do.

Proceed now to rate the counselor responses to the client statements below. After rating all the responses to a statement, determine your discrepancy from the authors' rating for each response, add them, and divide by the total number of counselor responses presented in the exercise. Analyze each response you rated inaccurately.

CLIENT STATEMENT 2
"With my visual problem, sewing is really hard for me. And the teacher had me sewing on a simple poncho while all the other kids were making blouses. How do you think that makes you feel?"

Your		*Discrepancy*
Rating	*Responses:*	*Score*
_____	1. "I guess you must have felt pretty embarrassed and inadequate about working on something a lot easier than the others."	_____

——— 2. "You must have felt pretty humiliated   ————
sewing on that poncho and could just
have crawled under the floor. I bet you
resented your teacher for being in that
situation."

——— 3. "You felt you could just kill your teacher   ————
for making fun of you like that."

——— 4. "I wonder if you told the teacher how   ————
uncomfortable you felt. I'll bet she'd
have understood."

——— 5. "You feel at a real disadvantage in that   ————
class with your visual problem. I guess
you must have felt you stuck out like a
sore thumb being the only one working
on a poncho."

——— 6. "You feel like you can never succeed in   ————
sewing with your visual problem."

——— 7. "Could you pretend your eyes are in that   ————
chair and tell them how you feel about
the problems they cause you?"

——— 8. "Your visual problem really caused you   ————
to feel uncomfortable in that situation."

Sum: ————
Average Discrepancy Score: ————

CLIENT STATEMENT 3

"I guess I just dread meeting new people; once I know them a
little bit I can do all right."

Your *Rating* *Responses:*		*Discrepancy* *Score*

——— 1. "You feel nervous when you meet new   ————
people."

——— 2. "It's all in your head. There's no reason   ————
to fear meeting new people."

——— 3. "If you'd try every day to pretend you're   ————
not afraid and practice meeting at least

one new person your fear would soon
disappear."

_____ 4. "When you get to know people, you're _____
not as scared."

_____ 5. "Even though you're comfortable when _____
you're with people you know, you get
butterflies when you meet strangers."

_____ 6. "It's really tough for you to meet new _____
people."

_____ 7. "You're very apprehensive about meet- _____
ing new people but you do okay with
people you know."

_____ 8. "Although you're more at ease with peo- _____
ple you know, you're really frightened
about meeting new people and afraid of
how you come across to them. In that situation, I gather part of you is saying,
'Gee, I wish I could get out of this,' yet I
have the impression another part of you
would like to overcome those fears."

_____ 9. "You feel some confidence with people _____
you know well, perhaps because you
know how you stand with them, but with
new people you're so afraid you might
goof up."

Sum: _____

Average Discrepancy Score: _____

CLIENT STATEMENT 4

"I feel strange when I enter a room with other people in it.
Everyone looks at me."

Your   _Discrepancy_
Rating   _Responses:_   _Score_

_____ 1. "Sort of feel strange when you enter a _____
room and everyone looks at you, do
you?"

——— 2. "How do you know they're looking at   ————
          you?"
——— 3. "Try in those situations to keep eye con- ————
          tact with people. I'm sure you'll soon
          find yourself feeling better."
——— 4. "I hear you saying you feel ashamed   ————
          when others stare at you."
——— 5. "I gather you feel very uncomfortable,   ————
          fearing others are looking at you crit-
          ically."
——— 6. "When you walk into a room with others, ————
          you sort of feel self-conscious and un-
          sure of yourself."
——— 7. "I'm not sure what you mean by strange. ————
          Could you tell me more about that feel-
          ing?"
——— 8. "It's hard for you to do that."   ————

                                       Sum: ————
                    Average Discrepancy Score: ————

CLIENT STATEMENT 5

"I always have had my parents telephone for me about appointments and other things. I might foul up if I did it myself."

Your   Discrepancy
Rating   Responses: Score
——— 1. "You depend on your parents to handle   ————
          a lot of things for you because you're
          unsure of yourself."
——— 2. "You know I'm wondering how you can   ————
          ever be independent when you lean as
          much as you do on your parents."
——— 3. "Am I getting this right? You've always ————
          doubted yourself and been so afraid of
          bungling things and looking stupid that
          you play it safe by depending on your
          parents. You know, I'll bet there's part

of you that says, 'Gee, I wish I could be
more confident and independent.'"

_____ 4. "How do you think your parents experi-   _____
ence the way you lean on them?"

_____ 5. "When you have to phone for appoint-   _____
ments or do other things, you find your-
self depending excessively on your
parents."

_____ 6. "I gather you're so afraid of blowing it   _____
and looking foolish that you avoid risks
by having your parents do things for
you."

Sum: _____

Average Discrepancy Score: _____

RATINGS FOR ASSESSMENT EXERCISES

Client Statement 1	Client Statement 2	Client Statement 3	Client Statement 4	Client Statement 5
1. 1.5	1. 3.5	1. 2.0	1. 2.5	1. 3.0
2. 2.0	2. 4.0	2. 1.0	2. 1.0	2. 1.0
3. 4.5	3. 1.5	3. 1.0	3. 1.0	3. 5.0
4. 1.0	4. 1.5	4. 2.0	4. 1.5	4. 1.0
5. 3.0	5. 3.5	5. 3.0	5. 4.0	5. 2.0
6. 2.5	6. 2.0	6. 2.5	6. 3.5	6. 4.0
7. 3.5	7. 1.0	7. 3.0	7. 3.0	
8. 1.0	8. 2.0	8. 5.0	8. 2.0	
9. 4.0		9. 4.5		
10. 4.5				

Homework Practice Exercises

Two brief homework assignments may help increase your
perceptiveness and awareness. First, for the next few days use the
skills you have just practiced and rate the level of empathy others
communicate in conversations. You will discover how seldom people
listen intently and acknowledge that they have heard another person and how refreshing and encouraging an occasional level-3.0
response can be. Second, observe the frequency with which you
yourself respond empathically in your conversations.

Guidelines for Communicating Reciprocal Empathic Understanding

To this point, the discussion has focused on the characteristics of empathic communication. We will now present specific recommendations on how to convey reciprocal empathy to clients.

ATTENDING AND LISTENING

To be empathic, one must first receive the client's messages, both verbal and nonverbal. It takes very active listening to tune into the client's personal meanings, views, and feelings. Initially the counselor should attend, listen, and concentrate on the verbal and nonverbal behavior and state of being of the client. The term *attending* refers to being receptively present, available, and involved with another person. Attending allows one to receive verbal and nonverbal messages, conveys respect and interest, and serves as a powerful reinforcer.

Eye contact. Attending means first of all observing keenly and looking at the client. Maintaining eye contact, however, does not mean staring fixedly into the other person's eyes. Rather, it is a natural being-in-touch with the other person, much of the time through eye-to-eye contact, which communicates warmth and caring as well as interest and understanding.

Exercises in nonverbal responsiveness. We encourage you to pause at this point and experiment with two exercises. First, invite another person to sit down with you and maintain eye-to-eye contact. Initially ask your friend to stare at you intently for a few moments. Be aware of your reactions. You will probably notice feelings of discomfort and self-consciousness. Next, ask your friend to look at you with indifference. Notice how the eyes and other facial features convey this lack of interest. Now be aware of your emotional reaction. Take a few moments to recall other times when you have experienced another's lack of interest. Last, ask your friend to show interest, caring, and concern in his eyes and face. Be especially aware of your feelings now as contrasted to those experienced earlier.

For the second exercise, look at yourself in a mirror. Note the difference in expression when you stare in an indifferent, empty way, and when you attempt to convey warm interest and caring.

Imagine the different impact which the two expressions may have on a troubled client.

Receptive posture. Responsiveness is further communicated when the counselor faces the client squarely rather than leaning away at an angle. Involvement is also conveyed by leaning slightly forward, toward the client. Be aware of any tension or tightness, and try to maintain an alert but relaxed posture that is comfortable and natural, rather than rigid. One should avoid closed postures, in which arms and legs are tightly crossed. Position yourself so that there is not too much distance between you and your client, and arrange your environment so that there are no barriers between you and the client and so that the atmosphere is as receptive and free of distractions and interruptions as possible.

Be fully present. Besides attending physically to the client, the counselor must also be fully present psychologically. This process requires considerable discipline in focusing your attention on staying in contact from moment to moment and accurately receiving the client. Your goal must be to listen and to understand how the client experiences and views life, rather than to be preoccupied with your own interpretations, notions about how to change the client, or thoughts about what you are going to say next. Remain in experiential contact with the client and avoid letting your mind wander or becoming distracted with your own thoughts.

Furthering responses. Responses that indicate that you are listening and that encourage the client's expression communicate your attentiveness. Minimal responses may include saying, "Yes," "Mm-hmm," "I see," or nodding your head or smiling. Repeating a key word or the last word or phrase of the client's or saying "and" or "but" with a questioning inflection also conveys "being with" the client. Numerous investigations document the powerful reinforcing effects of such counselor responses on client verbal behavior (Krasner, 1958, 1962, 1963, 1965; Salzinger, 1959; Kanfer, 1961).

In summary, the counselor should maintain at least a minimal level of attending, with frequent eye contact. Leaning away from the client should be avoided, and the counselor should endeavor to remain fully present psychologically. At those times when the counselor feels genuinely involved or when the client is engaged in self-exploration of personally relevant issues and feelings, the counselor's full and intense attending will strongly reinforce the client's behavior.

The baseline intervention in counseling is the reciprocal empathic response, by which the counselor attempts to acknowledge that he has heard the client's message and is with him. Reciprocal empathy is similar to what Carkhuff (1969) refers to as "interchangeable" responding. It is defined by level 3.0 of the Empathic Communication Scale, which is the minimally helpful or facilitative level (Anthony, 1971). Additionally, level 3.0 responses also include inquiries to expand or specify expression when the client has been vague.

Gendlin (1974) reports that many therapists practice "blind therapy"—that is, they are concerned more with trying to say something stunning than with being keenly attuned to the client and responding to him. We agree with Gendlin, who writes (pp. 217–218):

> Responding in a listening way is a baseline prerequisite for any other modes of responding. It is not just one of many ways, but a precondition for the other ways. It is for therapy what watching the road is in driving a car. One does many things—shift gears, look at signs, engage in conversation, think private thoughts. Driving a car is by no means nothing but watching the road. However, it is quite unwise to forego watching the road for any other activity. A glance now and then at something else is fine, even necessary to find one's way. Also, watching the road does not take all one's attention and time; one can also think and converse—*but watching the road has priority!* As soon as the situation out the windshield gets murky, the conversation must stop, one's thinking must cease, one must slow down and attend entirely to what's in front, until that becomes clear again. Unfortunately many therapists drive without watching the road. They don't even want to see it! They think they already know what is in the person just then.

An effective counselor must do many things besides conveying empathy to the client. He must be able to confront discrepancies, for example, but after making necessary interventions, he must return to "responding in a listening way" to discover where the interventions have moved the client, what impact they had, and what they opened. We encourage the reader to study varied theoretical approaches and counseling techniques to develop a wide repertoire of skills and interventions that may be drawn upon as they fit individual counseling situations. It is helpful to have some mastery of role-playing, psychodrama, behavior modification, gestalt therapy, transactional analysis, Adlerian techniques, and so forth. However, these skills are of little use if the counselor does not possess the basic skills of empathic responding, which are necessary to establish and maintain the prerequisite counseling relationship and to learn where other interventions leave the client.

The reciprocal empathic response (level 3.0) generally consists of acknowledging that the therapist has heard the client. This is done by expressing back to the client in new words the feelings that he expressed *explicitly* and also by including the *explicit* reasons, precipitants, or experiences underlying the feelings. Thus, in a stereotyped format, the reciprocal empathic response would be, "You feel _____," or more ideally, "You feel _____ because (or about, or since) _____." To respond in this manner, you must focus your attention on listening for feelings and for the meaning, content, and reasons for feelings. This example of a reciprocal empathic response tunes into the client's feelings and the experiences underlying the feelings.

> *Client:* "I try and try to be helpful to the kids and it never seems to work. George just lets me go ahead and then complains because I don't do better."

> *Counselor:* "You must feel discouraged and frustrated when your husband not only fails to support you, but actually complains about what you do with the children."

Reciprocal empathic responses should reflect the client's obvious and explicit feelings, meanings, and emotional intensity. The response should not subtract from the intensity expressed, nor should it communicate deeper feelings or meanings that are only implied. The goal of the reciprocal response is not to facilitate deep, new insights. Rather, it encourages self-exploration and facilitates trust and rapport by helping the client feel understood. Moreover, it helps the client identify his feelings and see them as causes of behavior, and it refines the counselor's understanding of where the client is phenomenologically. A common mistake is to respond only to the content or subject matter of the client's statement, simply parroting what has been said. Such content responses subtract or fail to acknowledge surface feelings that are present. Some counselors err in the opposite direction by consistently going too deep, inaccurately or prematurely interpreting implied feelings or material below the surface level of awareness.

LANGUAGE AND PHRASING

To be perceived as an understanding person, the therapist must respond in language the client will readily understand. Professional jargon is a barrier to communication and is to be avoided. In addition, many professionals tend to respond with stereotyped, repetitive speech patterns. In supervising beginning counselors, we have found that they commonly use a limited variety of communication leads. The same three or four response leads, such as, "You feel . . . ," and "I hear you saying . . . ," repeated over and over not only bore the client but also seem phony, unnatural, and contrived, since they may arouse resentment. Such stereotyped responding can draw more attention to your technique than to your message.

A repertoire of varied introductory phrases is vital. To help you expand your repertoire of possible responses, the authors have compiled the following list of empathically communicative lead-in phrases. To acquire the skill, you will have to do more than give the list a casual reading. You are encouraged to review and to use the list of response leads frequently while practicing the empathic communication training exercises found later in this and the following chapter. The reciprocal empathy response format ("You feel _____ because _____.") is merely a training aid to assist in focusing on the affect and content of client messages. The list will help you respond more naturally.

Empathic Response Leads

Kind of feeling . . .
Sort of saying . . .
As I get it, you felt that . . .
I'm picking up that you . . .
Sort of a feeling that . . .

If I'm hearing you correctly . . .
To me it's almost like you are saying, "I . . ."
Sort of hear you saying that maybe you . . .
Kind of made (makes) you feel . . .
The thing you feel most right now is sort of like . . .
So, you feel . . .
What I hear you saying is . . .
So, as you see it . . .
As I get it, you're saying . . .
What I guess I'm hearing is . . .
I'm not sure I'm with you, but . . .
I somehow sense that maybe you feel . . .
You feel . . .
I really hear you saying that . . .
I wonder if you're expressing a concern that . . .
It sounds as if you're indicating you . . .
I wonder if you're saying . . .
You place a high value on . . .
It seems to you . . .
Like right now . . .
You often feel . . .
You feel, perhaps . . .
You appear to be feeling . . .
It appears to you . . .
As I hear it, you . . .
So, from where you sit . . .
Your feeling now is that . . .
I read you as . . .
Sometimes you . . .
You must have felt . . .
I sense that you're feeling . . .
Very much feeling . . .
Your message seems to be, "I . . ."
You appear . . .
Listening to you it seems as if . . .
I gather . . .
So your world is a place where you . . .
You communicate (convey) a sense of . . .

FREQUENCY AND TIMING OF RESPONSES

When the counselor is actively responsive, the client is likely to feel understood, and the counselor is likely to be empathically accurate and not stray too far off the track. We recommend making frequent verbal and nonverbal responses (nodding, facial expressions, gestures) to the client's expressions and avoiding prolonged periods of remaining silent. It is a mistake to assume that you may respond only after the client has paused or stopped talking. If the client is expressing numerous feelings or jumping from one meaningful area of discussion to another, it may be necessary to interrupt. For example, the counselor might interject or intervene with: "I'd like to interrupt to check if I'm understanding what you mean. As I get it, you're feeling . . ."; or, "Before you get into talking about that, I would like to make sure I'm with you. You seem to be saying . . ."; or, "Could we hold off discussing that for just a minute. I'd like to be sure I understand what you mean. Would you expand on what you were just saying?"

Note this last intervention; we want to point out the importance of not pretending to understand when you do not. Similarly, we recommend that you avoid concluding prematurely that you understand. Empathic accuracy and responsiveness are achieved by eliciting full expression of feelings and by checking to see whether your perceptions are accurate.

CLARIFYING AND CONFIRMING

In "checking out," you verify with the client whether you are on target and have accurately grasped the client's meaning and feelings. When you are uncertain whether your understanding is accurate or after you have made a number of reciprocal empathic responses, it is helpful to ask the client for feedback about your accuracy. Periodically asking for confirmation in this manner communicates a respectful sensitivity and a desire to understand, builds rapport, and minimizes misperceptions or projections. Perception checking is an essential component of active listening and empathic understanding. It is not a sign of personal or professional inadequacy to admit that you are confused or uncertain.

Some examples of combined reciprocal empathic responding and checking out are: "Let me check if I caught what you meant.

You were really irritated not simply because she was talking to other people, but because of the way she went out of her way to avoid you. Is that it?"; or, "Kind of feeling fed up and you're just not sure it's worth the trouble. Is that the way you feel?" or "Do I understand you to mean that you see your sexual problem as really just a part of your general fearfulness in relating to people?"; or, "Then the way he treated you just confirmed your feelings of being deficient and lacking. Is that what you're saying? Did I hear you right?"

INTERNAL FRAME OF REFERENCE

The goal of empathic understanding is not to understand *about* the client, but to understand *with* the client. Diagnostic understanding and knowing about the client are not the same as seeing the client through his own eyes. Empathic understanding goes beyond an understanding of external, factual circumstances, and the counselor errs by focusing on understanding external circumstances alone. Rather, he should concentrate on the individual and the impact external forces have on him. An example of a response focused on the external is, "He was really mean to you." In contrast, an internally directed message is, "You were very hurt by his comment."

A technique we have found useful in conveying an empathic understanding with the client is to occasionally change your reflection from third to first person, speaking as though you were the client for a moment. The following example of a deeply empathic response illustrates how this may be done:

> *Client* (a physically handicapped, teenaged girl confined to a wheelchair): "I feel like I can't do anything. I watch my sister in her pretty clothes, dancing, dating. You just can't imagine how I feel inside." She breaks into tears. "I want to do what she can do."
>
> *Counselor:* "Sort of saying, 'I'm *so* miserable and my life seems so empty and drab. I want to be alive like my sister, but I feel so helpless.'"

FOCUSING WITH SPECIFICITY

It is very difficult for a counselor to understand a client who continuously communicates in an abstract, intellectualized, and

superficial manner about impersonal topics. Additionally, research shows that the client's depth of self-exploration and self-
experiencing is related to successful therapy outcome (Truax
and Carkhuff, 1967; Klein, Mathieu, Gendlin, and Kiesler, 1969).
There are times, therefore, when the counselor needs to guide the
discussion to specifics, to the exploration of the personal relevance
of experiences described, and to the feelings involved. Focusing
with specificity will also encourage the self-exploration necessary
for insight and problem solving.

The counselor should formulate interventions specifically
and concretely, even when responding to intellectualized and vague
statements from the client. For example, instead of saying, "You
appear upset," which is quite generalized and vague, it would be
much more helpful to pinpoint specifically the client's state of feeling and the environmental or internal referents of his expression
by responding, "You sound as though you feel just humiliated about
the way she said that to you, right in front of everyone." Labeling
specific feelings implicit in the client's statements also encourages
the client to be more concrete in his expressions. Effectiveness is
further enhanced by accentuating the personal relevance of the
client's comments, attempting not to reinforce vague and irrelevant expressions, and by providing some structure and limits
on discussion.

Even though a client may be motivated to work on a problem,
he usually experiences stage fright of a sort and some ambivalence
about exploring himself and the unknown. Therefore, he may avoid
fearful or painful areas and feelings, ramble, and try to keep the
discussion safer by not examining personal relevance or meaning.
The counselor will sometimes need to channel the discussion and
focus on circumscribed content areas. At such times, it is appropriate to request specific information, details, feelings, experiences,
and illustrations (what, how, when, where, and who questions). You
may ask the client to clarify or elaborate specific phrases, words,
or concepts so that you can understand him better. However, you
must take care not to fall into the role of interrogator or psychic
detective, thereby fostering passivity in the client. Although questioning and probing occasionally are required to facilitate self-
exploration and to elicit details and information necessary to

understanding, they tend to circumscribe the client's responses and, therefore, should be used sparingly.

The client is likely to be more receptive to questions preceded by reciprocal empathic responses because such responses acknowledge the client's prior message. Likewise, an empathic response to the client's reply to a question is recommended. Questions such as, "What do you feel right now as you talk about that?" when the client's feelings can be readily discerned are inept and tend to block communication. Questions intended to expand expression of feeling are appropriate, however, when the client's feelings are vague or ill defined. Again, however, it is recommended that such inquiries be preceded and followed by empathic reflections whenever possible. To illustrate, one might say, "I sense how wounded you feel. Can you help me better understand what she does that causes you to feel so hurt?" Keep in mind that interrogation and grilling are closely related and that they are psychonoxious rather than facilitative. Questions are often grossly overused by unskilled counselors and by those unwilling to struggle and to make the personal investment understanding their client requires.

A counselor must rely largely on his own experience as a guide to the need for more concreteness or specificity. However, focusing with specificity is generally particularly important in the early phase of counseling for eliciting essential information and formulating goals and in the later change-oriented stage for making homework assignments and deciding on steps to the client's goals. In the middle phase of counseling, generalization from specific incidents to patterns or themes often facilitates awareness of preconscious material, and concrete focusing, therefore, is somewhat less important.

What and how questions are generally the most fruitful. Why questions are usually unproductive, leading to intellectualization, justifications, and excuses instead of specificity. Examples of some questions and leads that focus with specificity include: "I'm wondering, what did you see or hear that led you to draw that conclusion?"; "What was it about his behavior that . . . ?"; "What does he do that causes you to feel . . . ?"; "How do you know? How can you find out?"; "What do you experience as you talk about that?"; "Could you give me an illustration of that so I can see it better through your eyes?"; "Would you talk a little more specifically about your feelings toward her?"; "How did that make you feel?"; "I'm a little puzzled as to . . ."; "Tell me more about . . ."; "Explore that a little more."

FEELING TONE AND INTENSITY

The reciprocal empathic response (level 3.0) accurately communicates back to the client the level or intensity of the feelings expressed. More is required, however, than merely selecting a word or expression to reflect the client's affective state. The counselor should also respond in a voice, tone, and intensity similar to the client's. Genuine nonverbal gestures and expressions commensurate with the client's feelings might also be used.

As an example, picture a man boiling with anger, teeth gritted and fists clenched, who pounds his leg as he says, "I'm so burned up over the way my boss lectured me I'd like to punch his lights out!" A counselor might respond, "You're just so furious you can hardly keep it all inside." However, even though the response includes an appropriately descriptive feeling word, it would hardly seem empathic if the counselor spoke it in a dull, lifeless voice, while sitting expressionless and motionless. Empathy demands that the counselor's tone and posture fit the fury the client has expressed.

SUMMARY OF RECOMMENDED GUIDELINES

1. Receptively attend to the client by maintaining eye contact and a responsive posture, by remaining fully present and in contact psychologically, and by making furthering responses.

2. Make your baseline counseling intervention the reciprocal empathic reflection, acknowledging the explicitly expressed feelings of the client and the reasons or experiences behind them.

3. Avoid professional jargon and stereotyped introductory phrases, and respond in language attuned to the client.

4. Respond frequently and do not be afraid to interrupt if necessary to check out the accuracy of your understanding.

5. Respond to the impact of events on the client (internal frame of reference) rather than to external facts only.

6. Be specific and concrete in formulating your responses, encourage the client to be specific, and ask questions as required to elicit feelings or information needed for understanding.

7. Respond in a voice, tone, and intensity commensurate with the affect expressed by the client.

Communication Exercises with Modeled Responses

These exercises are to help the trainee learn how to respond to clients with level 3.0, reciprocal empathic responses. It is crucial that a counselor be able to respond readily and spontaneously with reciprocal empathic messages. These exercises present a wide variety of statements and problems taken from actual counseling interviews. Read the client message, and formulate on paper a reciprocal empathic response (level 3.0) using the structured format, "You feel _____ because (or about, or since) _____." Incorporate words or phrases that identify the *explicit,* surface feelings expressed and the precipitants, or reasons, behind these feelings. It may be helpful to refer back to the description of level 3.0 of the Empathic Communication Scale. Next, translate the essential components of your structured-format response into natural language, as though you are speaking directly to the client. Make these responses as fresh, varied, and spontaneous as possible. Contrast your written response with the suggested, or modeled, response provided at the end of the exercises. Study the differences and become aware of the varied ways of formulating responses and of those aspects of your own response and of the model that you find most effective.

It is strongly recommended that you regularly refer to the Vocabulary of Feelings and the list of Empathic Response Leads to expand your response repertoire. We further encourage your regular use of the structured format prior to formulating natural responses. In our experience, the structured format increases perceptiveness to important aspects of the message.

The objective of these exercises is not deep, penetrating responses but the development of skills in spontaneously responding with reciprocal (level 3.0) responses. To foster skill acquisition, numerous exercises have been provided for trainee practice. This practice can become difficult, and at times you may grow tired or impatient. However, focused and intensive practice is necessary to acquire the skill. We recommend that you complete these exercises in a number of sittings spaced over a few days to reduce fatigue and to maximize learning. These exercises and others like them in this book will help you develop counseling skills that many persons have needed years of work experience to refine. Such skill acquisition, however, demands concentration, persistence, and scrutiny of your responses and the modeled responses.

To facilitate transfer of learning, practice making reciprocal level 3.0 responses occasionally in everyday conversation during the next few days. Avoid being preoccupied with this task, but endeavor to increase the frequency with which you acknowledge having heard someone and convey understanding. Observe whether people respond differently to you when you convey empathic understanding than they do when your conversation is of the typical variety.

CLIENT STATEMENTS

1. *High-school student:* "My history teacher sent me down here because I was arguing with her. I can't help it! Can't *you* do something about her? It's completely unfair and we all want to refuse to do it. She told us today that we have another term paper to do before the end of the term. We should just all go to the principal."

2. *Woman:* "I'm a very emotional person, but my husband is quite reserved. It took a long time before he could show any affection to me. You begin to wonder what's wrong with you."

3. "I guess when it comes right down to it, I don't know where I'm going in life."

4. *Teenage girl:* "I can hardly wait to finish school next month. The future seems so bright and exciting, I just want to hurry and start doing so many things!"

5. *Client of opposite sex:* "I have mixed feelings about you. I like you too much sometimes, but I don't want to like you. I'll get hurt."

6. *Man:* "No matter what I do, my wife always puts me down. She just wants to keep me under her thumb, like a child, her little boy. And I just can't take that. I hate that. Yet sometimes I do sense that a part of me likes how comfortable it is, being kept as a child."

7. *Minority-group member:* "Hell, I just want to be accepted as myself, as a person, for what *I'm* capable of doing! I don't want to just be hired because of my skin color. That's as phony and degrading as being excluded because of my color. Why can't they just accept me for who I am?"

8. *Woman* (in tears): "Everything is just bearing down on me to the point where I just want to. . . . I honest to gosh don't even

want my own children. I'm so rotten bogged down with responsibility, and I'm failing them, I can't give them what they need, and I, I'm just sick of it." Her voice cracks. "And yet I know I couldn't live without them."

9. *Man:* "For once I'd like to show my wife that I can do something without her push. I don't want her to know that I'm coming here for counseling; if she knew she'd try to take responsibility for it."

10. "I don't know where to go from here. A lot of things are going through my head, but I just can't get them out."

11. *Woman:* "I know I'm capable in my work, and when I was in school I was on top. But I really don't feel like much of a woman, you know, in a sexual sense."

12. *Woman:* "Today I just couldn't tolerate the kids a second longer. I love them and enjoy watching them, but they just irritate me so terribly. Judy is okay because she's kind of quiet and even-tempered. She never gives me any trouble. But Tom can absolutely drive me nuts. Sometimes I simply can't stand to be around him. I feel like smacking him. Everything he does seems to irritate me."

13. *Man:* "I think I know how my daughter feels about my wife. My wife comes on strong, and I don't know how to react either and I get angry."

14. *Woman:* "He (husband) just up and left and then says he wants to still be friends with me. He even said, 'Keep the ring, I can't buy another one if we should get back together again.'"

15. *Wife speaking about illiterate husband:* "I try to understand how he feels, not being able to read, but he constantly wants me to tell him what's in the newspaper or what else I'm reading. It's really getting to me. I'm always having to consider how much I should take time to discuss things with him."

16. "Our daughter didn't come home at all last night. I stayed awake all night but I didn't dare do anything. It seems like I'm always wrong if I try to do something. I don't know what to do anymore."

17. *Mother about teenage daughter:* "She didn't call—a friend just stopped by the house and said she was not able to get home. When we got there she was unconscious. We rushed her to the hospital and when we called this kid to find out if she had taken any drugs, he wouldn't tell us anything. We had to threaten to have the police pick him up."

18. "We've been coming here now for eight weeks, and it doesn't seem to help. I had hoped my wife and I could get back together again but now it seems hopeless. We just keep drifting farther and farther apart."

19. "My husband has always run everything. He has never asked my opinion on anything. I'm tired of just doing and thinking the way he wants me to. But, how can I do what I want when I have never learned how?"

20. "Every morning when I check and I find he has wet the bed again, I about lose control of myself—I just can't understand why it happens. We do everything possible to try to help him stop wetting the bed."

21. *21-year-old female:* "Things went great over the holidays, contrary to my expectations. I've felt much stronger. I spent most of my time with my family in Phoenix. For the first time I felt a caring without being controlled. For the first time I also felt Father loved me—in his own way."

22. "You don't know how relieved I am just to know I'm not crazy for having some of these feelings."

23. "My husband and I often disagree about how to handle his 14-year-old boy from his first marriage. I always lose the arguments. I guess I'm conscious of being only 21 when he is 38."

24. *27-year-old male:* "When I lose a chess game I have a reaction. First, I feel angry with myself for blundering. It's not like me to make rank blunders. I guess I feel humiliated, too. Typically, when I lose I want to start another game immediately."

25. *29-year-old married male:* "Sexually I'm unfulfilled in my marriage. Sometimes I've entertained thoughts of having sexual involvements with men. My wife and I can communicate about sex okay, but nothing changes. She seems unable to respond. She agrees it's a psychological problem. Her doctor told her that."

26. *17-year-old female:* "I want to include my father more in my life and be able to talk to him without feeling scared and crying. I'd like to be able to express myself, my viewpoint, and to disagree with him. But I feel nervous and upset around him. I froze up the other day when he put his arm around me."

27. "Every time I go in the house Mother nags me and Dad doesn't say anything about anything or seem to care. Sometimes I feel there is no point of going home."

28. *Married female, age 42:* "He presents things very logically but with no appreciation whatsoever of my feelings. It just seems pointless to try to get through to him."

29. "I think of my ex-wife and the struggle she has managing the children and I just can't go ahead with a new marriage right now."

30. *16-year-old female:* "They had some drug raids last week, and I was afraid a couple of my girlfriends would be busted. They've done some really stupid things lately. But I know how easy it is to get hooked. I was becoming dependent on speed when I decided I'd better quit. It seemed phony to me, taking drugs for kicks. When I quit, I was depressed for about two weeks. I was tempted last week when I was bored in school to take some drugs to catch up. Then I realized what a chance I'd be taking."

31. "Actually our fight was about sex. My husband thinks I'm frigid. Maybe I am in some ways. But he pushes me so hard. We can't seem to talk about things like this. I just feel I can't confide my feelings in him."

32. *A woman who has recently remarried:* "Sure, I'm saying I'll do it, but I'm scared as hell to have that 10-year-old of his come to live with us."

33. *Female, age 19:* "I don't know what's happening. I'm supposed to have a high IQ, and I'm going to the university on a scholarship. But I'm not really trying. I'm just getting by."

34. *31-year-old woman:* "Why must I be wildly enthusiastic about our sex life? Can't I participate because I see him enjoy it even if I don't have an orgasm?"

35. "I tried to do what we talked about last time and I felt worse afterwards."

36. *Male, age 29:* "I can't relax—I feel as though I should be doing something all of the time. But I don't like to think of myself as anxious. Rather I feel I have an uncontrolled drive to accomplish. I must be pushing all the time."

37. "There must be something wrong with me because I do love my wife, but I can't get over feeling it's unfair to be tied down so much."

38. *37-year-old male teacher:* "I have a lot of difficulty accepting compliments. A relative of mine told me about the profound positive impact I've had on one of my students. My thought was, 'How

can that be? You don't do anything to have an impact like that.'"

39. *27-year-old single female:* "I've been taking a class. The teacher has been talking about the joys of womanhood and how to catch a man. I've felt there are so many things standing in my way. It's always been hard for me to talk with fellows. The teacher says you have to reach out to fellows."

40. "Things are really terrible—it's just me." The client pauses. "Lately I've felt like five or six people. Nothing is consistent. My moods have been shifting all over the place."

41. *Man:* "I just can't seem to forget how I walked out on my ex-wife and kids. I had a girlfriend who seemed so much more exciting, and I guess I was tired of the humdrum and responsibilities. Now I can't imagine how I could have been so stupid. I feel so embarrassed about it that I can't even look people I used to know in the eye. Now I can't even locate her, and of course her relatives won't tell me where she's moved. I actually think I still love her. I don't know what to do, or how I can ever make up for it. I just don't know."

42. "I've been worried about going off my rocker. But I can't because it would be so terribly embarrassing to my family." Client pauses. "And they're all doing so well."

43. "I wish I knew what to do. I don't know whether to go back to my sales job or not. I get so nervous having to talk to people, but it is good money. I guess I could quit and try something else I liked more, but I'd have to start at the bottom and make less money. I don't know if I could stand doing that."

44. A middle-aged man has been actively discussing his feelings about his recent divorce, with the counselor responding empathically. Following the counselor's last response, there is a long silence as the man quietly stares at his hands.

45. *19-year-old college student:* "I had a talk with Fred and learned he is very dependent on me. It's kind of scary. Why would anyone want to lean on a nobody?"

46. *Man:* "I don't feel like I even have a vote in my own marriage. Janet likes to take care of all the bills and money, and she continually makes important decisions for us without consulting me. The other day she went out, with no discussion at all, and bought a new stereo record player and tape deck. She acts as though she weren't even married!"

47. *15-year-old male:* "In sports I've always been the guy who doesn't do anything right. I'm always the last guy chosen. They fight over who doesn't have to choose me."

48. "I find that I'm troubled by some very vague fears, doubts, and uncertainties. Yet, darn it, I can't see any reasons to account for these. Everything is fine in my marriage, I'm doing better than I ever have at work, and financially I'm comfortable. It seems like I ought to be happier than ever before."

49. "I want to be recognized for being competent, not for being blind. I'm offended when someone praises me for doing routine things that anyone could do. It makes me feel like I'm on exhibition."

50. "I feel like my husband undermines me. When I took an IQ test, my verbal IQ was 125. I told him and he said, 'That's kind of low, isn't it?'"

51. "I've felt unimportant and unneeded as though the only thing I've had to offer my wife is material support. She's such a competent person she really doesn't need me."

52. *Female, age 30:* "I have memories of my father playing the organ and staring at me with a blank look—as though I wasn't there."

53. *16-year-old female:* "Mother doesn't seem to care. If she'd just try to understand. She's a good person with everyone else. But we just can't seem to get along. I spend most of my time in my room."

54. *Female, age 21:* "In the past I've always done everything because I felt I had to do it, as though I was meeting someone's expectation. But when Bruce called Friday, I invited him to dinner not because he wanted me to, but because *I* wanted to."

55. *23-year-old woman:* "I'm in a terrible bind! I've fallen in love for the first time in my life, to the best guy I've ever known. And what's more, he loves me—he's crazy about me. He asked me to marry him. It's like a dream come true, but I'm not worthy of him. I couldn't marry him. A few years ago I had a child out of wedlock and gave him up for adoption. He doesn't know about my past, but I'm sure he'd find out. I just couldn't hurt him like that."

56. *Male college student, age 23:* "I don't know what I want to do with my future. I started out in school studying business. I didn't like that, so I switched and thought I wanted to be an architect.

I tried that for a while and changed again. Now I only have one se-
mester left until I graduate in education. But I hardly care if I finish. I already know I don't want to be a teacher. But I don't know
what I want to do. I took some vocational tests a couple of years ago.
I dug them out again the other day, but they don't help at all. I'm
really discouraged. I just don't know where to go with my life."

57. *26-year-old divorcee:* "I just can't understand. If I had been
the kind of person that he needed, he wouldn't have left me. Evi-
dently I lacked somewhere in filling his needs."

58. *28-year-old divorced woman* (in tears): "I'm not doing jus-
tice to the children. And it's bad for them to grow up in an atmosphere like I'm giving them. I'm so rotten unhappy all the time. I
can't seem to find myself." She sighs. "I'm never happy. I'm never
smiling anymore, I'm just miserable. And I hate myself for that."

59. *15-year-old Caucasian boy:* "To be really honest, I don't like
the Black kids in school. They're so different. They don't seem very
friendly. And I guess I'm actually afraid of them. I don't know what
to expect around them, or how I should act. But I'm always uncomfortable around them and scared I'll do something they won't like
and that they'll jump on me."

60. *44-year-old divorced woman:* "Well, anyway, I'm just trying
to level off and forget my past. I'm trying desperately just to close off
in my mind the hurt and everything that's ever happened to me
and just live from right now on."

61. "Now that my husband has left me, I get lonely and depressed much of the time. I wonder what is wrong with *me*—or is it
that *men* shouldn't be trusted?"

62. "I've really felt irritated with Gloria because she didn't
call. If I could get her alone long enough I'd ask what kind of game
she is playing. I learned she did the same thing with Barbara too."

63. *21-year-old female college student:* "Things just kind of went
the same this week. Nothing exceptional really happened. I went
to classes, studied a lot, wrote a term paper. I guess the only thing
of any significance was that I got asked out for tomorrow night."

64. "My wife and I fought again since we saw you last. She
got pretty bent out of shape because she said I haven't been helping
her around the house and she feels like a slave. She hit the roof because I didn't take out the garbage. That's what set her off, and she's
still mad."

MODELED RESPONSES

1. "Then as you see it, you're being treated unfairly and just feel mad, like rebelling."

2. "So in response to his not being too demonstrative, you find yourself starting to question if you're somehow lacking."

3. "Kind of feeling confused, without any direction."

4. "I can hear how excited and alive you feel—enthusiastic to get involved in some new activities."

5. "So on the one hand you find yourself feeling very warmly toward me, and yet fearful of feeling that way—maybe it will just lead to hurt."

6. "You seem to be experiencing some mixed feelings. When she responds to you like a child, you get mad, but you realize at times that it is comfortable or easy to be in that role. Could you help me better understand your meaning, that a part of you likes or is comfortable in the role of a child?"

7. "You seem to be feeling fed up with only being seen as a color or a minority, instead of accepted as a person . . . as an individual . . . as yourself."

8. "The pressure of all the responsibilities has just reached the point where you're feeling overwhelmed. You especially seem to be feeling deficient and like you're failing with your children."

9. "You appear to feel irritated just thinking about her pushing and taking responsibility, and you would like to prove you can do something on your own."

10. "Kind of feeling lost and not sure where to start. Maybe we could begin by checking what you are aware of feeling right this moment."

11. "So you've felt successful in school and work, but if I'm hearing you correctly, you feel lacking or uncertain about your own femininity."

12. "So you find yourself getting so uptight and angry over something either about Tom or the way he acts that it's all you can do to keep from exploding at him, and that's quite different from the way you feel and respond to Judy."

13. "You can understand how your daughter feels because you too have reacted by getting angry at the way your wife does things."

14. "You sound confused about what it means when your husband leaves, then gives you messages that he wants to continue the relationship and even maybe reestablish the marriage."

15. "Trying to be understanding doesn't really help you deal with the pressure felt from his constant expectation of you. You're really in a quandary trying to decide how to handle the situation."

16. "It certainly leaves you feeling helpless and inadequate when you're so uptight but feel like you dare not move any direction even in an emergency."

17. "Apparently it was distressing to be trying so hard to help your daughter and have this friend of hers be so uncooperative. I guess you were angry by the time you had to push him to get the information you needed."

18. "It's terribly disappointing to you after having such high hopes and watching the situation getting worse."

19. "You feel like a robot and resent your husband for being so dominating, yet you're torn because of fear or uneasiness about how you would deal with more opportunity to say what you think."

20. "You find it frustrating that despite all your efforts your child still wets the bed, and it's difficult to not blow your top."

21. "Hey, that sounds neat! It's really encouraging to you to feel more strength and to experience love and caring without being controlled. And that was really special—feeling your father's love for the first time."

22. "A burden has been lifted for you to know that you're not mentally ill just because you have those feelings."

23. "So being younger than your husband leaves you feeling uncertain and at a disadvantage when the two of you argue about his son. You feel frustrated always losing the argument."

24. "It's really hard for you to lose. Lots of feelings surge through you: anger and disappointment with yourself for goofing, loss of face, and, I guess, a determination to beat the other guy next time."

25. "So things don't get any better even though you talk and she acknowledges her hang-up. You just feel so frustrated and at times you find yourself having fantasies about sex with men."

26. "That sounds like a real dilemma. You want to get closer to Dad, be more open with him about all sorts of things. Yet you get pretty tense when you're around him, just feel tied up inside."

27. "Kind of feel picked on by Mother, then when your father says or does nothing, it's discouraging and you feel, 'What's the use?'"

28. "So you're feeling he's logical all right but he's also insensitive."

29. "When you think about your ex-wife's struggles in managing the children, you feel a concern and a real reluctance to consider another marriage."

30. "Sounds like having almost been hooked before, you realize how easy it could happen if you let down. It seems phony and stupid to you—still at times you find yourself drawn to it and have to remind yourself how much is at stake."

31. "So, as you see it, your problem is much broader than just sex. I gather you feel some real pressures from him and for some reason just can't share certain feelings with him—feelings about sex, for example."

32. "You agree on having his child come to live with you, but at the same time you're really dreading it."

33. "Am I getting this right? You're wondering what the devil's happening. Here you have a high IQ, all the ability you need—yet, for some reason, you're not doing any more than you have to, just a bare minimum."

34. "You see no reason why you should have to enjoy sex for any other reason than giving pleasure to him and wish he'd let you enjoy it in your own way."

35. "From what you've told me, I'm not sure if you're discouraged, angry, or just frustrated. Tell me what it is you're feeling right now as you think about it."

36. "So I gather it's sort of like you just can't let go of that push from within to accomplish. Almost like you feel compelled to push all the time."

37. "You're confused about how you can feel love for your wife and at the same time want more freedom."

38. "So you really felt uncomfortable when you heard that. From what you say it sounds as though you find it very hard to believe you can make such a positive impression on one of your students."

39. "So when you think about what you have to do in your relationships with fellows, you just see so many obstacles you won-

der if you're really up to it. Reaching out is really scary for you."

40.   "It's really been disturbing for you lately—just feeling *so* mixed up and confused—almost like you're not even sure of who you are at times."

41.   "I'm very aware of your remorse as you talk and of how foolish and ashamed you feel for leaving them. Right now you particularly seem up in the air as you realize, 'I still care for her, and yet it may be too late.'"

42.   "Sounds like you're afraid of falling to pieces and worried that if you did it'd be humiliating to your family. I sense your concern that you don't want that to happen."

43.   "It's a tough decision whether to take the risk of starting from scratch and maybe enjoying the work more or to stick with something nerve-racking but secure."

44.   "You don't seem to know quite what to say right now." Or, "You're very quiet. Could you share some of what's going on inside of you right now?"

45.   "So you really are frightened. Sort of like you're so unsure of yourself you don't see how you can support anyone else."

46.   "It really aggravates you when she takes charge of things. Not being considered leaves you feeling unimportant and left out."

47.   "I gather you're saying you weren't there when athletic talents were being passed out. It's embarrassing and you feel so left out and inferior when you're the last guy chosen."

48.   "The fears and doubts you experience really bother you and are puzzling, too. It seems like you ought to be happy and contented, but you can't seem to put your finger on what is happening to you."

49.   "You really feel singled out when people flatter you for doing things anyone could do. Just an angry, uncomfortable feeling and a wish that people would recognize you for your competence, not your blindness."

50.   "You feel your husband puts you down, even when you've done well."

51.   "Just feeling inadequate as a marital partner as though all you have to offer is what you provide materially."

52.   "You find some feelings stirring even now as you think of the way he stared at you without acknowledging you. I'm wondering what you're feeling at this moment as you picture that scene."

53. "Sounds like you're feeling misunderstood and hurt. It's even tougher because mother gets along with everyone else. You somehow just seem to clash, so you stay in your room."

54. "You're both pleased and encouraged over inviting him because *you* wanted to, not because you were expected to."

55. "So you found everything you've been looking and hoping for, but now you're afraid it can only be a dream because you feel you don't deserve him and don't want to hurt him."

56. "It's like you're saying, 'I'm about ready to throw in the towel; I can't see any way out. I've studied a number of different areas I thought I was interested in, I've taken tests, I've pondered it, and I'm still confused and in the fog.' That *must* be distressing."

57. "Let me see if I understand. For you, then, it comes down to a feeling that he left you because you couldn't meet his needs. You're feeling you must have a deficiency somewhere."

58. "Just find yourself feeling depressed and lost all the time, and then when you think of the impact that may have on the children, you worry and really feel crummy."

59. "You see them as so different that you don't know how to read or predict them. You're fearful that you'll upset them, but you're uncertain how to respond to them so that they won't get mad."

60. "You have such painful memories that you wish you could just erase your past and begin from here."

61. "Been feeling so all alone and down in the dumps since he left. And find yourself wanting to know what's wrong, asking, 'Am I the cause for what he did, or are all men just that way?'"

62. "Sounds like you're pretty fed up with her and feeling that in your relationship she better either shape up or ship out."

63. "You say the date was significant. I wonder how do you feel about being asked out?" (focusing in an effort to elicit feelings)

64. "So your wife's been on your back because she feels you haven't carried your share of the load this week. I'm wondering what's been going on inside of you during all this turmoil." (shifting focus from wife to husband's feelings)

Practicum Exercises

The following exercises are designed to facilitate further the generalization of empathic communication skills to counseling and other real-world settings. They may be used either after or along with the preceding exercises.

It is important for the trainer or instructor both to reduce the threat for students and to respond with sensitivity, empathy, and respect. The initial exercise allows trainees to receive feedback on their responses, yet reduces their personal vulnerability to a minimum.

EXERCISE ONE

This is known as the file-card exercise. The instructor either reads a written client statement or plays an audio- or videotaped client message. The trainees are then instructed to write level 3.0 responses on 3 × 5 file cards, which have been distributed earlier. Trainees are told to omit their names, and the completed cards are passed to the instructor. The instructor reads the responses to the trainees and asks them to rate the answers on the Empathic Communication Scale. In the initial ratings, it is helpful to ask the trainees to determine first whether the response is reciprocal, subtractive or additive and then to determine the numerical rating. The trainees can indicate their ratings by holding up the corresponding number of fingers. Half-step ratings like 2.5 can be indicated by holding up two fingers from one hand and laying a finger from the other hand atop them. By observing the group ratings, the instructor can roughly average the ratings, and he can also present his own rating to the group. Brief discussion to explicate the reasons for each rating should follow. This procedure allows feedback to be given to shape trainee behavior, but in an atmosphere in which anonymity reduces threat.

When responses to a number of statements have been rated and discussed, the instructor may begin having the trainees move closer to the ultimate goal of verbal response to a client by asking for *volunteers* to read their responses to the group instead of passing the file cards in. Again, the responses are rated and briefly discussed by the group. Now, as trainees gradually begin to risk some personal vulnerability by reading their own responses, the instructor will need to remain particularly mindful of giving feedback sensitively and in an atmosphere of caring, respect, and empathy. The trainer must be a model.

EXERCISE TWO

Following the file-card exercise, trainees should be ready to move closer to real life with the around-the-room exercise. Either the instructor or a volunteer trainee should role-play a client after spending a few moments creating a problem for therapy. Have members of the class or workshop sit in a circle. The client sits inside of the circle and begins by making a statement to one of the group members, who responds as the counselor. The counselor should pause for twenty to thirty seconds after the client's statement to formulate a level 3.0 response without rushing. After the counselor responds, the client moves to the next trainee counselor in the circle and makes a second statement, to which the second counselor responds. This process may continue until everyone in the circle has an opportunity to role-play the counselor.

After each counselor responds, the other group members should write their ratings of the response on the Empathic Communication Scale. These ratings and any notes explaining them may be shared briefly at the end, or if they are made on file cards and numbered, simply passed to the appropriate counselor. This procedure could also be audio- or videotaped.

EXERCISE THREE

The following exercise has been found extremely useful as the next step in training groups of no more than eighteen participants. In a group of twelve or fewer members, one half of the group is asked to volunteer as counselors; in a slightly larger group, a third may be asked to volunteer. The counselors are seated in a semicircle, with the instructor or a trainee volunteer seated in front of them to role-play a client. Other group members are assigned to be rater-observers for specific counselors. The counselors should be encouraged to respond at least three or four times to the client. They are instructed to respond spontaneously while the client interacts with them. The role-playing should continue for four or five minutes.

At the completion of the sequence, the rater-observers and the client should give specific feedback to each of the counselors. The feedback should include the ratings of the responses and specific reactions, both positive and negative, to posture, attending behavior, voice quality, and the nature of the response.

EXERCISE FOUR

With a larger training group, this exercise may be used as an alternative to Exercise Three. The larger group is divided into smaller groups of six to eight trainees, who then divide themselves into pairs. One partner in each pair role-plays a counselor, and the other plays the client. One pair at a time role-plays, while the remainder of the small group observes and rates. The counselor should focus on making level 3.0 responses, attempting to respond at least four or five times during the role-playing. After the client and the group give specific feedback, the roles are reversed. The exercise continues until each pair has played both roles.

EXERCISE FIVE

For this exercise, trainees are divided randomly into groups of three. One member of each triad is selected to be the counselor, another role-plays the client, and the third member is a rater-observer. The objective is still to respond only with reciprocal, level-3.0 responses. The observer should sit beside but slightly behind the client and use fingers to signal the counselor after each intervention, indicating the level of the response. After three to four minutes of interaction, discontinue role-playing and allow the client and the observer to discuss their impressions and to share feedback with the counselor. Specify times and ways that the counselor could have improved, and also share positive feedback. Audio- and videotape might again be used. Each member of the triad should have the chance to be the counselor. Afterwards, new triads may be formed and the practice continued. The instructor can move from triad to triad to give feedback during this exercise.

In role-playing exercises, trainee resistance sometimes arises. The instructor must remain responsive, empathic, and respectful, and not resort to defensive criticism or coercion. Much of the trainee's resistance may stem from fearfulness and feelings of ineptness and vulnerability. In behavioral rehearsal, trainees also frequently resist the limitation to only make empathic responses. It is helpful for the instructor to make it clear that conveying empathy is merely one of the interventions an effective counselor makes, but that for the purpose of refining the skill, practice is temporarily limited to empathic communication alone.

Chapter 6

ᵂᵂᵂᵂᵂᵂᵂᵂᵂᵂᵂᵂᵂᵂᵂᵂᵂᵂᵂ

Expanding the Client's Meaning: Additive Responses

Deeper empathic interventions go beyond what the client has explicitly expressed to feelings and meanings only implied in the client's statements and, thus, somewhat below the surface of the client's awareness. Consequently, these interventions add implicit material that the counselor infers from the client's message. Interventions rated at levels 4.0 and 5.0 on the Empathic Communication Scale accurately add what may have only been alluded to or hinted at by the client. For example, suppose a client relates how deeply he invested in a relationship with a girlfriend who later dropped him, leaving him intensely angry with her. A reciprocal empathic response by the counselor would tune into the explicitly expressed anger or resentment over the desertion. However, a little further discussion may show that just below the surface, implied and perhaps only vaguely recognized, lurk more vulnerable and tender feelings of deep hurt. An additive empathic response from the counselor would direct the client's attention to these deeper feelings.

Additive empathic responses that attempt to formulate what the client has not yet clearly conceptualized are mildly to moderately interpretive because they require the counselor's inference. A number of writers cite the interpretive nature of deeper empathic responses (Bergin, 1966; Truax and Carkhuff, 1967). The prominent psychotherapist Carl Rogers explains that he works at the edge of the client's awareness in an interpretive manner, seeking to bring feelings and meanings into consciousness by identifying them at the moment they are about to enter awareness. In describing the role of the therapist, he says, "He does not merely repeat his client's words, concepts, or feelings. Rather, he seeks for the meaning implicit in the present inner experiencing toward which the client's words or concepts point" (1966, pp. 190–191). Rogers suggests that empathy involves "sensing meanings of which he/she [the client] is scarcely aware, but not trying to uncover feelings of which the person is totally unaware, since this would be too threatening" (1975, p. 4). This sort of empathy, Rogers argues, is a necessary therapeutic tool, for unless the therapist dips "from the pool of implicit meanings just at the edge of the client's awareness," therapy cannot progress toward its goal (1966, p. 190). Speisman (1959) adds research validation that "moderate interpretations" are more effective than either deep interventions or superficial responses.

Thus, there can be little progress if the counselor intervenes only with reciprocal empathic responses. The client must be stimulated and assisted to become aware of feelings, of self-defeating perceptual, cognitive and behavioral patterns, and of purposes underlying behavior that he has previously denied to awareness, distorted, and not clearly conceptualized. With such insight, the client can translate awareness into constructive action and behavior change.

Timing Additive Interventions

Additive empathic responses can have a forceful impact and, therefore, should be employed prudently and discriminatingly. In the early phases of the helping relationship and initially in each counseling session, the counselor should focus on making level 3.0, reciprocal empathic responses. Deeper, additive empathic interventions are most likely to be facilitative only when three preconditions have been met.

First, a trusting therapeutic relationship needs to have been already established, in which the client feels understood, respected, and accepted by the counselor. Times when the client is experiencing negative feelings toward the counselor are poor ones for deep interventions. Second, the client should be volunteering personally relevant material and feelings and be attempting self-exploration on his own initiative rather than simply submitting to the counselor's probing. A client who is not trying to explore himself on his own is not likely to use or accept deeper insights. Third, a deeper intervention should be preceded by a series of reciprocal empathic responses. Responding in an acknowledging and listening manner prepares the client by creating a low-threat environment conducive to dropping defenses and examining the self. These responses also prepare the counselor by placing him on the client's experiential track, increasing understanding and documenting the tentatively held hypotheses of what may be just below the surface of the client's expression.

Deep, interpretive interventions add information to the client's perspective, but they require some time to integrate and they may be threatening. The counselor must give the client time to digest and assimilate the new learning, and he must listen empathically and acknowledge the impact of the message on the client. Thus additive interventions need to be interspersed with level 3.0 responses, not offered in rapid succession. The counselor must also time his interventions so that the material they concern is close to the client's awareness, increasing the likelihood of acceptance of the material by the client. Additive responses should not emanate from the counselor's narcissistic desire to dazzle the client with his insightfulness and wisdom. The counselor's inferences about underlying feelings, meanings, relationships, or purposes should remain tentative until additional evidence confirms their probable accuracy. Next, the counselor should determine whether the client can benefit from such awareness and whether he is ready to accept such feelings or conceptualizations. If the counselor endeavors to foster awareness of ambiguously perceived material still remote from the client's current awareness and experiencing, it is highly probable that the client will reject the response defensively. With such deep responses, the counselor always runs the risk of being inaccurate. A counselor who attempts to push a client rapidly into acquiring new insights will likely make numerous premature, inaccurate, and unempathic responses, which may shake the client's confidence, stimulate feelings of being misunderstood, and elicit resistance. Any ill-timed or overly additive empathic response that the client rejects, whether accurate or not, rates no higher than level 2.0 on the Empathic Communication Scale.

Further guidelines to timing the appropriateness of empathic responding will be presented in the form of indications and contraindications at the end of the chapter.

Evaluating Effectiveness

To evaluate the facilitativeness of an additive empathic intervention, or of any therapeutic intervention, one must listen carefully to the client's response. Gendlin concludes, "Sensitivity is not really a magical source for the right therapist response; rather, it consists in carefully noticing the client's *next* reaction to what the therapist says" (1968, p. 212). An intervention is probably helpful if the client's response is characterized by one of the following: maintenance of at least the same level of problem- or self-exploration; a release of emotion (unless the client is an emotionally overexpressive individual who constantly emotes); deeper exploration and self-experiencing in which there is greater involvement of feeling, spontaneous volunteering of more personally relevant material, and struggling to explore the self and the world more deeply; or verbal or nonverbal affirmation of the validity of the counselor's response.

A counseling intervention is most likely too deep, poorly timed, or off-target if the client reacts by: verbal or nonverbal disconfirmation; changing the subject; ignoring the intervention; becoming mixed up or confused; being more superficial, more impersonal, more emotionally detached, or more defensive; growing argumentative or angry rather than examining the relevance of the feelings involved. No matter how technically or diagnostically brilliant an intervention, it is most likely ineffective and inappropriately timed if it does not facilitate continued or deeper exploration.

By examining the client's behavior and level of self-experiencing immediately after interventions, the therapist can gauge his moment-to-moment effectiveness. Occasional inaccuracy or faulty timing need not be disastrous if one responds to the client's reaction in a listening, reciprocally empathic manner. Additionally, if an inaccurate or irrelevant statement by the counselor distracts the client from his own experiencing, the counselor must invite him to refocus on previously expressed feelings.

Identifying Underlying Feeling

Deep empathic responses help the client conceptualize and translate vague and undefined feelings and experiences into words and ideas. An additive response verbalizes and labels (Dollard and Miller, 1950) underlying feelings for the client, bringing them into focus and awareness, or accurately pinpoints a feeling that the client has mislabeled. In Chapter Four, we illustrated the difference between explicit and underlying feelings. In attempting the deeper empathy of levels 4.0 and 5.0 the counselor will need to respond to emotionally constricted individuals by conveying in his voice a somewhat greater emotional intensity than the client has expressed and to select words of feeling whose strength corresponds to the probable intensity of the client's actual underlying feelings.

Expanding Underlying Meaning

Additive responses draw attention not only to implied deeper feelings, but also to meanings at the edge of or just beyond awareness. Such responses help the client formulate material that may have been sensed, but has not yet been clearly understood. The counselor may need to concentrate extra attention on assisting the emotionally constricted, intellectualizing client to identify his feelings. However, the more intense the emotionality of the client, the more the counselor can focus on helping him conceptualize meanings without fear that this will lead to overintellectualizing defensiveness and repression of affect. Deeper empathic responses assist the client not only to become aware of underlying feelings but also to intellectually conceptualize meanings, relationships, patterns, purposes of behaviors and emotions, and implicit goals. It must be borne in mind that the identification of what someone is feeling in itself is not the ultimate goal of counseling. Intellectualization detached from experience is barren, for there is an organismic wisdom (Rogers, 1961) in people and they are wiser than their intellect. Similarly, experience without conceptualization is blind and unintelligible. Full experiencing integrates both feelings and thought. Thus the goal of deep responding is to facilitate awareness of both underlying feelings and underlying meanings. What is beyond awareness (preconceptual, unconscious, preconscious) is typically only vaguely sensed, felt, and experienced bodily. It has not yet been translated into understandable concepts, labels, and ideas that give it meaning and direction and make it subject to self-control and self-determination.

IDENTIFYING RELATIONSHIPS AND MAKING CONNECTIONS

One way of adding implicit meaning is by assisting the client to make connections so that he perceives relationships and associations. He may not be fully aware of the relation of certain feelings to his behavior, of environmental situations or stimuli to his responses, of beliefs to behavior, or of his own behavior to the behavior of others. Thus a counselor may focus on themes, similarities or parallels between different experiences or behavioral reactions to situations, or similar feelings or thoughts experienced at different times. For example, a counselor might respond, "As I've listened to you, it's as though you've gotten the same message from your parents and your wife: 'As a person you aren't worth much. Your only value comes from what you achieve and accomplish.'" Another example of an additive empathic response that associates or links similarities would be: "It sounds as though your feelings of resentment about your minister lecturing you really resembled what you used to experience with your father."

A counselor may link situations, feelings, or experiences that are contiguous temporally or environmentally. For instance: "You've talked about something similar a couple of times before. I've gotten the impression that whenever you're around an available man who isn't 'safe,' perhaps you begin feeling panicky and get drunk in order to relate to him." Not infrequently, thoughts or self-statements (things the client says to himself) may be associated with feelings or symptoms. Consider this response by a counselor: "I think I've become aware of something. You seem to hit these times of real depression and feeling worthless whenever someone has criticized you. I'm wondering if at those times you internalize that criticism and put yourself down too, by telling yourself how inadequate and rotten you are."

Another type of connecting additive response that might be made with clients experiencing anxiety or conflict is the goal-catastrophic fear association. Many clients fantasize that horrible, fearful things will happen to them if they act on their desired goals. Thus their desires and fears conflict. The client may not be completely aware of these catastrophic anticipations, yet they may control or govern him, leading him to avoid many things and to experience anxiety and immobilizing conflict. One of the common self-defeating catastrophic fantasies is the fear of being exposed as inadequate or deficient. Others include fear of failure or defeat, of losing prestige, of losing the support of others, of ridicule or disapproval, and of losing control. In the case of a boy who wants to go out with girls but who implicitly fears the catastrophe a real date might turn into, an additive intervention of this connecting type would be: "I sense how you long for a close relationship to a girl. Yet it seems that when you get to the point of wanting to ask for a date you're paralyzed—so frightened that you might get turned down or laughed at."

CONCEPTUALIZING PERCEPTUAL PATTERNS AND
IMPLICIT ASSUMPTIONS

Another method of adding deeper, implicit meaning and expanding awareness is to identify underlying, preconscious assumptions about the self, other people, or the world. Through past experiences, the client may have been conditioned to perceive himself, life, or people as a whole in idiosyncratic ways. The individual acts on these assumptions, which are typically beyond awareness, as if they were true, and they become the basis in his life for anticipating and predicting, setting goals, and behaving. Frequently such perceptual patterns or beliefs are overgeneralizations or exaggerations molded through unfortunate early experiences or models. Thus the spectacles through which the client views himself

and the world are distorted. Deeply empathic responses only identify and help conceptualize these implicit assumptions. If the
counselor goes further and explains that such perceptual sets are
distorted or unreasonable, he is no longer empathic because he has
shifted from the client's perceptual field to an external frame of
reference. Nonetheless, there may be instances in which it is helpful
to share differing perceptions of people or the world with the client.
The methods and times for sharing personal perspectives will be
considered in detail in Chapters Eight and Nine.

Ellis (1962, 1973a) and Shulman (1973) refer to many common
implicit assumptions that generate dysfunctional patterns of behavior. Some common examples of distorted self-definitions include: "I am a helpless, innocent victim"; "I am not feminine (or
manly) or attractive enough"; "I am lacking, not smart enough,
and, therefore, destined to fail"; "I am wicked"; "I am weak and
need to be led"; "I am so exceptional that I am entitled to my own
way"; "I am undesirable and no one could love me."

Some frequently encountered beliefs about people and the
world include: "Life is a dangerous, dog-eat-dog jungle"; "Life
doesn't give me a chance, and I'm destined to suffer"; "Outside
circumstances cause my unhappiness and I'm powerless to change
them"; "People are hostile and rejecting"; "Men (women) can't be
trusted"; "People are stupid, and you should take them for all you
can"; "Life is chaotic and completely unpredictable."

If a counselor were to become aware of an implicit perceptual
pattern, he might respond: "As you talk about yourself in relation
to women, it seems as though deep down you feel, 'I'm unattractive to women and not masculine enough.' Does that fit?" Another
possible response is: "There appears to be some real fearfulness
for you in allowing anyone to get close. Kind of like, 'If I trust anyone closer than arm's length emotionally, I'll get knifed in the
back.'"

VERBALIZING IMPLICIT GOALS AND IDEALS

A closely related manner of responding with additive empathy
is to help the client conceptualize implied ideals and goals. Much
like preconscious assumptions, these ideals are often distorted,
beyond awareness, and self-defeating. Again, however, deeper

empathic interventions aim only to identify these goals accurately and not to label them as distorted. Many times goals and directions for action are implicit in the client's expressions of self-dissatisfaction or in the insights he has gained. In additive responding, it is desirable for the counselor, whenever possible, to help clients see the directions implied in their statements and to explore their private goals and intentions. A structured response format facilitating this type of intervention is, "You feel _____ because _____, and you want to (or you wish, or you'd like to) _____." To illustrate: "I can see how inadequate you feel when you fumble around trying to talk with girls. And I also sense how badly you want to learn how to interact, and to begin dating."

Shulman (1973) and Ellis (1962, 1973a) identify many irrational and distorted goals and ideals. Common self-defeating goals that counselors may help clients see more clearly include: "To be worthwhile it is essential to be perfect, completely competent, and without flaw"; "I need to be loved and approved of by everyone"; "I must find the perfect (right) solution to every problem"; "I must please everyone and be a nice guy who never offends"; "I must be dependent on someone stronger to protect and lead me"; "I have to be the best and the first"; "I must be the center of attention"; "I must never yield or give in"; "I should retaliate and get even with the world."

Some common distorted ideals about what is important and desirable include: "The only thing worth being in life is a star"; "A real man is a tough guy who never takes any guff from anyone"; "A real woman should always be feminine, inoffensive, unassertive, and dependent"; "I should never lose control"; "I should always know the right answer"; "I should always have my own way"; "It is easier to avoid responsibilities and problems"; "I should be able to succeed and to be happy without discomfort or struggle."

SUMMARIZING TRENDS

Additive empathy may also be conveyed by summarizing and pulling together ideas, perceptions and feelings. In effect, the counselor helps the client take two or three pieces of a puzzle and fit them together to make a complete picture. For instance, implicit beliefs about the nature of people and the world, self-definitions, and underlying goals are often intertwined. Consider a situation in which a counselor discovers with a client that the latter perceives the world as a dangerous, unpredictable place and later finds that the client sees himself as deficient and inadequate. Subsequently, while exploring the client's desire to depend on someone stronger to guide and protect him, the counselor links this desire to the client's assumptions about himself and the world, thus joining these seemingly separate feelings. The counselor summarizes: "When you talk about always liking to find someone stronger to lean on, that really seems to fit with your feelings of being weak and lacking. Maybe kind of like, if you can find someone strong, they can take charge and be a buffer for you with that risky world out there."

Synthesizing previously disconnected elements or patterns fosters movement and lends a sense of direction to future therapeutic efforts. A summarizing empathic reflection might also be used to terminate an interview or to cap off a problem or content area that seems fully explored.

CONCEPTUALIZING PURPOSES OF BEHAVIOR AND FEELINGS

Deeper empathic responses may also include an accurate recognition of the underlying purposes for the client's behaviors, problems, or feelings. It is important, however, that such identification not derive primarily from the counselor's external frame of reference or from preconceived theoretical constructs. Deep empathy emanates from first listening keenly and accompanying the client into his private world and making tentative hypotheses about the meanings and purposes of his behavior. It is vital that the counselor control any impulse to share these hypotheses until he is certain that they are valid for the individual client, not for some theoretical client, and until the client demonstrates at least a vague awareness of the hypothesis and readiness to consider it.

Symptoms and behaviors serve a purpose and are directed to a goal, not impelled by instinctive drives. When a client starts to have a dim, indistinct sense of the possible purposes served by his symptomatic behavior or feelings, an additive empathic intervention may foster awareness of the ends toward which the behavior is directed. To help the client grasp the meaning of his behavior, the counselor must comprehend what problems and symptomatic behaviors accomplish for the client. To gain this comprehension one might ask himself, "What consequences follow from the symptomatic behavior, and what effects do these behaviors have on other people?" Both the counselor and the client might consider how the client's life would differ if the problem or symptom were magically taken away.

This last consideration often pinpoints the person or situation the behavior defends the client against (Dreikurs, 1954). If an alcoholic client, for example, indicates he would find a "nice" girl and get married "if only" he could stop drinking, a valid hypothesis might be that avoiding any attachment to females is one of the goals of his drinking. One of the authors counseled an alcoholic who responded in this manner. In time it was learned that he was terrified of entering a relationship with a woman. His catastrophic fantasies of rejection stemmed from being completely deserted by his mother when he was a small boy and were reinforced by his first wife's betrayal and rejection. Staying drunk protected the man against the threat of another involvement with a woman.

A college-age woman entered counseling complaining of recent attacks of anxiety and insomnia that seemed unexplainable. Exploration of what she would do and how life would be different if her symptoms were to vanish revealed that she would proceed with plans to marry her fiancé, which had been postponed because of the puzzling symptoms. It rapidly became evident that underlying fears and ambivalence about the marriage warranted exploration. In the meantime, her symptoms served as an excellent obstacle against the marriage.

The therapist must be familiar with common underlying purposes of symptomatic behavior. Adler concluded that most neurotic symptoms serve as protective safeguards for self-esteem or as excuses (Ansbacher and Ansbacher, 1964; see also Shulman, 1964, and Mosak and Gushurst, 1971). Thus many problems are a type of protection sheltering the individual against some feared catastrophe (for example, failing and being found inadequate, being used or taken advantage of, or being disapproved of, ridiculed, or rejected). These security operations may function to save face. Many individuals seek refuge in their symptoms or in illness and content themselves with what they could do, "if only." Others may save face by suffering with their guilt feelings. Although the guilt feelings are uncomfortable and cause complaints, they may demonstrate the client's high moral standards and good intentions to himself and to others. He may make no effort to change his behavior, but he can still preserve his self-conception and public image through his regrets and honorable intentions (Dreikurs, 1950). Another client may plead that sickness exempts him from responsibilities ("With these terrible headaches I just can't work"). Some people will create a self-fulfilling prophecy consonant with their ideas, so that they can maintain their self-perceptions, save face, and in effect tell their counselor, "See, I was correct after all." An example would be the person who subtly and unconsciously, by his own behavior, invites criticism and rejection so that he can maintain his self-definition as a rejected person. Still another client's supposedly busy schedule may allow him to evade demands at home by keeping him preoccupied with a distracting "sideshow"—or, as Shulman (1964, p. 219) puts it, "I can't take care of anything else until I have slain this dragon." This client's busy schedule may also serve as an exemption from responsibility, an excuse for failure, or as a way of postponing performance. For example, he might rationalize that his poor grades on final examinations in school did not genuinely evaluate his intellectual prowess because his schedule left him no time to study.

Symptomatic behavior may provide evidence of a client's strength or courageous heroism. Who could help but admire the character of a martyr who has made long-suffering sacrifices for her neglectful husband or the strength of a secretary who never yields her virtue despite the incessant sexual advances of her male fellow workers? Of course, no one is aware, least of all the client, that such obstacles may be constructed for the very purpose of demonstrating imagined moral superiority, heroism, or strength.

Neurotic behaviors can be used for offense as well as defense. Many symptomatic behaviors serve to manipulate people and to gain something. The goal may be to win attention, to overpower, to conquer, to coerce servitude, or to punish and get revenge (Dreikurs, 1948). For instance, some individuals incorporate into their life styles the role of weakling or perpetual child, thereby pressing others into serving them. Such persons employ such tactical weapons as indecisiveness, creating obstacles, forgetting, making mistakes, becoming confused, and playing stupid by constantly asking questions to encourage someone else to take responsibility for their lives. Thus the role of weakling may not only exempt one from the burdens of responsibility, but it may also be used to acquire service and power. Other clients play the role of dictator or bully and more overtly control, overpower, and manipulate people (Shostrom, 1968).

In sum, neurotic symptoms can serve either defensive or offensive goals. The defensive goals are essentially security operations for protecting the self. Common defensive goals include: to protect self-image, self-definition, and self-consistency; to defend against such feared catastrophes as failure or exposure; to save face (for example, "If only . . ."); to avoid or postpone a test or a performance; to demonstrate strength, courageous heroism, or moral superiority; to declare an inadequacy and to seek an exemption from responsibility by hiding behind that inadequacy; to excuse retreat or failure; to divert attention (for example, one's own attention with a "sideshow"); to avoid closeness or maintain distance. Offensive goals, on the other hand, aim at the manipulation of others for the purpose of some gain. Common offensive, or aggressive, goals are: attention and influence; power, conquest, dominance, and importance; retribution, punishment, retaliation, or revenge.

IDENTIFYING POSTURAL AND NONVERBAL MEANINGS

Nonverbal behavior may express many of the client's underlying feelings. An awareness of the messages conveyed through the client's gestures and postural cues assists the counselor in adding deeper feeling or meaning to the client's verbal expressions. As will be examined later, the counselor may focus confrontations on discrepancies between verbal and nonverbal expressions. A client's grimace, swinging leg, tapping finger, fidgeting, or odd rhythm of breathing may all communicate what is just below the surface of awareness or not put into words. There is a danger, however, in the common proclivity of counselors to interpret such behavior in a stereotyped manner from a purely external frame of reference. The same nonverbal behavior may have different meanings with different clients, and one must also take into account the entire context in which such behavior occurs. When one is uncertain of the meaning of a nonverbal behavior, a level 3.0 inquiry about that meaning is recommended. For example, level 3.0 responses that invite the client to be aware of his nonverbal behavior and to explore its meaning include: "Could you translate your frown into words?"; "Are you aware of the way you are sitting right now? I'm wondering what your posture is saying"; (to a client beginning to cry) "You appear to be hurting right now. Can you put what the tears are saying into words?" At other times, the counselor may be attuned enough to the client to discern the implicit meaning accurately, and he can try to verbalize the underlying meaning himself. For instance, one might respond, "As you talk about that, you look down as though you may be feeling pretty discouraged."

ASSUMING PERSONAL RESPONSIBILITY

When responding at additive levels, the counselor should, whenever possible, help the client internalize and accept his role in and personal responsibility for his problems. Frequently, the client will disown the problem and project responsibility for his difficulties onto others, safeguarding his self-image by maintaining the fantasy that he is an innocent victim of circumstance. Not uncommonly, when clients describe the attributes of other people, they are actually describing disowned aspects of themselves. Perls (1973) notes subtle word substitutions that clients often make to escape personal responsibility. For example, "it" and "they" are often substituted for "I," and "can't" is used in place of "won't" or "don't want to."

Acceptance of responsibility may be fostered through confrontation that focuses on word substitutions or through additive empathic responses. A structured response format for empathic responses that encourage the personalizing of responsibility is, "You feel _____ because you have not (or did not) _____." For example, "I sense how disappointed you are with yourself because you haven't followed through on your commitment."

Relational Empathy

The here-and-now encounter between counselor and client is the context in which much of the most valuable learning of counseling accrues. Although relational immediacy will be examined in depth in Chapter Nine, it deserves mention in passing here.

The counselor should be aware of the current experiencing of the client as he engages in self-examination. Additionally, it is important to remain alert to the immediate interaction, to acknowledge the client's here-and-now reactions and feelings toward the counselor, and to empathically recognize the impact of interventions on the client, thus providing a model of a sensitive, open relationship. The client's feelings about the counselor, the current interaction, and the entire relationship are frequently unstated. Additive responding, therefore, consists of accurate recognition of such implicit or suggested feelings. An example of such a response would be: "As we get together, you appear rather fearful of me, as though you're really afraid of how I must see you after learning so much about you."

Tentativeness and Phrasing

Additive empathic responses are usually phrased as tentative suggestions rather than authoritative pronouncements. Deeper interventions contain an element of inference and may be inaccurate. Tentative phrasing allows the client to reject inaccurate, premature, and threatening interpretations without feeling that he is disputing the counselor. Tentativeness may also allow a client to accept some parts of an intervention and reject others. Some useful qualifying phrases include: "It sounds as if . . ."; "I'm wondering if you're saying . . ."; "Perhaps . . ."; "Maybe . . ."; "I get the impression that . . ."; "Possibly . . ."; "Is it possible that . . . "; "Would this fit . . . "; "Do you suppose . . . ."

Strive for concise, simple responses without technical terms. It is most helpful to use personal, informal language that incorporates the client's own phrases and terms.

Ruesch (1961) commented that the task of the therapist is to choose gestures and words which will stimulate something that is alive within the client. The language of the counselor may go beyond merely labeling and objectifying experience to stimulating the further unfolding of the client's experience. The use of metaphors and sensory imagery to paint word pictures that can be seen and felt as well as heard stimulates deeper self-exploration. Rice recommends that the counselor convey to the client the imagery the message evoked: "For instance, a client has been talking about feeling utterly alone, trying to understand how everything can be going so wrong, and the therapist responds, 'You feel as if you are all alone in a cavern shouting, 'What's wrong! What's wrong!'" (1974, pp. 309–310). To a client who has been complaining of being used unthinkingly by others, the counselor could respond metaphorically, "You feel just like a doormat, don't you? Everybody steps on you and wipes their feet, but nobody pays you any mind."

Documentation

It is often helpful to the client for the counselor to document his additive responses. Citing situations or experiences previously discussed by the client that provide support for your conclusions encourage the client to accept the intervention. For example, a counselor might explain, "I've noticed that you've mentioned a number of times how important being independent has been to you. You've discussed that in connection with our relationship also. Is it possible that you resent George because what he did may have threatened your ability to be independent at work?"

Appropriateness of Empathic Responding

Any counseling intervention, whether an empathic response, a confrontation, or an authentic sharing of the counselor's feelings, should be appropriate to the particular situation. Ideally, the counselor should base his choice of response on empirically derived indications and contraindications rather than merely dispensing responses indiscriminately from a theoretical conviction about their overall importance and essentialness. Such an indiscriminate approach makes the counselor something like a physician who propounds one drug as the cure for all human afflictions and who prescribes that drug for everything from colds to cancer. Empathic responses, confrontations, or other counseling interventions or techniques are not necessarily helpful in all clinical situations. In fact, there are even times when empathic responses may be counterproductive.

A sore need exists for the development, testing, and refinement of guidelines for differential intervention. In particular, guidelines and research on when specific types of interventions may impede client progress are needed. Unfortunately, research documentation of indications and contraindications for different types of responses is sparse. In the absence of adequate guidelines, some suggested and tentative indications and contraindications based primarily on clinical wisdom are presented here. Because these guidelines are still rather general and unrefined, we offer them as guideposts for appropriateness, not as inflexible rules to be rigidly applied.

INDICATIONS FOR EMPATHIC RESPONDING

1. During the early phase of counseling and generally in the opening moments of subsequent interviews, reciprocal empathic responding is of crucial importance in conveying understanding and establishing a therapeutic relationship. The goals of the early and middle phases of counseling are to establish the relationship and to help the client acquire increased self-awareness and understanding. Reciprocal and additive empathic responding facilitates the client's self-experiencing and exploration, which lead to self-understanding. During the change-oriented stage of counseling, the counselor still employs empathic interventions, but he accords greater emphasis to ways of translating insight and understanding into behavioral changes. Additive empathic interventions are usually inappropriate in the early interviews, before a good relationship has been established, and in the opening moments of subsequent interviews.

2. Empathic responses facilitate emotional expression. Thus when the counselor needs to assess the role emotions play in a client's problems, responding with empathy is indicated. Empathic responsiveness is similarly called for when feelings need to be ventilated to release the tension of pent up emotions, such as grief, anger, or hurt. Empathic understanding of the stress associated with painful states of being similarly conveys emotional support to the client.

3. Empathic responding is generally indicated with an emotionally constricted client—that is, one who is out of touch with his

emotions—to facilitate the experiencing and expression of a broad-ened range of feelings. Reciprocal and additive empathic responses help the client become aware of and label inner experiences and feelings, leading to an understanding of the role emotions play in problems. In addition, getting in touch with feelings often pro-duces a liberating effect and adds to the client's zest for living.

4. Reciprocal and additive empathic interventions help improve the communication of clients who are inexperienced or inept in "feeling talk"—that is, those who lack an adequate vocab-ulary of feelings or whose communications are limited by dominant patterns of intellectualization or acting out. Empathic responsive-ness assists such persons to become aware of their emotions, teaches them skills for conveying their feelings to others, and sensitizes them to an awareness of feelings in other people. Thus empathic understanding models an important dimension of communication that may help the client improve his interpersonal relationships.

5. Working through client defensiveness, negativism, and hostility in the therapeutic relationship calls for empathic respond-ing. Empathic interventions create an ambience in which the client can risk expressing his negative feelings without the threat of retalia-tion. Moreover, empathic acknowledgement disarms the client's defenses and permits dispassionate exploration of the sources of negative feelings. Any defensive resistances or negative reactions to the counselor must be empathically recognized and examined. When such roadblocks exist, the counselor must concentrate his attention on relational empathy aimed at current interaction and feelings. The purposes for such resistance or negative feelings need to be illuminated and these obstacles resolved, or it will be impossible to explore more central areas of conflict constructively.

6. Empathic responsiveness fosters receptivity to confronta-tions. Used as a preface to confrontation, empathic messages serve effectively as lead-ins that lower defenses and, by communicating understanding and helpful intent, soften the possible negative im-pact of confrontation.

7. Responding empathically is indicated when deeper insight is needed to solve emotional problems impeding behavioral change. Accurate additive interventions facilitate self-exploration and ex-pand awareness of underlying purposes and patterns of feeling

and behavior that are self-defeating. Empathic responding is essential in helping clients victimized by problems such as anxiety reactions, tension states, and emotional blocking.

CONTRAINDICATIONS FOR EMPATHIC RESPONDING

1.   Additive empathic responses that focus on underlying feelings instead of cognitive relationships, purposes, and meanings are recommended with the obsessive-compulsive individual. Such persons separate intellect from feelings, tend to analyze rather than feel, and use rational processes to avoid emotional contact. This type of client tends to disguise and distrust feelings, seemingly under the motto, "Analyze and conquer." The obsessional client uses words to cloud, not to illuminate. Therefore, the counselor should focus especially on responding in fresh, metaphorical language and sensory imagery, seeking to stimulate deeper contact with emotional experiencing. Empathic interventions should concentrate on facilitating emotional contact and self-experiencing rather than on further analyzing meanings or purposes.

2.   Generally, the more intense the emotionality of the client, the more the counselor can formulate additive responses that conceptualize implicit meanings, relationships, patterns, and purposes without fear that these responses will lead to overly intellectual defensiveness and repression of affect. However, with emotionally overexpressive, histrionic individuals who ventilate melodramatically and talk incessantly, empathic responsiveness, especially that which focuses on the feelings present, may indeed foster cathartic and temporary symptomatic relief, but it may also defeat the aims of therapy by permitting, reinforcing, and thus perpetuating the client's dysfunctional mode of coping. Since such clients need more to encourage their rational processes than to express their emotions freely, they might be better directed to evaluate and analyze than to experience feelings.

3.   The counselor should proceed with great caution to additive empathy with very distrustful, paranoid clients. More time than usual must be allowed for the therapeutic relationship to be established. This type of client is particularly likely to misinterpret an additive intervention as a critical accusation, slight, or criticism, particularly if it is inaccurate or too deep. The counselor should

place greater emphasis on reciprocal, level 3.0 responding than on additive interventions, and greater than usual tentativeness should appear in his language. Accurate additive empathic interventions can be especially threatening for the paranoid client, who may see them as validating his conviction that the counselor is a mind reader or has special inside information. If the counselor offers additive responses, it may be particularly important for him to show precisely how he arrived at such conclusions or perceptions.

4. With the very withdrawn, schizoid client, it may take a longer time than usual until the counseling relationship is established well enough to allow additive interventions. With such seriously disturbed individuals whose grasp of reality is tenuous and whose perceptions are colored by projections, distortions, or delusions, empathic responding may actually reinforce distorted perceptions. Concrete responses that elicit the behavioral details of upsetting events serve therapy better in that they yield a picture of the situational context and assist in identifying distortions and projections. Empathic responsiveness to distorted material does not encourage reality testing in individuals with significant thought disorders.

5. Caution must be used in formulating additive interventions with severely depressed clients who are suicidal. Such a client may construe an in-depth identification of underlying negative patterns or self-defeating behaviors as criticism and as a confirmation of personal worthlessness, turning the insight into a weapon against the self. Generally, interventions in depth should not be used with severely depressed clients. Until their morale has improved, these individuals are largely unable to benefit from conceptualizing underlying feelings or from identifying connections between their depression and precipitating factors. With severely depressed clients, other methods such as drug therapy, hospitalization, or environmental manipulation intended to ease the depression should be used before the counselor tries to facilitate deep insight.

6. When discrepancies and inconsistencies in behavior are present in the middle phase of therapy, empathic responding may be inimical to the therapeutic objectives. At such times, confrontations tempered with empathy and warmth will likely serve therapeutic aims more effectively than empathic responding.

7. After the early contacts with individuals who are strongly antisocial, nonconforming, alienated from societal values, and who act out on impulse, continual empathic responding is generally not helpful. Action-oriented techniques need to be introduced sooner than usual. Active confrontation may communicate more understanding to such clients than empathic responsiveness, which they may interpret as weakness. Being overly responsive to the expressed feelings of these clients may leave the counselor open to easy manipulation.

8. When the counselor's feelings and experiences in the counselor-client interaction persistently distract his ability to "tune in" with the client, authentic, self-disclosing responses may take precedence over and be prerequisite to further empathic responding.

9. Whenever the client realistically needs factual information essential to problem solving that the counselor can supply, empathic responding is contraindicated.

Communication Exercises with Modeled Responses

To assist you in expanding your capacity to respond with additive empathy, we have provided forty-five exercises with modeled responses. These exercises involve a wide variety of statements and problems, most taken from actual counseling interviews. After reading each message, formulate on paper the additive empathic response you would make as the counselor. You may wish to use the structured format provided in Chapter Five before translating your response into conversational language. In formulating your response, consider feelings implied but not explicitly stated in the message as well as feelings that probably lie at the edge of or somewhat beyond the client's awareness. Avoid deep interpretations that go well beyond the client's level of awareness.

After completing each exercise, compare your response with the authors' modeled response following the messages. Keep in mind that the modeled response is only one of many possible responses. Compare your response to determine how your response differs. Note especially the varied ways of formulating responses and consider those aspects of your own and of the modeled responses that impress you as most effective.

CLIENT STATEMENTS

1. *22-year-old male:* "I don't think I've ever been satisfied with things as they are. I daydream a lot—you know, just make up situations in my mind. I guess I have kind of an artistic temperament. I really am quite self-centered—you know, immersed in myself. I envy people who aren't self-conscious."

2. *35-year-old married female:* "My husband gets mad over my reminding him to make an appointment to see the doctor about that lump in his groin. But what do you do? When I remind him, he doesn't say anything; he just gives me the silent treatment. So then I don't say anything either. To tell the truth, I'm afraid of what I might say at that point—that I might regret it."

3. *29-year-old female schoolteacher:* "The tiniest things happen and I fall to pieces. It's been even worse this spring, the past three months. I get to feeling the kids I teach are against me, like they hate me. Yet I know better than that. On the last day of school I almost fell apart; that was when I called for an appointment to see you."

4. *Female college student, age 19:* "I recall my parents arguing when I was 14 and I was dating a guy 18 years old. Mother got tired of being blamed and told my dad he was raising a fag (the client's brother). Then Dad yelled at her that she was raising a whore." A short pause, and she looks at floor. "I guess I, ah—I guess I thought of myself as a whore after that." She begins to cry.

5. *25-year-old Black mother to White female counselor:* "Back home in the South, Whites only talk to Blacks when they want something. I like to see you and yet find myself feeling uneasy about it."

6. *17-year-old female:* "I wish my relationship with my school counselor weren't a counselor-student relationship. It would be neat if she were just a friend. The idea she is paid to be nice upsets me."

7. *22-year-old female:* "Everything I do well, I do alone." She pauses. "In dancing I don't follow well. If I feel someone is standing over my shoulder, I don't do well."

8. *26-year-old female to male therapist:* "I've always wanted a challenge in my relationships with men—to have a man really fall for me and then drop him."

9. *34-year-old female:* "I always felt my tennis partner had cuter outfits. She always was trim and looked better. I didn't play

well in singles. I always felt I needed my partner. When I won the singles match, I couldn't believe it. I thought the other person was off form."

10. *Female, age 22:* "I'm very sensitive to having anyone upset with me. Mother is all I've got. Sometimes she gets mad and stays mad for two days. I just about come unglued."

11. *16-year-old female:* "I get a feeling of restlessness and can't stay home for more than an hour. I have trouble staying in school, too. I get to feeling caged and have to get out."

12. *17-year-old female:* "One of my aunts is one of my 'other mothers.' She always thinks she knows everything. If I say something like a teenager, she preaches to me. She's really old-fashioned. My 'other mothers' are like a bunch of old hens who have to keep their eyes on me."

13. "I've thought of spacing the interviews further apart because I've been doing so well. But I feel that treatment is a controlling force. I know if I get upset I'm going to have to talk about it. I wonder how much of my improvement may be due to the policeman effect of treatment."

14. *16-year-old female:* "After school Ginny and I talked with Mrs. Edwards, the school counselor. She said if Ginny and I were going to be together a lot we should bring out each other's good points. She asked us to identify our strengths and weaknesses. But Mrs. Edwards began by pointing out my demanding and bossy nature. I thought she was really insulting. When I went home that night, I went right to bed. I felt I was dying bit by bit. Mrs. Edwards has been so negative—so much of it lately."

15. "I've never felt good about any of my achievements, as though I should have done better. I'm a good seamstress but I feel anyone else could be too, if they tried."

16. "I went to the party and actually it was fairly informal. But I felt uncomfortable, as though I had to play the expected role. I found myself evaluating what others were saying and wondering what they were thinking about what I said."

17. "I've seen myself as just common, like I would let anyone use me or do what they want to me."

18. "I'm a private person. I don't like to discuss my personal experiences. I think I'm afraid of not expressing myself right."

19.   "I talked with Dr. _____ about my gastrointestinal problem. You can't believe how blunt he is and how he contradicts himself. He infuriates me! But I just sit there and take it."

20.   "I feel my life is controlled by his work and his hours. He tells me what to do and I accept it, or else."

21.   *25-year-old single female:* "Sometimes I abhor myself for being so dependent. I've wanted to center my life around another person—to be loved completely. The feeling is overpowering at times. Sometimes the feelings have led me into situations with men that I've felt very ashamed of."

22.   "I'm pleased that I quit drinking, but I have the feeling I've never been able to just be me. I'm always doing things because other people expect me to."

23.   "I've tried to love her, believe me I've tried, but every time I start getting some good feelings for her she begins to nag me about some little insignificant thing, and the hassling really turns me off."

24.   *23-year-old woman:* "I'm in a terrible bind! I've fallen in love for the first time in my life, to the best guy I've ever known. And what's more, he loves me—he's crazy about me. He asked me to marry him. It's like a dream come true, but I'm not worthy of him. I couldn't marry him. A few years ago I had a child out of wedlock and gave him up for adoption. He doesn't know about my past, but I'm sure he'd find out. I just couldn't hurt him like that."

25.   *30-year-old, divorced woman:* "I know whenever I see somebody I'd like to really date, I can't seem to, um, get them to call me or get their interest, or whatever. And they even go to the point of getting my name and phone number, and then I never hear from them. And I don't understand this, you know, it's blowing my mind."

26.   *34-year-old man:* "I don't feel like I even have a vote in my own marriage! Janet likes to take care of all the bills and money, and she continually makes important decisions for us without consulting me. The other day she went out, with no discussion at all, and bought a new stereo record player and tape deck. She acts as though she weren't even married!"

27.   *30-year-old divorced woman* (in a tired, weak voice): "I'm just tired of rejection, because you take so much and you just get tired of it. But I don't know how tired I am because if he (her ex-husband) said the right words I'd be back in his hand again."

28.   *16-year-old girl:* "I'm going to leave home. No matter what
I do I'm always wrong. My mother keeps telling me my dresses
are too short, that I'm going to get in trouble with boys. I can't stand
it any longer. I'm going to run away."

29.   "I've just never really fit in. Growing up I was always in
the way, in everyone's hair. I've always felt on the outside, alone
and left out."

30.   "I can't be friendly to people. I have to wait to see if
they like me first."

31.   *Middle-aged parent:* "I feel like my son is using some kind
of drug. He's been doing poorly in school recently and acts really
funny. But I don't know what I should say to him. I'm confused."

32.   "Sometimes I feel just high as a kite, and other times
totally demoralized."

33.   *36-year-old man:* "No one—not people at work, not my
friends,—no one even takes me seriously. I can tell people something serious, and they think I'm just joking around."

34.   "Even when I've had doubts about myself or in what I
could do, I've never expressed them to anyone, so everyone thinks
I'm one hundred percent self-sufficient. And that isn't how I feel
at all."

35.   *Woman:* "All day I have to take care of the kids, and when
my husband comes home, I think at last I can carry on a conversation with an adult. And all he wants to do is stay home and watch
television."

36.   "I don't know if I'm getting any better or not. About
the only thing I look forward to is the lift I get when I take my
medication."

37.   "I had a crying session after our last interview. I'm that
way whenever I get sympathy. I don't want sympathy. Never in my
life have I confided in one person. Could it become a crutch?"

38.   *25-year-old:* "I'm feeling pretty upset right now. Our interview time is shot, and I've sluffed off a problem I had last night.
I'm angry with you too for letting me do it."

39.   *18-year-old female:* "Last week I decided to go to the university. I made that decision because Ginny (client's girlfriend) said
she thought I'd be happy there. She seems to have a power over me.
I guess I'd do most anything she'd ask."

40.   *19-year-old female:* "My sister called me from Stockton and

told me Dad is going to get married in January. I have such mixed feelings toward him. I pity him yet I also feel hostile. I think I'm afraid of being shut out of his life and want him to stay single. I can't accept his being affectionate with other women."

41.   "I feel like I have nothing in common with others, like I'm not worth anything. I feel so lonely but I don't want to depend on others. That's a sign of weakness and I don't want to be a weakling."

42.   *57-year-old female, depressed:* "Sometimes I have good thoughts about Mother—yet sometimes I wonder what will happen to me because of the hard things I said to her. Mother was very controlling and didn't want me to go anyplace, and I had my own family to look after. Even though she was partially crippled with her arthritis, she could have done more for herself."

43.   "I see myself as needing ego building from others. Yet I seem to be attracted to men who are critical and tear me down."

44.   "I'd like to be able to talk with Mother more easily. I can talk to Dad a little easier. Mother always seems busy; she brushes me off a lot. My brother is a lot better at getting things from her. I'm not very good at asking for things."

45.   *Twenty-five-year-old man:* "I guess there are really two parts of me. I don't want to go back to prison again. I hated it. And I love my wife and son. I don't want to hurt them again. I've hurt them enough. But stealing is the only way I know to get by. I don't have a trade or nothin'." He pauses. "I don't know of any other way I could give them all the things I want them to have. Stealing is the only thing I know how to do. When it comes right down to it, I've failed at about everything else I've ever done. As much as I love Sherry and my little boy, I won't put them through it all again. If the thief in me wins out, I'll cut them loose and let them try to find a good life for themselves. I know I'd be miserable, but I'd do it."

MODELED RESPONSES

1.   "You know, listening to you I get the impression that you're really pretty unhappy with your life and because of that you imagine situations you'd like to be in. You sound really discontented about your preoccupation with yourself, as though you're saying, "'I'd really like to get more involved in the real world with other people.'"

2. "I gather you're just bewildered about what to do. On one hand, you're worried about him, yet when you try to get him to see the doctor, he ignores you. It sounds as though you've about reached the end of your rope and are afraid you'll blow your top if you even talk with him. And you don't want that to happen. Could we think together about some alternative ways of approaching him?"

3. "Mmm! So even the little things have been getting to you. Sort of like you've barely been able to hold on. You're feeling panicky even now, I gather, afraid of falling completely apart. An urgent feeling of 'I've got to get hold of things,' and you're hoping that counseling can help you do that."

4. "It must have cut to the core when you heard your dad refer to you as a whore. And I gather after that *you* began to think of yourself in that light. You know, I'm wondering if perhaps that's how you're seeing yourself even now, as just sort of cheap—even worthless. Those feelings, just so painful. You don't want to feel that way about yourself."

5. "So you're having two different kinds of feelings toward me. Part of you feels toward me as you felt toward Whites in the South, very distrustful and wanting to avoid me. That's understandable, because life's experiences have taught you to be careful of Whites. Yet another part of you feels differently, actually wants to like me and to see me in a different light. Those feelings pull you in opposite directions, and you want to come to terms with them."

6. "From what you say, I gather you'd like to have a closer relationship with your counselor. You're not really sure how you stand with her, and you'd like to be special to her in your own right, not just because she's a counselor."

7. "Apparently, though you're perfectly capable when you're alone, being observed by another person makes you very uncomfortable, as though you're afraid of blundering and appearing inadequate."

8. "Let's see if I'm understanding you. It sounds as though you're wanting to hurt men by rejecting them when they've grown to care for you. I have the impression you have some real bitterness toward men. I wonder if you may be seeking to strike back at men for some hurt you've experienced in the past."

9. "Sounds like you felt inferior to your partner and so lacking in confidence that it amazed you when you won in singles. I get the definite impression that somehow you developed a pattern of underestimating yourself and always comparing yourself unfavorably with others."

10. "Just so distressing to have someone displeased with you and you're painfully aware of how much you depend on Mother. When she stays angry, I gather it's almost as though you feel abandoned by her."

11. "So when you're confined for very long, the tension builds up inside, as though you'll explode if you don't get out. I wonder what goes through your mind in those situations."

12. "So I gather you resent this 'mothering' from so many people. It seems to you they're intruding into your life, as though they have to protect you from yourself. You don't feel you need that, and you wish they'd stop bugging you."

13. "Sounds like you're feeling pulled in two directions. You think you're doing better, and part of you is feeling more able to handle things independently. But another part of you is afraid that you're still not strong enough—as though you're questioning whether you've really grown enough to stand on your own or whether your strength is just borrowed from me."

14. "Wow! It sounds like you just felt devastated by her criticisms. You just felt so belittled and so hurt and then gradually got more and more depressed. You just feel so demeaned by Mrs. Edwards and wonder what to do."

15. "I'm getting the impression that you somehow always feel you fall short of your expectations. Even when you do something well, you underrate it. It's as though you see yourself as so deficient that you can't believe anything you do really can amount to much."

16. "So you really didn't enjoy yourself. I gather you just couldn't let go, you know, relax and be yourself. Like if you let go others might disapprove. You're so conscious of that that you're on guard, keenly aware of yourself and others."

17. "Gee, that sounds like a painful way to think of yourself, almost as though you feel you have so little to offer you have no right to expect much from others—just try to please others at any price and expect nothing more than a few crumbs in return."

18. "That fear of making a goof—you know it sounds as though you feel so unsure inside that it's frightening to open up much. If you lower the barriers, you feel you'd be vulnerable to being criticized and disapproved of."

19. "Sounds like you really get burned up with him. You know, you really sound pretty disgusted with yourself, too, for letting it happen and then just keeping the anger bottled up. You're fed up with the whole situation and would like to find a different way of dealing with it."

20. "You're getting pretty sick of being dominated by him. You'd like to be your own person, yet you're afraid what might happen if you stand up for yourself. I wonder what it is you fear might happen if you stood up for yourself."

21. "So you're saying that when you've yielded to that almost desperate need to feel close to and loved by a man, you've at times paid a heavy price of guilt and pain. You'd like to have that closeness you've been seeking but not feel at the mercy of the need for it."

22. "Though you're happy to be sober, there's still a sense of not being whole, of something missing. Really feeling frustrated with yourself because you want to be your own person and do things because they fit for you, not just be pleasing others all the time."

23. "I guess you're feeling frustrated and bewildered because when you start feeling close to her, she seems to push you away. You really seem discouraged and to be wondering, 'What the hell can I do?'"

24. "You've found your dream. One part of you wants to let it come true, but another part of you feels unworthy and is pulling away, frightened that if he knew he might reject you. And the fear of that possibility is almost more than you can bear."

25. "You're really not only bewildered, but frustrated with yourself because you can't seem to hold the attention of the men you meet. You're getting to the point where you just *have* to understand what's wrong and what you yourself might be doing to discourage them."

26. "I sense how powerless and insignificant you've been feeling, like you are almost useless and just along for the ride with Janet. But you sound sick and tired of sitting in the background and watching. You'd like to start casting your vote."

27. "You've experienced the pain of being pushed away long enough that you're just *sick* of being hurt, yet you're really vulnerable to being rejected again because you still haven't let him go despite the divorce. I guess I wonder if you must not feel you have little value as a person, given the way you're willing to endure such pain."

28. "You really appear to be feeling a lot of hurt over the way she doesn't seem to believe in you or feel good about you. It's so painful that you're just about fed up with the situation, but you really do seem to care about her and wish that it could be better between the two of you."

29. "Just feeling cut off from the world, isolated and insignificant all of your life. Like being locked out and abandoned, and longing but not knowing how you could get in and relate to people."

30. "I wonder if your pattern then is to stay rather aloof, because you sound pretty apprehensive about initiating contacts and feel a great deal of risk in trusting people much until you can be sure they won't reject you."

31. "But I hear much more than just confusion over how to approach him. You also sound terribly frightened, both about what you may find out and about what might happen."

32. "Just soaring sometimes, and buried in a black hole at other times. That swing between those extremes is alarming to you, and I sense you are feeling that somehow you must get yourself on a more even keel."

33. "So your world is a place where you feel trapped in the part of a clown, with everyone laughing, but with no one taking you seriously as a real person. And you convey a sense of feeling powerless to break out of that role, and yet you sound damned dissatisfied with it."

34. "So despite the outward impression of great adequacy and confidence, inside you're actually feeling rather deficient and full of questions about your abilities. And I gather you're frightened of how people would react if they knew how you feel. Maybe feeling very vulnerable right now in letting me see more of you."

35. "So you feel isolated all day, and instead of the anticipated relief when he comes, you still feel abandoned and neglected. You're just getting fed up with it and want somehow to reach him, to have some companionship with him."

36. "You sound pretty discouraged and depressed, as though life seems empty and meaningless to you. You'd like to gain some zest for living, but it looks pretty bleak to you right now."

37. "So it's a new and in some ways a frightening experience to share with me some of those feelings you've kept inside. I think I'm hearing you say you're afraid you may become dependent if you continue sharing. But I think I may be hearing something else, too, that you've had a longing to have a close relationship—the kind that would permit you to share more of your personal feelings."

38. "So you're feeling angry inside right now, frustrated and mad at yourself for not using your time better and mad at me for permitting it. You know I feel bad that we weren't focusing on what seemed most important to you. Next time perhaps we could explore what was happening that you held back on discussing that particular problem."

39. "That power that Ginny seems to have—you know, I'm wondering if something else is happening—if perhaps you're strongly influenced by Ginny and perhaps others too because of some feelings you have about yourself. Sort of like you trust the judgment of others more than your own. I'm wondering if you've somehow learned to fear making a wrong decision and find it less risky to depend on someone else."

40. "It's really distressing to you when you think of his getting married. Even though your relationship with him hasn't been the best, still it remains very important to you. You seem to fear that what caring he now has for you will be lost forever if he remarries. That's so painful for you to think about."

41. "So you're really caught in a bind. On one hand you feel so isolated and hungry for relationships. But on the other you feel different from others—as though no one could possibly care for you. And you seem to be struggling with another conflict. Admitting to yourself you need and want more involvement with others is like admitting you're a weak person, and you can't accept that. I have the impression you've had to deny that need in yourself. At least you feel some strength in your isolation, but your fortress is such a lonely place. You'd like to get out of it."

42. "When you think of Mother, you find yourself pulled by these opposing feelings. Part of you feels guilty, even dreads being punished for some of the things you said to Mother in anger.

Yet another part of you feels angry. Even now you resent how unreasonable she is to make her demands with no recognition of your own and your family's needs."

43. "Just find it confusing, and you're wondering how to cope with these contradictory forces. Part of you wanting, even craving perhaps, relationships with men who will give you approval and reassurance—you know, build you up. Yet you find yourself drawn to men who are quite the opposite. You'd like to come to terms with these feelings and get out of your self-defeating pattern."

44. "So in a way you seem to be saying, 'If I am going to have better communication with her, I'm going to have to risk myself more.' But that's been tough for you to do in the past. Perhaps we can explore further what happens inside of you that seems to hold you back."

45. "The possibility of cutting loose your family and ending up back in prison sounds like a really bleak picture, especially because you really care for them. One part of you wishes you knew how to take care of them by being straight, but another part of you sounds really helpless in figuring out how to provide for them without stealing. You're afraid you just don't have what it takes or know how to make it."

Practicum Exercises

These exercises help consolidate the learning from the past three chapters. Used either along with or after the written exercises, they provide behavioral rehearsal closely approximating actual counseling situations. In the experience of the authors, practice through role-playing is necessary to refine empathic communication skills and to facilitate generalization to actual interpersonal exchanges.

EXERCISE ONE

The first practice in additive empathic responding is the filecard exercise presented at the end of Chapter Five. The instructor presents a client statement, and the trainees write an additive response on file cards, omitting their names. The cards are passed in, the instructor reads them one at a time, and the group rates each response and discusses it. It is recommended that following the rating and evaluation of five or six responses, some exercises be undertaken in which the instructor has volunteers read their responses to the group for rating, feedback, and discussion.

EXERCISE TWO

Divide the training group into triads whose participants will assume the roles of counselor, client, and rater-observer. The client is instructed to assume the role of a person seeking help for an emotion-laden problem. The counselor should be instructed to make at least four or five level 3.0 empathic responses before attemping an additive empathic intervention. The roleplaying sequence should continue for about five minutes, and then the client and the rater-observer should share feedback and ratings with the counselor. Roles should be exchanged until all trainees have had at least one opportunity to be the counselor. Tape-recording or videotaping is highly recommended in the feedback process. To broaden the learning experience and to provide extended practice, the entire group can be sorted into triads several times.

Homework Assignment

To assist in consolidating and refining empathic communication skills (as well as the varied skills discussed in other chapters), the trainee who is involved in practicum, internship or actual work experiences should regularly audiotape or videotape interviews. The trainee can then rate his own responses on the tape. He can also practice by stopping the tape after the client makes a statement, carefully formulating and writing a response, then comparing the written response to the actual response he made in the interview. The effects of this exercise often startle and enlighten the learner, emphasizing the need for further skill development.

Chapter 7

Relating to Clients with Respect

The counselor's respect for the client is essential in setting the stage for behavioral change. Affirmation of the self as a worthwhile individual is a universal human need, and the counselor must be able to respond positively to that multifaceted need if he is to be an effective helping person. Respect for and unconditional acceptance of the client provide the therapeutic climate most conducive to growth and change. Once the client has experienced the respect and good will of the counselor, he can open himself to reflect on and change his social and psychological situation. Until the client feels accepted as someone worthwhile, he will have little motivation to cooperate actively in counseling. Thus the helping person must create an atmosphere that verbally and nonverbally communicates to the client that his individuality, his uniqueness, his wishes, his thoughts, and his behaviors are respected as inviolate parts of his self over which he alone has undisputed jurisdiction. Respect for the client communicates full recognition of the client's right to be what he is or desires to become with full acknowledgement that only from his wishes, strengths, and effort is change possible or likely.

The facilitative quality of respect subsumes many facets of the counselor's feelings, beliefs, attitudes, and behavior, and these attributes collectively determine whether the client will experience full respect for his personal identity, uniqueness, and individuality. Respect comprises four vital elements, each of which will be discussed in this chapter: demonstrating a commitment to understand the client; conveying acceptance and warmth; affirming the client's worth and uniqueness; affirming and nurturing the client's strengths, potential for growth, and capacity to solve problems.

Levels of Respect

The Respect Scale is presented below, followed by examples and explanations of its varying levels. The reader is encouraged to commit to memory the essential characteristics of each level of the scale and to refer to it while studying the examples and completing the exercises later on.

RESPECT SCALE*

Level 1.0. Verbal and nonverbal responses communicate overt disrespect, or negative regard, declaring the other person's feelings and experiences unworthy of consideration. The helper may make himself the focus of evaluation, actively disapprove of behavior, impose his own values or beliefs, dominate the conversation, challenge the accuracy of the other's perception, or depreciate the worth of the other by communicating that he is incapable of acting constructively or functioning appropriately on his own.

Level 2.0. The helper communicates little respect for the feelings, potentials, or experiences of the other person. He may ignore what the other says, respond in a casual, passive, or mechanical manner, and withhold himself from involvement. He may decline to enter into a relationship or display a lack of concern or interest.

Level 3.0. The helper communicates a positive concern and respect for the other person's feelings and his ability to act constructively and express himself. The counselor suspends his own

*Adapted from scales of respect, nonpossessive warmth, and unconditional positive regard to be found in Carkhuff, 1969; Gazda and others, 1973; Rogers, Gendlin, Kiesler, and Truax, 1967; Truax and Carkhuff, 1967.

judgment of the other and communicates an openness or willingness to enter into a relationship.

Level 4.0. The helper affirms the worth and value of the other person by his efforts to understand and by his communication of very deep respect, concern, and care. He is open and willing to invest himself enough to risk receiving potentially hurtful feedback in order to further the relationship. His responses enable the other person to feel valued as an individual and free to be himself.

Level 5.0. The helper communicates the very deepest respect for the other person's worth, value, and potentials as a separate individual who is free to be himself. He communicates his caring for, valuing, and appreciation of the other as a unique person. After the relationship is well established, respect may entail challenging the other person to achieve his goals and take responsibility for himself. Expectations and personal reactions such as disappointment and irritation may be expressed provided they are couched in good will and helpful intent. Encouragement and praise may also be shared.

EXAMPLES OF LEVELS OF RESPECT

Client Statement 1

Twenty-year-old female: "You're right, you know, about my being late today because of some feelings about our interview last week." She pauses briefly. "Remember, we'd been talking about how I—uh—how I've been so unsure of whether Tom (a boyfriend) really loves me. Well, I know it might sound crazy but I got this—this awful feeling of being all alone—you know like no one really cares about me. And then I got to thinking about you, that you only see me"—her chin quivers, and she looks at floor—"because it's your job—that I'm just another client"—she chokes up—"and you could care less about me. I about decided not to come today."

Level 1.0 response. "Those feelings really get in your way, don't they? You know after six interviews it's pretty upsetting to me that you're still unsure about my interest in you, especially when I've made special arrangements to see you two different times."

Explanation. The counselor's message conveys negative regard for the client and implied criticism of her feelings. The counselor also shifts the focus to his own sense of frustration, indicating that the client's feelings not only are inappropriate but also reflect ingratitude for the "special arrangements" made on her behalf. As a consequence, the client would tend to experience the counselor's acceptance as conditional upon her trusting him, even though trust is not the client's feeling at the moment. Moreover, the counselor's response would tend to reinforce the feelings that brought the client to therapy in the first place: that no one really cares about her. Such responses often contribute to premature termination by the client.

Level 2.0 response. "Sounds like we're going to have to explore those feelings further. My impression is that you're experiencing some feelings of transference in our relationship."

Explanation. The counselor's response doesn't totally ignore the client's feelings, but it fails to convey an awareness of the significance of the feeling as experienced by the client. It indicates some interest in exploring the feelings, but this interest tends to be negated by an inappropriate interpretation which, although it may be accurate, rejects the client's feelings as invalid. Moreover, use of the term *transference* may convey disrespect by taxing the client's ability to understand or criticizing her for ignorance by implication. The client would tend to be puzzled by such a response and would find it even more difficult to risk sharing such feelings in the future.

Level 3.0 response. "Those are certainly painful feelings you've been struggling with. I'm pleased you decided to come today, even though it was difficult for you. Perhaps we can explore together where those feelings are coming from."

Explanation. The counselor conveys awareness and unqualified acceptance of the client's feelings, an expression of positive regard, a commitment to help, and an encouragement of further self-expression.

Level 4.0 response. "Those feelings of doubt you've experienced toward Tom and toward me are very painful, even now as you share them with me. It's been a real struggle for you—part of you caring and wanting to believe that Tom really loves you and that my concern for you is genuine, another part perhaps fearing no one could really care and not wanting to take any more risks. But I'm glad you came today. I'd have felt bad if you hadn't come because you thought I didn't care. That's not at all where I am in my feelings toward you. I wonder, though, if I've done or said something that would raise doubts in your mind about my feelings toward you."

Explanation. The counselor communicates a deep appreciation of the client's feelings. He indicates a high level of respect both through expressions of caring and through his willingness to explore the possibility that he may have unknowingly contributed to the client's feelings of insecurity.

Level 5.0 response. "I'm very concerned that your doubts have been putting you through so much pain you've even thought of not coming. You know your fears that you're just another client I have to see don't really represent my true feelings at all. I do have choices about whom I see, and it's important to me that you know I see you because I value you as a person. It took some real courage on your part to come today and to risk sharing these feelings with me. I'm pleased you came and risked sharing them."

Explanation. The counselor conveys a deep level of respect by recognizing and accepting the client's pain and by expressing his awareness of the courage manifested in her decision to come. The counselor's expression of valuing the client and of seeing her by choice (which is true) deepens the respect. Such a deeply respectful response may lower the client's defenses and increase the likelihood that she will risk more.

Client Statement 2

Thirty-seven-year-old male: "When I think of what I've put Ardith (his wife) through these past five years, with my drinking, chasing broads, ignoring the children, staying out all night—hell, I don't know why she even wants me. I don't deserve her. I'm not worth—you know what I am? I feel like a piece of shit. Yeah, that's exactly how I feel."

Level 1.0 response. "So you've really put her through a lot, haven't you? You know, not many women would put up with what she's gone through. You're pretty lucky to have a wife like that."

Explanation. Ignoring the feelings of remorse and worthlessness, the counselor focuses on the client's previous behavior, clearly conveying disapproval and negative regard. The counselor's depreciating response will probably reinforce the client's guilt and shame. Such a response undercuts encouragement and constructive action.

Level 2.0 response. "It sounds to me as though you may have a problem with alcoholism. Alcoholics Anonymous has been helpful to many people with drinking problems. Are you acquainted with A.A.?"

Explanation. Again the counselor ignores the feelings expressed by the client, but he communicates no negative regard. The worker's intent in referring to alcoholism and A.A. may be helpful, but his conclusion is premature, and the client will not perceive this labeling as a reflection of respect. Premature conclusions convey no commitment to seek to understand and thereby indicate a lack of respect.

Level 3.0 response. "So you're feeling crummy about yourself and the trouble you've caused Ardith. But underneath all of that, I sense that perhaps you're saying you want to get yourself straightened around and regain some respect in the eyes of others and, equally important, some self-respect."

Explanation. Positive concern and respect are conveyed by an expressed awareness of how "crummy" the client feels about his previous behavior and by reference to his unexpressed desire to make constructive changes. The counselor does not pass judgment on the client's past actions.

Level 4.0 response. "You're really feeling down on yourself, just feeling completely worthless. Yet, despite all the anguish and pain for you and your wife these past five years, perhaps there's some reason for feeling hopeful. You seem to want to pick up the pieces and build a better life for yourself and your family. That's a big task, but you have a lot of strength to draw from, and if you wish I can perhaps be helpful to you in tackling the problems."

Explanation. The counselor conveys deep respect in his effort to understand the client's feelings. He demonstrates additional respect by crediting the client with the desire "to pick up the pieces" and the strength he needs to do it and by expressing helpful intent in the last part of the message.

Level 5.0 response. "I can sense the anguish you feel over the pain you've caused your wife and family. I know how that must hurt. But I see some real reasons for feeling hopeful. You seem to be facing your problems head-on now, even though it's tough. Right now, you're probably feeling pretty overwhelmed, and it's going to take some real courage on your part. But I sense some real strengths. If you can hang in there, taking it just one day at a time, I believe you may be able to rebuild your life gradually and regain the respect for yourself that you seem to have lost."

Explanation. A very deep level of respect for the client's worth and his ability to meet the problem is conveyed by a sensitive and realistic perception of his anguish. The expression of hope and of belief in the client's strength will help the client feel the counselor's support, which is vitally needed in this instance.

Exercises in Assessing Levels of Respect

These exercises are designed to refine your ability to discriminate different levels of respect in preparation for practice in communicating respect. Five messages are given, followed by several possible responses. Using the Respect Scale to assist you, rate each response in the space provided at the left of the counselor response.

CLIENT STATEMENT 1

Man, speaking angrily: "You're supposed to be my counselor, and I thought what I told you didn't go out of this room! Somebody has been telling my fiancée ugly rumors about me, and I think it must have been you. Do you have anything to say for yourself?"

Your Rating		Responses:	Discrepancy Score
_____	1.	"You're enraged that someone would tell your fiancée such things, and you really wonder if I am responsible."	_____
_____	2.	"Sorry, but it wasn't me. I don't even know who your fiancée is."	_____
_____	3.	"That's ridiculous. You're getting paranoid."	_____
_____	4.	"What did your fiancée tell you?"	_____
_____	5.	"That must have been distressing, but you ought to know me well enough to know I'd never do a thing like that. I wonder why you don't trust me more."	_____
_____	6.	"I can see how angry you are about the gossiping. I'm not aware of having said anything about you to anyone, and certainly I wouldn't want to damage you in any way. Could we talk about it more?"	_____

_____ 7. "Hey, hold on a minute. I know you're   _____
upset. Gee, I would be too about some-
thing like that. What possible reason
would I have to do such a thing?"

Sum: _____
Average Discrepancy Score: _____

Check your ratings with those provided on page 182. Determine the difference, disregarding whether it is positive or negative,
between each of your ratings and the authors' ratings, and enter
the differences in the blank to the right of the responses. Then add
the differences between your ratings and the ratings provided for
the ten responses. Divide this sum by 7 (the number of responses).
This is your average discrepancy score for the first exercise, which
provides a guide to your ability to discriminate the levels of respect.
The goal is to achieve an average discrepancy score of 0.5 or less
by the end of these exercises. After each exercise, study the responses you rated differently from the authors, refer to the Respect Scale, and try to pinpoint the reason why the authors rated
it as they did.

Proceed now to rate the responses below. After rating all the
responses to a client statement determine your discrepancy from
the authors' rating for each response, add them, and divide by the
total number of counselor responses presented. Continue to analyze
each response for which your rating was inaccurate.

CLIENT STATEMENT 2

Thirty-eight-year-old female: "I'm sure glad that Gladys told
me about you. I've been at my wit's end trying to figure out how to
straighten out my teenage daughter. I've been hoping someone
could tell me who to see who'd have some answers."

Your _Rating_	_Responses:_	_Discrepancy_ _Score_
_____	1. "I hope I can justify your confidence in me."	_____
_____	2. "If it's answers you're seeking, you've come to the wrong person. If you want	_____

help in growing yourself, maybe I can
help you."

_____ 3. "Sounds like you've felt pretty over-   _____
whelmed with your daughter and are
hoping I can help. Teenagers can certainly be challenging at times. I'm not
sure whether I have any answers, or
whether anyone does for that matter,
but I'm surely willing to join you in
searching for some more effective
ways of coping with your daughter."

_____ 4. "What seems to be the problem with   _____
your daughter?"

_____ 5. "It's been my experience that problems   _____
with children usually can be traced to
poor parenting practices. If you go
ahead with me, we'll be focusing on
how you interact with your daughter."

_____ 6. "Just really felt at your wit's end."   _____

_____ 7. "I can sense the frustrations you've   _____
felt, in trying to cope with your daugh-
ter. It sounds as though you've felt at
the end of a blind alley with no place
left to go. It's been my experience that
there are no simple answers to problems of this nature, but I'd like to explore the problem further with you to
see if we can understand it better and
together come up with some helpful
ideas."

Sum: _____
Average Discrepancy Score: _____

CLIENT STATEMENT 3

Forty-year-old male to male counselor: "I'm feeling really
uptight right now!" He pauses. "I know I should really talk with you
about this sexual problem of mine that's really caused trouble in our

marriage. But," and he purses his lips, "damn, it's really hard. You'll probably think I'm a pervert or something and I don't think I am."

Your Rating		*Responses:*	*Discrepancy Score*
_____	1.	"This is really tough for you, I know. I gather you're concerned I'm going to jump to a wrong conclusion that you're a pervert. I know how painful it must be for you."	_____
_____	2.	"Try me!"	_____
_____	3.	"Many people have sexual problems of one sort or another, but I know that's probably no comfort to you. I can sense your discomfort in sharing such a personal problem. But I want you to know that I'll make an honest effort to understand."	_____
_____	4.	"People tend to be self-conscious about discussing sexual problems. You'll find it's not really that bad once you get talking about it."	_____
_____	5.	"I'm glad you've finally decided to talk about it. Now we can stop spinning our wheels."	_____
_____	6.	"You've really had misgivings about discussing this. You're feeling on one hand that you need, perhaps even want, to discuss your sexual problem, yet you're afraid to for fear that I'll condemn you. I'm pleased you've brought it up, and I promise you I won't condemn you or jump to any conclusions. I respect you for risking by telling me this much, and I assure you that if you choose to reveal more about your problem my interest will be in attempting to help you with the problem."	_____

_____   7.   "Oh, I've talked with lots of people   _____ about sexual hang-ups before. You don't need to worry."

_____   8.   "How do you mean, pervert?"   _____

_____   9.   "What makes you think I'm that   _____ narrow-minded?"

Sum: _____

Average Discrepancy Score: _____

CLIENT STATEMENT 4

Black male parolee to white therapist: "You tell me you want to help me. You damn honkies are all alike. Don't try to give me that jive about wanting to help me. I wouldn't give you the time of day. Man, don't think I'm here because I want any help from you. I'm here because that honky parole officer told me if I didn't get my ass over here they'd throw me back in the joint."

Your Rating		_Responses:_	_Discrepancy Score_
_____	1.	"You're mad as hell. It really burns you to have to see me, especially when you feel I'm trying to jive you. I guess I'd feel the same way if I didn't have any more choice than you have."	_____
_____	2.	"Hey, how come you're pissed off at me? I didn't send you here!"	_____
_____	3.	"Sounds like you don't want to go back to prison. What did you do that your parole officer threatened you if you didn't come here?"	_____
_____	4.	"You're pretty ticked off about having to see me. You wouldn't be here if you had it your way."	_____
_____	5.	"The way it sounds to me you're lucky not to be back in prison now."	_____
_____	6.	"I can understand your resentment at having to come and your feeling that there isn't a chance in hell I'll under-	_____

stand or even want to understand. Maybe I can't help, but I'm willing to listen if you're willing to take a chance with me."

_____ 7. "What's this crap that all honkies are _____ all alike? You know, you've got a chip on your shoulder the size of a log. You don't know anything about me other than my skin color, yet here you are raking me over the coals."

Sum: _____
Average Discrepancy Score: _____

CLIENT STATEMENT 5

Fourteen-year-old girl: "In our family it seems like I never get to talk."

Your Rating		*Responses:*	*Discrepancy Score*
_____	1.	"Tell me about what your family is like."	_____
_____	2.	"Must feel kind of left out. I wonder what you could do to be heard?"	_____
_____	3.	"That must really be unpleasant for you. But you ultimately have to accept the responsibility for not getting to talk. You need to assert yourself and speak up."	_____
_____	4.	"That must be discouraging to feel like you don't have a say and not be listened to. I'd be interested in what some of the things are you wish you could say."	_____
_____	5.	"Never? Isn't that a little bit of an exaggeration?"	_____

Sum: _____
Average Discrepancy Score: _____

RATINGS FOR ASSESSMENT EXERCISES

Client Statement 1	Client Statement 2	Client Statement 3	Client Statement 4	Client Statement 5
1. 3.0	1. 2.0	1. 3.0	1. 4.0	1. 2.0
2. 2.0	2. 1.0	2. 2.0	2. 1.0	2. 3.0
3. 1.0	3. 3.5	3. 4.0	3. 2.0	3. 2.0
4. 1.5	4. 2.0	4. 2.0	4. 3.0	4. 3.5
5. 2.0	5. 1.0	5. 1.0	5. 1.0	5. 1.0
6. 4.0	6. 2.5	6. 5.0	6. 4.0	
7. 2.0	7. 4.0	7. 2.0	7. 1.0	
		8. 2.0		
		9. 1.0		

Guidelines to Responding with Respect

Since trustworthy empirical research on respect is as yet lacking, no hard and fast rules telling the counselor precisely how to use respect in therapy can be laid down. The following guidelines, however, come from accumulated clinical wisdom, and they provide good rules of thumb by which the concerned practitioner can judge and improve his own performance.

COMMITMENT TO UNDERSTAND

The counselor's primary mode of conveying a commitment to understand the client is, of course, through his communication. As has been emphasized previously, these communications are complex, involving numerous and often subtle behaviors that the practitioner may not even be aware of. Though one will not always fully understand the client's messages, the client will usually infer the counselor's desire and effort to understand from his verbal and nonverbal messages. Obviously, the content of verbal messages plays a key role in communicating understanding.

Since empathic responding is one important way of conveying a commitment to understand, helping persons who respond with high levels of empathy generally communicate moderate or high levels of respect as well. The counselor also conveys a commitment to understand by asking the client to elaborate on messages that are unclear or lack enough detail to be understood. You will note several such inquiries among the modeled responses that follow the exercises at the end of this chapter. Examples of inquiries aimed at elaboration are the following: "I'm not sure I fully understand what you meant by that . . ."; "Could you tell me more about that? I don't think I have a full picture yet"; "I'd like to understand all of your feelings about that. Could you . . ."; "I'm a little confused by what you meant just then. Could you elaborate a little?"; "Let me see if I heard you correctly. I thought you were saying you feel. . . ."

People appreciate the efforts others make to understand, and those efforts leave them feeling respected. Care must be taken, however, to avoid the common mistake of concluding prematurely that one understands when, in fact, one knows too little to understand. Ironically, the words *I understand* mean just the opposite when the client's feelings and situation have been inadequately explored. Inwardly the client is likely to think, "How could you understand? I haven't told you that much!"

In demonstrating respect through a commitment to understand, avoid interrupting (except for valid reasons), arguing, discussing topics of interest to you but irrelevant to the client, or attempting to persuade the client that your beliefs, values, or solutions are correct. Remember that respect involves showing both courtesy and regard for the client's views and feelings through attentive listening and checking out if you indeed have understood accurately. Respect does not necessarily mean agreeing with or condoning the client's beliefs or behavior, which the client may well disapprove, but it does mean valuing the client as an individual and championing his right to choose how to believe and behave.

CONVEYING ACCEPTANCE AND WARMTH

Respect, as we define it, requires that the helping person develop an accepting, nonjudgmental attitude toward the client, irrespective of the nature of his problem, behavior, or personality. Experienced helping professionals who have seen many persons with diverse problems generally are much less judgmental than neophytes. One basic reason for this is that seasoned practitioners have learned through experience that the more deeply one understands the life experiences of another, no matter how appalling his behavior might seem, the more understanding and accepting one becomes of that individual. To avoid evaluating clients, the counselor should keep in mind that the essence of his task is to understand and to help, not to judge the client and his behavior.

In developing an accepting and nonjudgmental attitude, we recommend that you develop an immunity to being embarrassed, shocked, dismayed, or overwhelmed by another's behavior, however offensive it may seem. Most counselors may someday expect to encounter problems associated with child abuse and neglect, rape, incest, wife-beating, sexual deviations, crime, and other types of behavior generally regarded as repugnant. Immunity, we hasten to add, is not at all the same as indifference, which runs counter to empathy and respect. Rather we mean that you should avoid untoward emotional reactions to clients, many of whom have a gross lack of self-respect that would only be reinforced by a response of shock or embarrassment.

A counselor can convey acceptance by saying, "You sound almost apologetic for feeling the way you do. It's okay to feel that way; I can accept those feelings." The statement, "I respect your point of view, and I can accept how you feel," also conveys respect, as does, "You know, all of us, when we examine our lives, find things that we have done that we deeply regret. But maybe the important thing is to be able to benefit from our mistakes and to learn from them. You're probably wondering about my reactions to you in light of what you've done. I guess I'm not concerned as much with what's happened in the past as with where you are going with your future."

Also of great significance in conveying respect are the nonverbal forms of communication, over which the helping person has relatively little conscious control. A blush, a frown, a sneer, a lifted eyebrow, a look of shock or scorn or dismay, a vacant stare—these and a host of other facial expressions may tell the client much more about our feelings toward him than our words do. Likewise, looking out the window, filing one's fingernails, cleaning a pipe, or otherwise channeling one's attention away from the client conveys a lack of interest and respect. Obviously, such behaviors are to be avoided. Yawning is another behavior that the client may interpret as indicating a lack of interest and acceptance. Yawning, however, is not under conscious control and may result from sitting too long or from fatigue. When such is the case, a simple apology and explanation convey respect and keep the client from drawing erroneous conclusions.

Facial expressions can convey disrespect in the form of criticism, disapproval, shock, or condemnation. Potentially destructive to the relationship, these nonverbal communications are readily perceived by most clients, many of whom are highly sensitive to criticism or rejection in any form. If a discrepancy exists between the counselor's verbal and nonverbal communication, the client is more likely to attach credence to the latter than to the former. People learn through life's myriad transactions that nonverbal cues indicate others' feelings more accurately than do spoken words. To avoid facial expressions, postural cues, and related behaviors that convey disrespect, we recommend that you strive to develop fully those beliefs and attitudes toward troubled fellow humans that preclude the negative feelings and hence the problematic facial expressions. Trying to conceal untoward feelings by carefully controlling facial expressions is not only unlikely to succeed but also has the undesired effect of distracting the counselor's focus of attention from the client to his own behavior.

The personal quality of counselor warmth also strongly influences whether the client feels accepted and, therefore, how he responds. Intonation and tempo of speech do much to communicate warmth. Although warmth is an elusive and nearly indefinable quality, it is generally agreed that the speech of a warm person is calm and relaxed, not only conveying warmth but also fostering a relaxed, nonthreatening climate, thereby tending to diminish the client's tension and anxiety. The warm person speaks in a well-modulated voice and with inflections that correspond to the dynamic changes of mood and intensity during an interview. Monotonic speech is often considered a sign of boredom and hence of low respect. Speech that is rapid or staccato tends to have an excited quality that excludes warmth and respect.

Although the pitch of one's voice may be largely beyond control, much can be accomplished, if need be, to increase the warmth conveyed in speech. Keep in mind that feeling warm about someone does not ensure that that someone will perceive your warmth. We encourage you to seek feedback about the degree of warmth you project. Small groups of three to six students can provide good learning experiences in this regard. Two students role-play a counselor-client interview, while the others in the group watch. After several minutes, the client and the observers provide the counselor with feedback about the warmth he conveyed and with suggestions on how to increase his warmth. This exercise helps not only the counselor but also the other students, who should aim for carefully respectful communication. You may also use audio-recorders for feedback and for improving your speech. It is common for trainees, and experienced practitioners for that matter, to be taken aback when they discover discrepancies between how they really come across and how they thought they came across in a given interview. You can enhance the warmth in your communication, as many others have, by expanding your awareness of your speech patterns and by modifying undesired patterns through practice.

At this point, further clarification regarding the nature of warmth and a word of caution are needed. Warmth is not to be confused with strained efforts to smile and be friendly. Excessive friendliness should be avoided, because it frightens some clients and offends others, who view it as unwarranted, insincere, or seductive. Remember that respect permits the client to maintain a comfortable distance. Avoid pressuring for an intimacy the client may not be prepared to accept. A warm, pleasant demeanor, combined with demonstrations of interest and concern, is welcomed by those seeking help. Effusive friendliness is not.

AFFIRMING WORTH AND UNIQUENESS

Respect also involves an affirmation of the worth and uniqueness of each human being, however much he may differ from us. Such an affirmation is difficult, though, because we tend to value most those who think, feel, and behave as we do. The most effective helping persons, however, have learned to "embrace the alien" (Reid, C., 1972)—that is, they welcome opportunities to relate to different individuals, and they feel enriched by experiencing the uniqueness of other persons. Open to contrasting beliefs, values,

and life styles, the helping person is not only flexible about himself, but he also cherishes the freedom and opportunity of others to
think for themselves and to choose their own ways of living. Relating with respect to widely varying types of individuals requires
freedom from prejudices about race, sex, ethnicity, age, religion,
belief system, socioeconomic level, life style, physical characteristics (including length of hair and body odor), and past and present
behavioral patterns. Before you can overcome prejudices, you
must first, of course, be aware of them. Unfortunately many people lack this awareness, assuming instead a self-righteous belief
that they lack prejudices entirely. No more open to experiencing
themselves than to experiencing people who are strikingly different,
they tend to alienate others, who perceive and respond negatively
to the subtle manifestations of their prejudices. Never really able
to come to terms with their prejudices, such therapists can do far
more harm than good.

Fortunately, if one is willing to assume the "risks," there are
steps that can be taken to overcome prejudice. Research indicates
that extensive interaction with those from whom one differs in
some basic characteristic (race, for example) tends to dissolve prejudice and to supplant it with positive feelings (Rokeach, 1968).
Encounter groups provide opportunities for interaction with different types of people, and we recommend them both for expanding awareness of one's own feelings and prejudices and for achieving
greater understanding of diverse individuals and one's impact
on them.

An example of a counselor response that affirms the worth
and uniqueness of an individual is, "You know, you're right; I don't
see it that way, but that's okay. I respect your point of view and I
think it's fine for us to differ." The counselor might also say, "I
want to share with you an impression I've gained in our time together. You've been willing to risk sharing some deeply personal
and painful feelings, and that takes real courage. I really appreciate
this quality in you." Or, "I can see you're wondering what I'd do in
your situation. You know, what I'd do might be all wrong for you.
What is important is what fits best for you." A similar message
appears in, "I don't care how other people view it or feel about
it. What *you're* thinking and feeling is what really matters."

AFFIRMING STRENGTHS AND PROBLEM-SOLVING CAPACITIES

The counselor manifests respect for the client by adopting a strength-oriented perspective. Looking for positive qualities and undeveloped potentialities rather than limitations and prior mistakes or failures will help one perceive the client in terms of what he might become rather than in terms of past behavior. This does not mean one should overlook past behavior or become an idealist. Rather, we recommend a realistic but positive perspective. Perceiving and conveying respect for strengths, potentialities, and changes achieved through counseling tend to mobilize the client's hope and to promote his motivation, both of which are indispensable to the helping process.

Another basic determinant of respect is rooted in the helping person's belief about the human capacity to change. The conviction of course must be based on reality in the sense that the client's situation can in fact be improved and that the client has the capacity required to make the improvement. Otherwise the helping person may be engendering false hope that can culminate only in discouragement, disillusionment, and perhaps bitterness and cynicism. Fortunately, however, most problem situations can be bettered to some degree, and the large majority of clients have the capacity to effect changes in their lives.

One reason why belief in the capacity of others to change is so crucial is that the person's perception of himself and of his situation tends to be strongly colored by relevant feedback from others. Beliefs others convey about a person's chance of success or failure in a given venture influence that person to adopt a similar outlook. The resulting attitude, then, is a powerful force in shaping the motivation and effort the person invests, which determine to a great extent the outcome of the venture. Thus a self-fulfilling prophecy is set in motion. If a person believes there is little chance of changing his life situation as he desires, his belief is likely to produce ineffectual efforts at coping and little or no change. The power of the self-fulfilling prophecy on the client's expectations is documented by research (Aspy and Hadlock, 1967; Morgan, 1961; Rosenthal and Frank, 1956; Rotter, 1954). Respect for the capacity of others to solve their problems and to make desired changes in their lives thus is based not only on humanistic values but also on hard scientific evidence.

Your perception of the helping role and the helping process also has much to do with the level of respect you achieve in your relationships with clients. Those who consider it their place to provide solutions or to dispense advice will tend to assume responsibility for solving the client's problems and to place the client in a dependent role. Obviously, such role perceptions demean the client by failing to recognize his strengths and by relegating him to a position of passive cooperation—or passive resistance, as more often occurs under these circumstances. Moreover, the client is done a disservice by being denied the opportunity to gain in strength and self-respect as he struggles with the problem at hand. Fostering dependency tends to leave a person weaker rather than stronger and in the long run does more harm than good.

The type of relationship most conducive to the client's growth is an equal partnership, not an arrangement that accords superiority to the counselor and inferiority to the client. Both are joined in mutual effort to search for a solution to the problem, but final responsibility for decisions and for action must reside with the client. The counselor, thus, plays a facilitative role in helping the client *help himself*. The counselor assists the client in gaining a broader perspective of his problem, understanding himself and others better, and considering available solutions and their consequences. In final analysis, however, the client must choose for himself and implement his own plans.

When the helping relationship has evolved to the point that the counselor's good will is no longer in question, the counselor can convey high levels of respect by holding the client to the expectation that he assume increasing responsibility for dealing with his problem. In some instances, confronting a client with his procrastinating tactics, facing him with his patterns of avoidance and evasion, and refusing to accept his explanations that problems he has brought on himself are due to external causes convey high levels of respect. Such confrontations recognize and value the client's potential for utilizing latent strengths and thereby becoming more responsible and independent. In this phase of the helping relationship, acceptance of the client may at times be somewhat conditional. That is, the counselor does not accept the client's tendency to perpetuate the use of patterns that both have identified, explored, and labeled as dysfunctional. Rather, when the client commits himself to a course of action, he is expected to keep his commitment. If he evades responsibility by resorting to typical patterns of rationalization or blaming others, the counselor may express disappointment, irritation, or frustration because the client is letting himself down, clinging to outmoded and ineffectual ways of coping. The counselor conveys respect by expressing belief in the client's ability to translate his insights into action and to endure the uncertainty and anxiety inevitably associated with change.

An example of a counselor response that affirms the client's strengths, potentials for growth, and problem-solving capacity is, "I know from what you've said that you have a lot of doubts about yourself. I can accept that, but I want you to know I believe that if you really put your mind to it you can accomplish the goal we just discussed." The counselor places proper responsibility on the client by saying, "I can't presume to know what is best for you, but I'm sure willing to think with you and to help you discover what would be best." Or, "It sounds as though plenty of others have freely given you advice about what to do. I could do that too, but it wouldn't be helpful. My goal is to help you think through a solution that makes sense to *you*." And when depression at future prospects rears its head, the counselor can explicitly recognize the client's strengths: "When you feel as depressed as you've been feeling, it's natural to have the feelings of hopelessness you just expressed. Depression tends to make us view things in the worst possible light. But as I consider the many accomplishments you've made during your life, I can see a lot of strengths that you're blind to right now because you're feeling so depressed. My goal is to help you rediscover those strengths and to put them to work in getting out of this pit of despair you've gotten into."

OTHER FACETS OF RESPECT

Respect also involves courtesy, physical arrangements, privacy, and confidentiality. A comfortable office and interviews conducted free of telephone calls and outside distractions are basic. Common courtesy manifested through appropriate social amenities and thoughtfulness are so elementary that elaboration seems unnecessary. Keeping information about the client and his situation confidential is a primary responsibility of any helping person, and confidentiality is the unquestioned right of clients. Violating this right is both disrespectful and unethical.

Situations That Challenge Respect

All helping professionals, however well-intentioned, encounter early in their experience certain behaviors or situations that severely test their capacity to relate with high levels of respect. Actually these behaviors are also commonly encountered in other walks of life, where they usually cause difficulties in interaction and elicit reactions low in respect. Because high levels of respect are requisite to successful counseling, however, it is vital that counselors develop an awareness of their own patterns of reaction to these behaviors and evolve patterns of response that preserve the client's self-respect and promote growth.

We have identified five types of situations that most frequently cause difficulty for counselors. Since counselors differ widely in personality, counseling styles, and response patterns, our five categories include situations that cause no problem for certain counselors and exclude situations that are particularly challenging to others. We have already discussed the category involving clients of varying race, life style, and values. Now we will examine the other four.

PROVOCATIVE BEHAVIOR

The first of the challenging situations, offensive behavior, may consist of aggressive, verbal abuse, as is often encountered, for example, in working with delinquent youths or criminals in correctional settings. Offensive behavior may also involve aggressive challenges to the counselor's integrity, competence, or motives. The counselor's natural reaction to offensive behavior in whatever form is to feel defensive and to respond protectively. When one is attacked, accused, or blamed unfairly, the tendency is to counter with anger, to set the other person straight, or, in effect, to blame the blamer. Defensive reactions or counterattacks, of course, are counterproductive, since increasingly sharp exchanges escalate the conflict and may destroy the helping relationship. To avoid responding defensively, it is helpful to keep in mind that the client's provocation, though directed at the counselor, usually springs from some other source. An angry outburst, for example, may be a displacement of general frustration unrelated to the counselor, as often happens with a person who is incarcerated, or may simply manifest supersensitivity combined with a low threshold for anger. In other instances, a client may have lifelong feelings of resentment toward figures of authority and may be reacting negatively to the authority of the counselor's position and not to the counselor as a person. No matter what the source of a negative response from the client, the counselor must explore and resolve the bad feelings lest they undermine the helping relationship. Guidelines for managing this and similar nuances of the relationship will be found in Chapter Nine.

Whatever the dynamics behind the provocative behavior, a defensive response by the counselor only repeats the pattern of response that the client has typically experienced, and hence the response is antitherapeutic. Mastery of his own natural defense reactions permits the counselor to feel unthreatened by the provocative behavior and to respond facilitatively. Empathic responses convey both respect and understanding, and tend to expand the client's expression of his feelings, thereby producing a cathartic release of the negative feelings. By cutting into and draining off the emotions, empathic responses can defuse the situation, permitting a more rational exploration of the factors that underlie the client's feelings.

Approaching negative, hostile feelings empathically is difficult for the counselor who has not already evolved effective ways of dealing with his own negative feelings. The findings of an important research study (Bandura, Lipsher, and Miller, 1960) indicate that counselors who avoid expressing negative feelings in social interaction tend also to avoid negative expressions from the client by changing the subject, ignoring the feelings, or by similar avoidance behaviors. Unfortunately, such counselors leave the client to struggle alone with the negative feelings, which have the potential, if left unresolved, of undermining the helping relationship. Thus self-awareness is essential to dealing effectively with provocation. Trainees who have great difficulty managing anger in themselves or others may need personal therapy. Skillfully led sensitivity-training groups can also be of great value if group members actively try to expand awareness of their responses to anger. Classroom exercises for dealing with provocative behavior and other challenging situations are described at the end of this chapter.

SELF-EFFACING CLIENTS

The second challenging situation arises with individuals who are self-effacing and dominated by feelings of self-depreciation and worthlessness. These individuals tear themselves down, constantly apologize for themselves, and court the favor of others, including the counselor, by flattery and ingratiating behavior. Such clients have minuscule self-respect, and it is crucial, therefore, that the counselor respond with high levels of respect.

The counseling problem coming from self-effacing behavior lies in the self-fulfilling prophecy, since self-depreciating behavior tends to invite depreciation by others. Likewise, trying continually to please at the expense of self unwittingly invites being taken for granted, if not exploited, by others. The cycle may be perpetuated in counseling if the counselor is not alert to it. It is not uncommon, for example, for counselors to be tardy for appointments, to cut interviews short, or to change the appointment times of self-effacing clients first when schedules must be juggled. Lacking assertiveness, such clients typically acquiesce even though they experience inconvenience, hurt, disappointment, and resentment.

The counselor demonstrates high levels of respect by helping the self-effacing person believe in his right to expect more from others, including the counselor. Empathically being in touch with, eliciting, and accepting the negative feelings that lie beneath the client's obsequious behavior also convey respect and help the client learn experientially that he is valued quite apart from complying with the real or imagined expectations of others. Most importantly, if the counselor is courteous, empathic, and conveys the expectation that the client has a perfect right to respect and he holds the client to that expectation, he will foster self-respect and assertiveness. In effect, the self-fulfilling prophecy still comes into play, but it works for the client, not against him.

DEPENDENCY AND HELPLESSNESS

The third category, excessive dependency, is related to self-effacing behavior. Both patterns involve strong elements of self-doubt and often, therefore, exist together in the same individual.

The excessively dependent client attributes to the counselor an infinite wisdom and an omnipotence that contrast with his own feelings of helplessness and impotence. As a result, the client looks to the counselor to solve his problems, imputing to him the magical powers of a wizard. Unfortunately, some counselors also make the mistake of overestimating their powers and underestimating the strengths of their clients; indeed, therein lies the threat to responding with high levels of respect. Fostering or reinforcing dependency, as mentioned earlier, conveys disrespect for the potential or actual strengths of the client and promotes weakness rather than strength.

It frequently occurs, of course, that many clients, after failing to cope with their problems, seek help precisely because they feel overwhelmed and helpless. In such instances, the counselor's immediate task is to mobilize the hope, motivation, and active participation in the search for a solution needed for problem solving and growth. The client who has actively participated in exploring problems, planning goals, and deciding upon strategies has much more invested in the process and, therefore, is more likely to follow through on the plan of action than is the person who has passively observed the counselor's diagnosis and presentation. Again, we emphasize that to avoid minimizing the strengths and inner resources of the client, you develop a strength-oriented perspective and expect responsible, independent behavior from your clients whenever feasible. We are not recommending that you refrain from acting on behalf of your clients or avoid helping them with certain tasks. Such help is in fact desirable if it is likely to foster independent action in the future. Counseling relationships entail dependency needs, as do all human relationships. Emotional support is often a crucial need of the client, and the counselor who ignores this need or who expects independent action before the client has mobilized the necessary strength also conveys disrespect. Our plea is that the counselor be judicious in rendering such assistance, weighing the consequences to determine if the help is in the client's best interest.

EMBARRASSMENT AND HUMILIATION

The threat to responding with respect to embarrassing or humiliating revelations should be readily apparent. When the client reveals such problems, he is keenly sensitive to the reactions of the counselor, fearing that he may be condemned. It is readily under-standable, in light of societal attitudes, that it is very painful for clients to discuss such problems as exhibitionism, incest, cruelty, or infidelity. If the counselor appears shocked, uneasy, or appalled, the client will interpret such reactions as rejection or condemnation. Such reactions, as we discussed earlier, are extremely destructive and virtually negate any possibility of developing or sustaining a positive, trusting relationship.

Skill Development Exercises with Modeled Responses

These exercises involve messages from clients in actual inter-views. As you read each one, note particularly which of the four vital elements of respect appears germane to the situation. Note also whether the message involves one of the situations particu-larly challenging to the counselor's capacity to respond with re-spect. Next, assume you are the counselor working with the client. Following the guidelines presented earlier, write a response to the message that attempts to convey a high level of respect. After you complete each exercise, compare your response with the modeled response that follows the exercises. Bearing in mind that the mod-eled response is only one of many possible responses, analyze it and compare it with your own. Careful completion of these exercises at your own pace will improve your capacity to respond with respect to the many, varied, and challenging situations encountered in counseling work.

CLIENT STATEMENTS

1. *17-year-old female, twelfth interview:* "I screamed my head off at Mother yesterday—called her every name in the book. I never do anything for her, and she's always doing things for me. I don't know how she can stand me. I'm no good for anything."

2. *35-year-old female, initial interview:* "Before I tell you about my problem, I need to know if you're a Catholic. My problem with my husband centers around our religion."

3. "You know, I've thought and thought, weighed all the pros and cons, even listed them on a sheet of paper, and I still can't decide whether to take that job or not. What do you think I should do?"

4. "I don't think you are really very interested in me as a person, only as some object to analyze."

5. *25-year-old male, early in first interview:* "I want to make it clear at the beginning that I'm not coming to see you because I'm crazy or mentally disturbed or anything like that. But I heard that you help people make decisions and I'm really in need of advice right now."

6. "I've just been completely at odds with myself lately. I'm hoping you can help me sort out this mess."

7. *19-year-old female college student, in first interview, after three minutes of elaborating conflicts she is having with her fiancé:* "Well, those are the details kind of summed up. It all just leaves me completely mixed up. I'm frightened of getting married while we're having these kinds of problems. But I really do care for Bob, and I know it would just crush him if I put off the wedding or break it off completely. I really need your advice. Nancy (who referred her) said you've done a lot of marriage counseling. From all of your experience how do these problems sound to you? Would it be better to break it off or does everyone have these kinds of problems?"

8. *Middle-aged male after a few months of counseling:* "I wish I had the know-how and skills to keep this job. Then maybe I wouldn't worry myself into such a frenzy that I make stupid errors. I think sometimes I make mistakes just from trying too hard. I just can't compete with most people. It's futile."

9. *Middle-aged man, during twelfth interview:* "My girlfriend is pressing me for a decision as to whether or not I'm going to get a divorce. My wife says I have to give up the girlfriend or get out. I'm completely up in the air. Some of my friends encourage me to leave her, others tell me I'm crazy to hang on to her. I'm not ready to decide what I want and I don't know which way to turn. What's your advice?"

10. *43-year-old woman, during first interview:* "There's something I really need to talk to someone about, but it's so hard to tell anyone."

11. *22-year-old female:* "My dad tells me that Fred is all wrong for me. Aunt Sara thinks that Fred is really a neat guy. My friends say I'd be making a real mistake not to marry Fred. Gad, I don't know what to do, and Fred's getting tired of waiting."

12. *21-year-old single male, second interview:* "I hope you can

help me overcome my problem with masturbation. And don't tell me it's not a problem just because 95 percent of the males masturbate. I'm fully aware of that fact. The point is I want to overcome the rotten habit irrespective of what other guys do."

13. *33-year-old male, twenty-seventh interview:* "I've about given up on myself. I feel like I'm not even trying to change. I don't know why you bother with me. You must be getting sick and tired of seeing me week after week."

14. *26-year-old female, initial interview:* "I talked to the pastor about my marriage. I've prayed about it. I've talked to my doctor. Nothing has helped. I'm about at the end of my rope. If you can't help me, I don't know what I'll do. Can you help me?"

15. *20-year-old female, third interview:* "After I'd gone to bed with Harvey a number of times, he wanted me to go to bed with his buddy, Jim. I didn't really like Jim and told him I didn't want to but Harvey insisted on it so I finally agreed to go out with him. After I slept with him I just felt dirty, like a tramp. After that I felt it really didn't matter and I must have slept with—oh, forty or fifty different guys, I guess, anyone who flattered me and seemed interested. Now I just feel like how could I think of marrying a decent guy. Who'd want someone like me?"

16. *19-year-old male, twenty-fifth interview:* "I've about given up on myself. I must be a lost cause. All my fears of people have returned. I've been afraid to come here today and wouldn't have if Mother hadn't twisted my arm. All week I've felt sorry for myself, just trapped in the house, and so mad at the world I've been miserable to live with. Mother doesn't know what to do. One time she'll sympathize. Then she'll scream at me and tell me I'm acting like an ass or a spoiled brat. I think I'm just hopeless."

17. *15-year-old student to school counselor, fourth interview:* "I can't talk to the teacher. She doesn't like me—she thinks I'm just a goof-off. She wouldn't believe me if I told her I really do want to try in her class."

18. *47-year-old female, initial interview with 25-year-old female marriage counselor:* "I had really expected someone older. Are you married?"

19. *15-year-old female in correctional institution, first interview, in anger:* "I'll tell you what you can do to help. You can help me to get out of this damn place!! I was supposed to go home over the

last weekend, but Nelson (the previous counselor) broke his promise. Can you get me out of here next weekend?"

20.   *14-year-old male, in trouble and failing academically in junior high, speaking contemptuously:* "I could care less if they catch me shoplifting. Maybe they'd send me to prison. I'd like that. It'd be neat. I'd figure a way to break out. I'd show 'em they couldn't keep me."

21.   *19-year-old female to counselor, 2 days prior to his scheduled departure for a two-week vacation; she looks at the floor:* "What if I can't hack it while you're gone? What if I slash my wrists? Would it make any difference to you? I'll bet you wouldn't even be upset."

22.   *27-year-old, single male, fifteenth interview:* "I'd really like to take that job at _____ but I don't know how I'd get back and forth. I don't drive, and frankly I don't want to learn. I've always been afraid I'd get in an accident and kill someone. Everyone bugs me about learning to drive."

23.   *36-year-old male who is extramaritally involved, second interview:* "No one accepts my feelings and how much this relationship (with girlfriend) means to me. It's as though they expect I could say it's all over and forget it."

24.   "It was my money and my hard work that got the business where it is today. I want my son to profit from my work, but I can't tolerate his drinking. I think I've got a right to set some expectations about his private behavior."

25.   "He's my grandson as well as their son, and I ought to have some say about what's happening to him."

26.   "It's hard to sit by and see your married kids make blunders and not want to interfere."

27.   "I don't know how to say this, but I'm afraid you wouldn't want me to even consider getting an abortion."

28.   "I was about to call you last weekend, but I decided I had to get by without bothering you."

MODELED RESPONSES

1.   "You're really feeling rotten about yourself today, just feeling worthless. That's such a painful way to feel. But I'm wondering if we could talk about what happened yesterday, what led up to your explosion."

2.   "Understandably, then, you wonder if I could under-

stand your specific problems. I've worked with members of your religion before and seemed to understand their problems. I can assure you I'll do my best to understand yours, too, and if I need clarification, I'll be sure to ask. But *your* feelings are what really matter. Do you feel you can risk sharing your problems with me?"

3. "I can tell you've really been going through a struggle. At best, it's a darn tough decision to make. But in the final analysis, I think the most important consideration is that it be *your* decision. What might fit for me might be all wrong for you. It'd be easy for you if you knew in advance the right decision, but many times there are no right and wrong decisions. It's what makes the most sense to you after you've considered all the factors."

4. "Then you're kind of feeling that I'm mainly interested in you as just some case or object to study, rather than personally concerned about you as an individual. Could we discuss that a little more? I'm uncomfortable being seen that way, and I'd like to understand how I've come across to leave that impression with you."

5. "If I'm understanding you correctly, you feel a real need to talk to someone right now, but certainly wouldn't want me to look down on you as being crazy or deficient in some way. That's certainly understandable."

6. "I'd like to better understand what that conflict is like for you. Would you help me see it through your eyes?"

7. "I certainly see the dilemma you're caught in. I can't presume to know what is best for you, but I'm surely willing to think with you about this and to help you discover what would be best for you."

8. "Just feel hopelessly inept and deficient. You know, I really get frustrated when I hear you put yourself down that way. I like you, and when you seem to sell yourself short and just give up I feel badly. I believe you have more strength than you give yourself credit for." (*Explanation:* This response is a strength confrontation that can be made because the relationship is well established. The same response early in counseling would be inappropriate and perhaps destructive.)

9. "I can see how mixed up you are, but it sounds as if many others have been willing to give you plenty of advice about what to do. I'm most concerned about helping you decide what direction fits you best."

10. "I can see that you're uncomfortable right now and that it may be painful to talk about it. If you can take the risk of sharing it with me, I'll listen and see if I can help."

11. "It's really confusing when so many people are telling you what you should do. You can't possibly please them all. But, you know, the most important person of all to please is *you*. You're the one who has to live with your decision. I'm interested in knowing your feelings."

12. "So if I understand you, you're saying you're not content just being one of the pack. I can appreciate those feelings. It's important to you to measure up to your own standards, not someone else's. I'll do my best to help you accomplish your goal, though, in all honesty it's a tough habit to break, as you well know."

13. "You really sound discouraged with yourself and concerned that I might be getting disgusted with you. I guess I'm more concerned that you're feeling defeated. I know the sledding has been rough for you over the past weeks, but I hope you can hang tough for a while yet. I'm a little confused, though, about your statement that you're not trying to change. I'd like to hear more about what's happening inside you."

14. "So I gather you're feeling pretty desperate, as though I'm your last hope. At this point, I know very little about your problems and can only assure you I'll do my best to be helpful. A lot, of course, will depend on the nature of your problems and your willingness to work on them. Let's talk more about your marriage."

15. "It sounds as though you felt you'd lost all your value after you slept with him, as though you had nothing to lose. Even now it seems you're feeling pretty worthless. But, you know, as bad as you feel about your past behavior, the important thing is not to let past mistakes bog you down. You're probably wondering about my reactions to you in light of what you just told me. I guess I'm not as concerned as much with what you've done as with where you're going in the future."

16. "Just feeling so dominated by those fears. On one hand feeling boxed in and wanting to get out. On the other hand, so afraid of people you don't dare venture out. I've come to really respect you over the time we've spent together and to believe that you have more strength than you give yourself credit for. But it's

as though you're just at the mercy of those fears, until you make the decision to face them head on, painful as that may be."

17. "Sounds like it'd be pretty scary for you to talk with Mrs. Williams. Like you feel she has it in for you. It's possible she may see you in a different light if you were to talk with her. Sure, it'd be hard, but I believe you could do it if you make up your mind. And if you'd like, I'd be glad to help you prepare to talk with her."

18. "You seem surprised and probably a little disappointed at seeing a younger person. You're wondering if I've had enough experience to really understand your problems."

19. "You're pretty burned about last weekend, I can tell. I gather you're wanting to go home pretty bad. We can talk about next weekend, but first I'd be interested in knowing what led up to the cancellation of your visit last weekend."

20. "So you'd feel you were succeeding in something, at least, by proving they couldn't keep you in prison. From that I sense you haven't given up on yourself altogether. But in other ways you seem so discouraged, like you've given up in hoping you can get better grades or make friends. Is that kind of close to how you feel about yourself?"

21. "You know you're dead wrong about that. I'd feel very badly. I can see that you're angry about my going and maybe feel I'm deserting you. But, Jennie, I want you to know that even though you may not feel it right now, I believe you have the strength to tough it out until I get back. If things get too rocky, you can call _____ (an associate). He knows about you and wants to help if things get too rough." (This response assumes the counselor's expressed assessment of the client's strengths is honest and accurate).

22. "I can accept your feelings of not wanting to learn to drive. Still it sounds as though your fear forces you to pass up some real opportunities. It's certainly your decision not to learn to drive, but in a way you're letting that decision be made on the basis of fear. If you'd like to work on mastering those fears, I'd be happy to explore that with you."

23. "I can see that you feel others are discounting strong feelings that are important to you. As I see it, how you feel is of great importance in deciding what you should do about your girlfriend, and I would like to understand better how you do feel about her."

24.   "I can sense your caring for your son both in your desire that he benefit from your business and your worry about his drinking. Could we think together about how you might express your feelings to him without offending or alienating him?"

25.   "Your interest and commitment to be helpful to your grandson are surely commendable. Perhaps we can think through how your concern can most effectively be expressed."

26.   "Your restraint in not interfering reflects a lot of strength on your part, especially when you're deeply interested in what is happening to someone you love. It really is difficult to know how and when to help when you see them making blunders."

27.   "I can sense your hesitation, and I'm pleased you're able to express your fear about my reactions. Your feelings and wishes are important to me as we think about what is best for you."

28.   "I want you to know that I'll respect your judgment as to whether or not you should call. It's a credit to you that you want to be able to be independent and not lean on me too much."

Practicum Exercise

To expand self-awareness and the ability to respond with respect in challenging situations, role-playing is suggested. Triads are again recommended, with the participants assigned to rotating roles of client, counselor, and observer. In the role as client, imagine yourself very angry with the counselor for some reason. Get in touch with your anger, and then express it heatedly. Observe how you feel about expressing your anger and also note how the counselor reacts. Observe and contrast the differences in your reactions when the counselor's responses are defensive and when they are empathic. In enacting the counselor role, observe your feelings at attacks by the client. Respond defensively at first and note the effect on the client's behavior. Next, respond with empathy and again notice the effects on the client's behavior. In the role of observer, note carefully the nature of the feelings expressed by the two role-players as well as cues to unexpressed, subtle, or unconscious feelings. Note the direction of the interaction when the counselor changes from defensive to empathic responses. After each scenario has been played out, change roles until each participant has had an opportunity with all the roles. When you are finished role-playing all of the parts, discuss your experiences and observations. Next, repeat the same procedure with the person playing the client taking the following roles:

1. A self-effacing client who is unclear about what counseling involves. He would like to ask the counselor to explain more but is very hesitant, apologetic, and afraid the counselor will be displeased.

2. An excessively dependent mother (father) who is distressed because she (he) believes the teacher of her eight-year-old son is being unduly harsh with him, causing him to hate school. She would like the teacher to be aware of the situation but is overwhelmed at the prospect of approaching her. She wants the counselor to intercede on her behalf because she is afraid of the teacher and of bungling the situation.

3. A client with homosexual attractions that he (she) has not acted on. He wants to discuss the problem with the counselor but finds it extremely embarrassing.

Chapter 8

‭❧❧❧❧❧❧❧❧❧❧❧❧❧❧❧❧❧❧❧❧❧‬

Relating to Clients
with Genuineness

Relating to clients with authenticity (genuineness), as defined
in Chapter One, would have been abhorrent to most therapists
less than fifteen years ago. At the time, "benevolent neutrality"
(Tarachow, 1963) and "controlled emotional involvement" (Biestek,
1957) were promoted as the therapeutic qualities most conducive
to insight and growth. The rationale for this position derived from
psychoanalytic theory, which postulates that the development and
analysis of the "transference neurosis" are central to therapeutic
work. Relating to the patient as a neutral observer rather than as a
"real" person, the analyst generally avoids disclosure of his own
feelings, views, and attitudes, thereby fostering an interpersonal
climate wherein the patient will "transfer" to the analyst unresolved
feelings, attitudes, and desires rooted in earlier relationships with
significant others, most often the patient's parents and siblings.
The role of the psychoanalyst thus is to assist the patient in reexperi-
encing and analyzing feelings from the past. The cathartic release
of past feelings through "abreaction" and the insight gained from
analyzing projections onto the analyst help the patient discern

archaic emotional and behavioral patterns and "reconstruct" his personality into a form that allows at least some measure of freedom from the paralyzing effects of outmoded defense mechanisms, distorted perceptions, and dysfunctional interpersonal patterns.

In recent years, serious questions have been raised by many theoreticians, practitioners, and researchers about the desirability and therapeutic advantage of relating to clients in such a depersonalized manner. One cogent argument against the practice is that clients need experience in relating to real persons and that the therapeutic encounter should provide such experience. The detached relationship offered by psychoanalytic therapists, by contrast, has no counterpart in the broader arena of social relationships and, therefore, has little transferability outside therapy. It has been argued further that depersonalized helping relationships are highly ambiguous, making the client anxious because he never knows how he stands with the therapist. Although a certain amount of anxiety may be conducive to therapeutic work, some clients have low thresholds for such anxiety and are therefore regarded as poor candidates for psychoanalytic therapy.

In recent years, humanistic theoreticians and practitioners, particularly those with existentialist leanings, have taken a position counter to the traditional psychoanalytic concept of a helping relationship. May (1969), Frankl (1962), Colm (1966), Rogers (1961) and others posit the hypothesis that authenticity, or genuineness, on the therapist's part fosters a climate of trust, provides an authentic human encounter, and facilitates reciprocal openness—in short, it provides an experiential, growth-producing human relationship that equips the client to begin and to cultivate rich and satisfying relationships with others. Jourard (1971) employs the term *transparency* to denote the quality of authenticity he believes therapists should offer.

Perhaps the most compelling argument for authenticity is the research evidence cited in Chapter Two, which documents the relationships between genuineness, or authenticity, and positive therapeutic outcomes. On the basis of this research, authenticity has been included in this volume as an essential therapeutic ingredient. Other research findings pertaining to guidelines to the effective use of authenticity will be discussed later in this chapter.

The Authenticity Scale*

As with the Empathic Communication and Respect Scales, level 3.0 on the Authenticity Scale represents the minimally helpful level. The reader is encouraged to refer back to the definitions of the levels when studying the examples and in completing the rating exercises below. Before proceeding, however, the reader is advised to review carefully the definition of authenticity presented in Chapter One.

LEVEL 1.0

Either a considerable discrepancy exists between the counselor's overt response and his actual feelings and thoughts, or his only congruent responses are negative and retaliatory. Likewise, striking discrepancies occur between verbal content and voice quality or other nonverbal behaviors. The counselor is guarded, attempts to conceal feelings, and responds evasively or defensively even to direct questions. He may speak with detachment or ambiguity. Any self-disclosures he makes appear to emanate from the counselor's needs and are irrelevant or inappropriate to the client's needs at the time. The counselor avoids self-disclosures that would be appropriate and helpful.

LEVEL 2.0

Incongruence exists between the counselor's behavior and feelings, and self-disclosure is shallow and minimal, with the counselor withholding appropriate responses. Rather than being genuinely himself, the counselor responds from an artificial, contrived, and sterile "professional" role, altogether lacking in spontaneity. Instead of making appropriate self-disclosures, the counselor seems to hedge or cover up for either personal or pseudo-professional reasons.

LEVEL 3.0

The counselor shows no incongruence between behavior, statements, and feelings, but does not make truly authentic re-

*Adapted from earlier versions of similar genuineness or congruence scales presented by Carkhuff, 1969; Gazda, 1973; Kiesler, 1967; and Truax and Carkhuff, 1967.

sponses that convey his feelings. The counselor is not defensive or insincere; neither is he spontaneously, enthusiastically, or intensely involved. Listening and attending, reflecting, clarifying, questioning, and accepting ("uh huh," "I see") responses often typify this level. The counselor shares personal reactions and feelings toward the client vaguely and superficially.

LEVEL 4.0

The counselor's responses and personal feelings are congruent, but he may have some hesitancy or discomfort in expressing them. The counselor voices feelings and reactions, both positive and negative, concerning the client and his situation when they are pertinent to the client's experiences, concerns, or struggles or to the counseling interaction. It is clear that the counselor is being himself. He expresses negative feelings in a nondestructive way that strengthens the relationship.

LEVEL 5.0

The counselor is openly and freely himself in the relationship, interacts spontaneously, expresses feelings on his own initiative, and is appropriately responsive to his inner feelings. The counselor openly shares positive, negative, and ambivalent feelings when they are relevant to the client's needs or the helping situation. He shares negative feelings and reactions in a constructive manner that facilitates exploration by both parties.

Examples of Levels of Authenticity

CLIENT STATEMENT 1

A thirty-seven-year-old married mother of five in her first interview: "Before I go any further, I have to know what your stand on abortion is."

Level 1.0 response. "I wonder why you're putting *me* on the spot. If you're pregnant, it's your feelings that matter, not mine."

Explanation. The response is guarded and somewhat defensive, revealing nothing of the counselor's feelings. The counselor need not always answer questions about his values or point of view, but in this instance he fails even to reveal his reasons for choosing not to answer the question. The client may be expected to feel "put down" and to respond by being less open in subsequent exchanges.

Level 2.0 response. "That really is a loaded question. Abortion is a pretty delicate subject for many people. Tell me, how do you feel about abortion?"

Explanation. In this response, the counselor is not defensive, but he avoids revealing his feelings by shifting the focus back on the client. The client's feelings, of course, are the central concern, but to elicit those feelings, the counselor must model openness, which he fails to do here.

Level 3.0 response. "So you're very concerned about how I stand before you share some of your feelings. I gather you're pretty uncomfortable about revealing your own feelings until you know something about how I might react. I know it's a touchy subject for you, but I'll do my best to understand."

Explanation. The counselor's response is not phony, defensive, or guarded, but it does not reveal his feelings. Rather, the reflective response keeps the focus on the client, which is generally appropriate. In responses at a higher level of authenticity, however, some risk by the counselor often prefaces a refocus on the client and sets the stage for a richer response by the client.

Level 4.0 response. "That's a touchy question to respond to, but I appreciate your wanting to know my stand. I guess I haven't really taken a stand one way or the other. There are so many sides to the matter, and I can't see it in terms of black or white. I've done a lot of thinking about it and just haven't come to a final conclusion. My position is that each situation is highly individual and that the important thing is what fits best for each person. How do you see it?"

Explanation. Evidencing no incongruence or phoniness, the counselor acknowledges his own struggle with a complex issue. The sharing of his position also entails elements of strong respect and makes no attempt to impose beliefs on the client. The client will tend to feel comfortable enough to risk sharing her own beliefs as a result. (It is assumed that the counselor's response *is* congruent with his inner feelings.)

Level 5.0 response. "You know, I find that a tough question to answer. I've asked myself the same question and have struggled with a lot of pros and cons. On the one hand, I respect the right of women to make their own decisions about their lives. On the other hand, I wonder if the developing embryo doesn't have some rights too. But I guess in final analysis the most important right is the right people have to explore their own feelings and make their own choices. You probably asked about my stand because of a struggle you're having. Let's talk about that."

Explanation. The counselor's response is open, genuine, and spontaneous. After sharing his own feelings freely, the counselor shifts the focus back to the client. The client may be expected to appreciate the candid response and to speak only in answer.

CLIENT STATEMENT 2

The following statement occurs at the conclusion of a conjoint marriage counseling session. The effectiveness of the interview was hampered by the crying and whining of an infant whom the parents brought along because their babysitter failed them at the last minute. The counselor found it difficult to maintain focus because of the distractions the infant created, and he felt frustrated during much of the interview. The mother says, "I hope you weren't too upset by the baby's fussiness today. She just seems to have the colic."

Level 1.0 response. "Don't worry about it. It didn't bother me at all."

Explanation. The counselor's response is clearly incongruent. Since the mother's perception of the counselor's discomfort probably prompted her question, she is very likely to consider his response phony.

Level 2.0 response. "Oh, it wasn't all that upsetting. I can understand your babysitter problem. You surely have a cute baby."

Explanation. The counselor does not entirely deny his frustration and discomfort, but he definitely holds back feelings and diverts the focus by first talking about the babysitting problem and then paying a compliment. Again, the client will perceive the counselor as guarded.

Level 3.0 response. "Thanks for your concern. I could see the baby was uncomfortable and really a handful to you. Was it upsetting for you?"

Explanation. The counselor neither conceals nor reveals his feelings of discomfort and frustration. In that sense, he was authentic, but he demonstrated no genuineness. Instead, he turned the focus back to the client.

Level 4.0 response. "I appreciate your concern. Actually I was distracted somewhat by the baby and found it a little frustrating because I wanted to be more in tune with the two of you. Still, I realized you couldn't help it with the bind you were in because of your babysitter."

Explanation. The counselor's response is congruent with his inner feelings, yet the expression of frustration conveys both respect and a commitment to be helpful. The client may be expected to appreciate this honesty and respect. The counselor's response fosters a climate of openness.

Level 5.0 response. "Say, you must have really tuned into my feelings. I did find myself distracted and frustrated at several points and wishing the baby wasn't here. My upset wasn't with you, though. I knew you couldn't help the situation. I just felt frustrated because we weren't able to accomplish as much as we might have."

Explanation. The counselor freely acknowledges negative feelings but in a constructive manner. He admits the feelings, but avoids blaming or criticizing the clients for the difficulty.

Exercises in Assessing Levels of Authenticity

The following exercises in rating responses for authenticity are to help the reader learn how to discriminate the degree of authentic communication in preparation for exercises in authentically communicating one's feelings. The two client statements are followed by possible counselor responses. Refer to the Authenticity Scale and rate each response in the space provided to the left of the response. After you have completed each exercise, compare your ratings with those provided on page 214. Determine the difference, disregarding whether it is positive or negative, between each of your ratings and the authors' ratings, and enter the difference in the blank to the right of the responses. Then add the differences and divide this sum by 10 (the number of counselor responses). This is your average discrepancy score for the first exercise, which gauges your ability to rate different levels of authentic responses. The goal is to achieve an average discrepancy score of 0.5 or less by the end of the two exercises. After each exercise, study the responses for which your ratings differ from the authors', examine the rating scale, and seek to discover why the authors rated them as they did.

CLIENT STATEMENT 1

The client is a single male, age twenty-three. Still dependent on his parents and lacking in responsibility, he has had difficulty getting himself up in the morning before 10 A.M. Although he had defined this as a problem behavior he wished to change, he has been tardy for several appointments scheduled for 11 A.M., each time apologizing and pledging voluntarily to be more responsible the following week. He arrives for his fourteenth appointment at 11:25. The counselor has been waiting and feels some irritation and disgust. In an embarrassed manner, the client says, "Gee, I'm sorry about being late today. I slept in and almost forgot our appointment until my mother reminded me. I hope it didn't put you out."

Your Rating		*Responses:*	*Discrepancy Score*
_____	1.	(Angrily) "To tell the truth, I'm just plain disgusted with you. You keep saying you want to change, but you don't do anything about it. I've about had it with you."	_____
_____	2.	"Well, I must admit I've been waiting for twenty-five minutes. But let's get started and make the most of our remaining time."	_____
_____	3.	"You know, you've been late several times recently. What do you think that means?"	_____
_____	4.	"I'll have to admit I'm feeling irritated with you. I don't like having the feelings, but waiting week after week is frustrating. More importantly, though, I'm concerned about the effects on you. When you're late, our time is shortened and you're really no closer to the goals you've set for becoming more responsible."	_____

_____   5. "Why should I be put out? It's your   _____
              time and your mother's money. You
              can use it any way you like."

_____   6. "You're uncomfortable about being   _____
              late and wonder if I'm upset with you."

_____   7. "No, I'm not put out with you, I'm just   _____
              concerned that half our time is already
              gone."

_____   8. "Put yourself in my shoes. How would   _____
              you feel?"

_____   9. "To be frank, I am somewhat put out.   _____
              You've been late several times recently
              for the same reason and I'm wonder-
              ing what is happening. I guess I feel
              frustrated because you don't seem to
              be making any progress and I feel
              handicapped in helping when half of
              our interview time is wasted."

_____   10. "Well, I guess I'm a little bothered. I   _____
              wonder what your theory is as to why
              you're late so often."

Proceed with the second exercise, which follows. After rating
all the responses to the client statement, again determine your discrepancy scores from the authors' ratings for each response, add
them, and divide by eight (the total number of counselor responses
presented). Analyze each response you rated inaccurately.

CLIENT STATEMENT 2

This situation involves the sixth interview with a twenty-four-
year-old client of the opposite sex. In previous interviews and earlier in this particular session, the client has engaged in active
self-exploration and has revealed some past situations about which
the client feels ashamed. The counselor feels positively toward the
client, seeing many strengths and assets. The client explains, "Right
now I'm really feeling embarrassed. I guess I would like you to think
well of me, and yet you're finding out so many terrible things without a chance to see anything good about me."

Your Rating		*Responses:*	*Discrepancy Score*
_____	1.	"After revealing so much about yourself, you seem quite fearful about how I'm reacting to you."	_____
_____	2.	"In my work I'm used to hearing many, many such things. You don't need to feel embarrassed."	_____
_____	3.	"I can appreciate your discomfort and concern about my reactions as you reveal so much of yourself. In the past, when I've risked and shared some very personal things with others, I have at times felt rather vulnerable and apprehensive about how they then saw me. I want to share with you that I like you and feel very positive about what you're accomplishing here."	_____
_____	4.	"I don't really think my feelings are that important to what we're doing. What seems most important is your great concern over having people like you and with the impression you're creating. I wonder if this is a pattern you have with others as well as with me."	_____
_____	5.	"As a counselor I try to be objective and not allow my personal feelings to interfere."	_____
_____	6.	"You indicate that I haven't had a chance to see anything good about you. I'll have to disagree. The way that you strive to understand yourself and make some changes tells me a lot. I see a lot about you that I like and feel very good about what you're doing for yourself."	_____
_____	7.	"I can tell you're very concerned about	_____

how I'm reacting to you. How do you
fear I may be reacting?"

_____ 8. "In our last session, as you were work- _____
ing on something, I remember admir-
ing how hard you were struggling with
yourself. I have a lot of respect for you
and the way you are struggling to
grow. I perceive you as having a lot of
strength, and although we've focused
on things you're dissatisfied with, I've
also gained the impression that you've
got a lot on the ball."

Sum: _____
Average Discrepancy Score: _____

RATINGS FOR ASSESSMENT EXERCISES

Client Statement 1		Client Statement 2	
1.	1.0	1.	3.0
2.	3.0	2.	2.0
3.	3.0	3.	5.0
4.	5.0	4.	1.5
5.	1.5	5.	2.0
6.	3.0	6.	4.0
7.	1.5	7.	3.0
8.	2.0		
9.	4.0		
10.	2.0		

Types of Authentic Responses

Occasionally a client will put the counselor on the spot by accusing him of taking sides with another person or of being disin-
terested, displeased, irritated, critical, or unfeeling; by raising
doubts about the congruence between the counselor's expressed
and actual feelings; or by questioning the counselor's competency
or the appropriateness of a certain response. At such times, the
client's verbalizations may have strong emotional overtones of

anger, resentment, or hurt. In these instances, the counselor's response is crucial for it will determine whether the client sees the counselor as open to negative feedback and honest in sharing personal feelings and as a person to whom the client can safely reveal his own negative feelings.

Whenever the client puts the counselor on the spot, the counselor's natural response is defensiveness, anger, or a similar negative reaction. Responding negatively, however, merely inflames the situation. Or, as the aphorism goes, "Nastiness begets nastiness." Paradoxically, in such situations, the "more human" response is not the natural response. Instead, the counselor must master his natural anger and accept the client's negative message as possibly valid and valuable for understanding the relationship. Thus negative client messages are viewed not as personal attacks, but as opportunities for elucidating the dynamics of the client's behavior, expanding the client's self-awareness, and fostering increased openness and trust in the helping relationship. Responding nondefensively both models openness for the client and demonstrates new patterns of responding that the client can apply in life situations when others verbally attack or criticize him.

A common way to communicate authentically with clients is to reveal personal experiences, interests, meanings, and attitudes external to the counseling relationship. This method includes, for example, appropriate sharing of aspects of one's past experiences and history and disclosing selected information about one's relationships to others such as spouses, children, or parents. When these responses are relevant to the client's concerns, properly timed, used sparingly and discriminately, brief, and communicated in a manner that does not put the spotlight on the counselor, they may be helpful. Such responses convey the counselor's humanness and openness, and they often help the client perceive himself as similar to others rather than as a deviant misfit.

An illustration of such a self-disclosure is: "I want you to know that I'm aware of your turmoil and how hard it is for you to set some limits with your mother. I've had to go through some similar pain in my own growth process, and I know how terribly uncomfortable it can be. I remember once when I felt very much that way when I was struggling with. . . ." The counselor can use his own relationships as a baseline: "If I said that to my wife, I think she'd feel very hurt. I wonder if your wife might also feel hurt." Sometimes past experiences are uniquely relevant: "I sense your concern as to whether I can understand the problems you're having with your Indian foster child. I worked on a reservation for a couple of years and have had a keen interest in Indian culture. I'm not sure that means I can understand the problems you're having, but let's give it a try."

Another type of authentic response, which is also central to relational immediacy (discussed in the next chapter), is the sharing of here-and-now affective and physical reactions to the client or situation. This type of sharing tends to deepen the encounter between counselor and client and provides a model of openness and humanness. This category includes conveying warmth and caring, disclosing troubled feelings, and exploring and elucidating the meaning of the physical sensations the counselor experiences. This type of response, like all attempts at authenticity, may be ineffective or destructive when made indiscriminately, and guidelines for constructive responses are provided later in the chapter.

The following exchange, which occurs during the eighth interview, illustrates a revelation of feelings and experience.

Client: "Life has been pretty empty for me. I've never really had a relationship with *anyone* who cared much about me." His voice cracks, his chin quivers.

Counselor: "It's very painful for you right now as you're aware of that emptiness. I wonder if those feelings include me—that you're afraid I don't care much about you."

Client (looking down): "Well, I've wondered."

Counselor: "That seems natural, given your past experiences. It's important to me, though, that you know that I feel a closeness to you and have a lot of care for you. I wonder if you can sense my feelings right now?"

The counselor can use his own reactions to the client as a way of enlightening the client on how he affects others. For example, "You know, it was hard for me to tell you how your defensiveness tends to drive people away from you. I was aware of feeling apprehensive that you might get defensive and feel I was just criticizing you." In much the same vein, the counselor shares his physical reaction to the client's plans and proposals: "As you started talking about reconciling with your husband, I noticed my stomach knotted up.

As I try to understand my reaction, I guess I'm really frightened at the thought that you might destroy yourself by risking his abuse and violence all over again."

Another type of sharing of self consists of openly expressing one's personal perceptions, ideas, reactions, and formulations. As was pointed out in Chapter Two, the early phase of counseling focuses on understanding the client and establishing a relationship. When this has been accomplished, however, the counselor may participate much more openly as a real person in his own right, rather than as a mere listener and mirror for the client. The counselor who is guarded and withholds most of his perceptions deprives the client of a valuable source of learning. The client's perceptions and thoughts are often distorted or irrational, and the counselor can be especially helpful by serving as a candid feedback system. Once the client perceives the counselor as understanding, non-judgmental, trustworthy, and motivated by helpful intent, the counselor should be willing to reveal thoughts and perceptions and to risk vulnerability much as he expects the client to.

An example of this type of authentic responding is: "I get the impression that you do things on the spur of the moment, impulsively, without thinking first about the consequences." To a burly male client, the counselor might share this reaction: "I experience you as a very warm person with a lot of caring about people. Yet, somehow you seem a little embarrassed about that, as though it's not manly to have those feelings."

Mental images and associations are another part of oneself that can be shared with another. However, one can readily think of examples of images or spontaneous, here-and-now associations that cannot be shared constructively. As with the other types of authentic responses, mental imagery must be judicious and well-timed. The reader should be thoroughly familiar with the guidelines for authentic responding presented later in this chapter. When these cautions are observed, however, therapist imagery may enrich counseling, stimulate productive exploration by both parties, provide creative and useful feedback, model self-awareness, and add some zest and humor to counseling. In fact, spontaneous and humorous imagery often provides the client with creative perspectives and symbols, which facilitate awareness in a fresh and vital way. Although the counselor does not share all of his fantasies and spontaneous associations with the client, sharing them selectively often deepens understanding for both counselor and client.

With a fearful and withdrawn client who avoids close relationships, the counselor creates an image of the client in the social universe: "As you were just describing the way your relationships have been, and your relationship with your wife, I had an image of you as a balloon in a world inhabited by porcupines. Have you ever felt that way?" Alienation or abandonment summons a picture of loneliness: "When you were talking about being left out, I had a mental image of you, all alone at home, enviously looking out the window and seeing everyone else alive and enjoying life, feeling so alone and yet wishing you were a part of it." A spontaneous reaction to a revelation by an ex-convict assumes its own imagery: "When you mentioned moving back to Iowa, the word *prison* flashed in my mind like a neon light. I thought to myself, 'If he goes back there with his old cronies, he'll end up back in prison.'"

An authentic response involving the counselor's sharing of some of himself may also convey empathic understanding. Although this response is recommended only infrequently, the counselor may express his own feelings or reactions to a situation and then determine whether the client has similar feelings. Such a message is still another form of additive empathic response, assuming, of course, that the counselor's feelings accurately reflect the client's. An example of such a response is: "I just listened to all the effort you went to in cleaning the house, preparing a banquet, and doing everything in your power to please your husband. Then you described how, instead of being appreciative, he blew up over your spilling a few drops of wine on his salad. You said you felt you'd made a mess of things and apologized. Yet, just listening to you, I found myself feeling indignant about his behavior. I wonder if you didn't feel some anger yourself?" A similar message is conveyed by this response: "I can sense how infuriated you were when that happened. But I wonder if you felt even more, because as I've just been listening to you, I became aware that if someone who mattered responded to me like that I'd feel deeply wounded, very hurt."

Feelings can also be expressed nonverbally. For example, in a group-therapy setting when the therapist is deeply involved in working with an individual or is feeling particularly close to someone, he might move to a chair or onto the floor near that person, with or without verbal explanation. Reaching out and touching a client is another example of this type of sharing. Such responses are much more appropriate in a group context than in individual counseling, and they must certainly be used discriminately and cautiously to avoid misinterpretation. Further guidelines concerning this response will be discussed in the next section.

Guidelines for Authentic Responding

Since indiscriminate authentic responding can be destructive, the counselor must observe guidelines to the effective use of authenticity. One vitally important guideline is that high-level authentic responses be avoided until the client demonstrates a readiness to respond positively to self-disclosures by the counselor. Trust and rapport in the relationship are prerequisite to such self-disclosures. If the counselor reveals personal feelings, views, or experiences prematurely, the danger exists that the client will perceive him as someone who seeks to influence, to direct, and even to pass judgment or who wants to shift the focus away from the client's problems. Thus early self-disclosures by the counselor generally threaten the client and lead to emotional retreat at the very time when the major goal of the counseling process is to reduce threat and defensiveness, thereby encouraging open self-exploration. Likewise, the counselor's frame should not be shared until the client demonstrates that he feels understood and trusted. Once such an interpersonal climate has been created, the client will be more receptive to considering and using a differing frame of reference.

The client's reactions to authentic responses by the counselor cannot be safely predicted until the counselor has interacted with the client enough to become well acquainted with him. One partial indication of the client's readiness is self-initiated exploration of problems and feelings related to the self and to the relationship. Only when this indication appears along with a nondefensive response to the counselor's tentative and experimental self-disclosures should the counselor conclude that the relationship is strong enough to risk truly authentic responding. Even then, the counselor will need to be keenly alert to possible negative reactions. Should the client so react, the counselor will need to respond empathically to the feelings and to desist temporarily from further self-disclosures.

In assessing the client's readiness, several other factors are relevant. When the client manifests negative feelings or reactions to the counselor, authentic responding is generally contraindicated. Exploration of the negative feelings and of their source must take precedence over authentic responding in the interest of reestablishing a climate conducive to mutual trust and openness. In some instances, however, the counselor may appropriately disclose his awareness of the strain in the relationship and of his desire to understand and relieve it. For example, he might say, "I can sense that you're upset about something that has happened in our relationship. I'd like to understand more about your feelings and the part I play in them. I'm sensing that your feelings are getting in the way of our working together more effectively."

Another guideline pertains when the patient is a severely disturbed schizophrenic. Gendlin (1967) found that the counselor must be active and authentically share his own experiences when a typically withdrawn, schizophrenic patient is silent and not interacting with the counselor or is verbal but focusing on some esoteric topic external to his life situation and difficulties. Betz (1967) likewise found that therapists who are active, spontaneous, and open are more successful in helping schizophrenics than are therapists who are passive, detached, and emotionally uninvolved.

An additional guideline concerns clients who are not psychotic but whose diminutive self-esteem or weak reality-testing limits their capacity for trust and readiness to engage in self-exploration. Because such clients have a marked tendency to misinterpret the motives of others, authenticity must be employed cautiously, sparingly, and with the utmost delicacy.

As the counseling relationship gains in trust, the counselor's openness and spontaneity can properly increase. The counselor must, however, bear the importance of appropriateness in mind. Being authentic does not mean having license to act out or express oneself indiscriminately. The purpose of counseling is to meet the client's needs; the counselor's primary goal is to help the client, not to be disclosing and authentic. Authentic responding should not place the spotlight on the counselor and seek to meet his needs. Authentic responses should have a definite goal and purpose, should be relevant to client needs, and should not distract from the current focus. The counselor should not ramble on with details about himself; rather, he should succinctly share his feelings, disclosures, or perceptions and then return the focus to the client. Unfortunately, some counselors are so narcissistic that they relish being the center of attention and impulsively blurt out their feelings or views without regard to appropriateness or timing. There is a marked contrast between such impulsiveness and true authenticity.

Moderation in authentic responding is usually associated with positive outcomes. A study by Truax and Carkhuff (1964), which we cited in Chapter One, reveals that genuineness increased beyond a certain level is not related to greater facilitation for the client. There appears to be a curvilinear relationship between the frequency and depth of authentic counselor disclosures and expressions of personal feelings on the one hand and positive therapeutic outcomes on the other. It seems likely that closed and enigmatic counselors as well as indiscriminately open, inappropriately revealing, and attention-seeking counselors are all ineffective. One study (Murphy and Strong, 1976), for example, shows that a client may perceive a counselor who frequently discloses being personally similar to the client as suspect and as having ulterior motives. In a psychotherapy-analogue study, Simonson (1976) found that university students in an initial interview reveal more to a warm counselor who discloses only brief, impersonal, and general demographic information than to a warm counselor who makes personal disclosures. He concludes that therapist self-disclosure can be counterproductive, especially early in therapy. Giannandrea and Murphy (1973) similarly report that subjects are more likely to continue in counseling when the counselor makes only a moderate number of self-disclosures.

Increased counselor expressiveness is usually appropriate when the client focuses on impersonal, superficial, and external events. At such times the counselor's activity and authentic expressiveness may facilitate the client's self-experiencing and relevant self-exploration. However, when the client is already engaged in relevant self-exploration and is in close contact with his own experiencing, authentic responses by the counselor tend to distract him. At such times empathic responsiveness is more appropriate than authenticity, and the counselor should take care not to make authentic disclosures that pull the client away from ongoing experiencing.

The counselor should seek to be in touch with his feelings in the relationship, particularly when he experiences difficulty relating to the client. In such instances he should engage in introspection to determine whether the troubling feelings originate in the client, in himself, or in the nuances of the interaction. If the client suggests or asserts that the counselor has certain feelings, the counselor should be open to considering that possibility and not be defensive or incongruent. If, after exploring the feelings, he determines that the client's perception is invalid, he should convey that fact to the client and explore how the client arrived at his conclusion. If, however, the counselor determines that the client's perception is correct, he should tactfully acknowledge the feelings and discuss them with the client.

It is often helpful for the counselor to engage in introspection to increase his awareness of current feelings and reactions to the client. Periodically, particularly when the relationship is troubled or the client seems bogged down, the counselor is encouraged to attend quietly to his own inward, physical sensations and experiences. Gendlin (1969) describes a "focusing technique" that may be very helpful for increasing self-awareness at such times. In employing Gendlin's technique, the counselor should attend to feelings, allow pictures, brief fantasies, new words, and associations to arise to consciousness. Certainly he does not share all of these experiences with the client, but some may be appropriately shared, and the counselor's awareness of them may be facilitative.

When the counselor experiences persistent feelings toward the client, he should seek not only to understand them, but to determine whether they may be constructively shared. When strong negative feelings (dislike, anger, repulsion, disgust) toward the client are present, they should not be expressed until the counselor has explored them enough to know their source and range. Like the client, the counselor may experience feelings that are transferred from past relationships to current relationships (countertransference). The counselor should also engage in introspection when he feels physically attracted to or sexually aroused by a client. Disclosure of such feelings may confuse or overwhelm the client, or it may elicit feelings of arousal or attraction, complicating the relationship and changing it from professional to personal. It is not uncommon, however, for seductive clients to elicit feelings of attraction, and examining them in the context of the relationship may help the client gain awareness of behaviors that cause difficulties in other relationships. (The process of examining here-and-now feelings and using the immediate relationship for learning will be examined in more depth later in Chapter Nine). Besides exploring problem feelings, the counselor should consider the possible impact, both good and bad, of disclosing such reactions. Finally, the counselor should consider ways to share such feelings facilitatively.

If negative feelings persist even after self-exploration, it may be helpful for the counselor to express them tactfully and with restraint. However, no constructive purpose is served by impulsively expressing anger. Yet, feedback to the client about how some aspect of his behavior is abrasive, offensive, or alienating to others may be very helpful if conveyed in the context of good will and helpful intent. However, the counselor must be careful not to conceal labeling, blaming, commanding, or criticizing under the guise of genuineness and authenticity. When sharing personal feelings or perceptions, the counselor should *remain experientially descriptive rather than evaluative*—that is, he should describe the feelings and be responsible for them, not shift that responsibility onto the client. For example, rather than stating, "You are _____," the counselor does better to say, "I experience you as _____," or "I'm feeling _____ about you." Feedback should also be highly specific, not general. A useful format (adapted from Dyer, 1969, p. 169) is, "When you did this _____ (describing the action), I felt _____ (describing your current inner experiencing)."

In responding authentically, the counselor must take care not to intimidate, coerce, or emotionally blackmail the client to take certain actions. Moreover, the counselor should avoid using self-disclosures of feelings or circumstances similar to the client's to influence, give advice, or otherwise manipulate the client to act according to the counselor's will. For example, a counselor might attempt to influence the client to follow a certain course of action by relating, "I had that problem once and I solved it by. . . ." In manipulating the client through self-disclosure, the counselor may unwittingly foster dependency, discourage the client from thinking issues through for himself, or engender resentment.

When furthering the self-exploration of one's feelings toward a client, the counselor may discover a complex range of inner feelings. This expanded awareness and experiencing of personal feelings may be very beneficial in unraveling emotions that might otherwise confound one's ability to relate constructively to a client. *Being authentic requires more than merely sharing superficial and easily identified feelings.* To aid in expanding self-awareness, we heartily endorse Gendlin's recommendation to recognize "the inward side of a feeling."

According to Gendlin (1967), the inward side of a feeling is the deeper aspect that reflects the positive motivation we experience toward our clients. Expressing the inward side of feelings safeguards the client's self-esteem, whereas expressing outer feelings poses a threat. For example, if the counselor feels bored with or angry toward a client, rather than express these feelings (the outer edge) that imply criticism or blame, he seeks to determine and to express deeper aspects of the feelings by asking himself, "Why do I feel this way?" In seeking the answer, he will discover that behind the boredom lies a positive desire to hear more personal and relevant information that can facilitate progress in therapy. Likewise, behind the anger lies disappointment in being unable to be more helpful to the client. If we similarly analyze such feelings as impatience, irritation, criticism, or disgust, we will discover that the inward side of these feelings will consist of a desire that the client have a better and more fulfilling life, a desire that can be shared safely and beneficially.

When self-exploration widens the range of emotions, it may be helpful to share that range rather than only one aspect of the feelings. Frequently, conflicting or ambivalent feelings are present. Dyer (1969), for example, cites an instance of feeling so angry that he could punch the client in the nose and simultaneously experiencing guilt about that feeling. He shared with the client his anger, his wish not to feel so, and his desire to resolve the feeling through discussion. As another example, rather than telling a client simply, "I'm displeased because I think you've been avoiding discussing a troublesome area for you," one might share his multiple emotions: "I'm aware of feeling displeased because for some time you've avoided talking about your drinking, which seems really to be a source of problems to you. Yet I'm also aware that your avoidance in part relates to me, and I'm concerned about introducing this topic because I know you may resent me for bringing it up. And yet, it seems to be a real source of trouble to you, and I'd feel I was letting you down if I permitted you to continue avoiding it."

Being authentic means relating spontaneously and naturally, as contrasted to relating according to a contrived professional role. Certain qualifications, however, warrant mention. To help the client understand the counselor, it is important for the counselor to attune his vocabulary to the level the client can readily grasp. Many counselors err by using words and phrases unfamiliar to their clients. Fearing embarrassment and a demeaning exposure of a lack of education or verbal skill, a client who does not understand may well not ask the counselor to clarify what he has said. Using understandable language thus not only facilitates understanding but also avoids possible blows to the client's self-esteem.

Another qualification relates to the expression of feelings of warmth and caring that often occur naturally in any deep human encounter. A natural response is to touch, embrace, or physically express the closeness. In our judgment, however, it is prudent to exercise restraint in such physical contact. An occasional hug or squeeze of the hand, or arm on the shoulder may be appropriate with clients who are depressed or under great stress. However, the counselor best expresses his care not through physical contact but through a commitment to understand and a willingness to journey into the painful and often frightening world of another's experience, maintaining all the while respect for and acceptance of the other. Verbal and nonverbal communication, exclusive of physical contact, adequately express a full measure of caring appropriate to the helping relationship. Moreover, physical contact, however innocent, can be misinterpreted by the client and may engender anxiety, fear, or sexual feelings, all of which are antithetical to the purposes of counseling. After any physical contact, therefore, the counselor should specify the motives for his action. As we noted above, brief touching and similar nonverbal expressions are more appropriate and less subject to misinterpretation in group contexts than in an individual interview because the presence of other group members acts as an emotional buffer and a behavioral constraint.

If a counselor is frequently inclined toward physical contact with his clients, introspection or professional consultation may be indicated. Physical contact should emanate from the client's needs, not the counselor's. It may be helpful in assessing one's motives to ask oneself if one experiences such inclinations equally toward both sexes, toward old and young alike, and toward both physically attractive and unattractive clients of the opposite sex.

An aspect of authenticity that some counselors often overlook deals with what might best be termed professional honesty. Halleck (1963) writes about professional dishonesty in work with disturbed adolescents, including false promises of confidentiality and failing to deal with frustration and anger. Counselors are tempted to invite the client to trust and share, reassuring him that whatever is shared will be kept in strictest confidence. Professional honesty, however, involves also sharing openly the realities of the situation and not misleading the client under the guise of wanting to be helpful. As Halleck observes regarding disturbed adolescents, "The worker cannot guarantee confidentiality to the patient since he is not the agent of the patient. The worker has obligations to the child's family, his clinic, his agency, or his institution. . . . To imply [that] this guarantee is extended or to extend it with the full knowledge that it is not meant to be kept can result in development of situations that inhibit communication. It does not take a very clever adolescent to understand that the worker has primary responsibilities to his agency and to the community. . . . If professionals do not let him know this, he will perceive their behavior as dishonest, and his communications to the adult world will be diminished" (p. 51). Regarding feelings of frustration and anger, Halleck maintains that "it is almost impossible to work with adolescents for any period of time without becoming periodically angered. It is dishonest and unfair to the worker and to the adolescent to deny, rationalize, or displace this anger. It belongs in the therapeutic situation and should be communicated with as much restraint, tact, and honesty as the worker is capable of providing. To do less than this establishes a basically dishonest pattern of interaction and precludes the possibility of the adolescent's experiencing positive emotional growth" (p. 53).

When a client seeks to elicit personal information from the counselor in an apparent effort either to shift the focus and thereby evade painful self-examination or to redefine the relationship as a social one, disclosures by the counselor are generally counterproductive. One may respond with minimal self-disclosure, thereby conveying openness, followed by exploration of the motivation behind the client's attempted distraction. The counselor, for example, may explain that he is not attempting to hedge but that the reason for asking the question may be more important than the answer. If the client offers no explanation and the counselor has reason to believe that he understands the dynamics behind the client's tactics, he may offer a tentative interpretation.

If the client asks how the counselor feels toward him (for example, "How do you feel about me?" or "How do I compare with your other clients?"), authentic self-disclosures may be premature or inappropriate. The counselor does better to explore the feelings underlying the client's inquiry and to share his own feelings somewhat, if that sharing is appropriate. Such questions often emanate from personal insecurity and self-doubt. Empathic responding and focus on the immediacy of the relationship thus are more appropriate than authentic self-disclosure in such instances.

These cautions should not be taken to mean that counselors should generally avoid answering personal questions. Many, if not most, of the personal questions clients ask have no ulterior motive, and a straightforward answer may be entirely appropriate. However, the counselor should not feel obligated to answer all such questions in the service of authenticity. If the counselor feels uncomfortable about answering a personal question or for some reason deems it inadvisable, he may simply decline to answer, explaining his reason for doing so.

After an authentic disclosure, the counselor is encouraged to use empathic communication to tune in to the client's response to the disclosure. This approach minimizes negative effects from inappropriate, poorly timed disclosures. The counselor is likely to pick up negative reactions to authentic disclosures by routinely listening carefully and responding empathically afterwards. Similarly, when an authentic response by the counselor is unproductive, it is advisable to pick up where the interview left off before the authentic response.

In the next chapter, we turn to relational immediacy, which is an integral part of authenticity in helping relationships.

Chapter 9

♦♦♦♦♦♦♦♦♦♦♦♦♦♦♦♦♦♦♦♦♦♦♦

Examining Here-and-Now Feelings and Interactions Within the Counseling Relationship

Relational immediacy involves the examination of here-and-now interactions and feelings within the counseling relationship. This examination is critical to the helping relationship because the feelings that flow back and forth between counselor and client determine whether an effective helping relationship will evolve and be maintained during the course of counseling. Moreover, the patterns of feeling and interaction within the relationship provide a rich source of information about the client's patterns in broader social relationships.

The counselor-client relationship is a social microcosm, a miniature world in which the client's interpersonal behavior and conditioned perceptual sets and distortions are manifested. The client often re-creates in the here-and-now counselor-client interaction the very problems that plague and defeat him in his other relationships. Thus the counseling relationship provides an interpersonal context wherein the client's overlearned, habitual patterns become evident to the alert counselor. The meaning the counselor attributes to these patterns depends on his theoretical bias. From Alfred Adler's perspective, the client recreates his life style, moves toward his familiar mistaken goals, and uses his usual safeguarding security operations. According to Karen Horney's conceptual framework, the client can be expected to resort to his usual interpersonal style of moving toward, against, or away from the counselor. Using Shostrom's (1968) grid illustrating primary manipulative styles of relating, the counselor can expect a client whose style is that of a controlling "calculator," a dependent "clinging vine," or a critical "judge" to live out his style of coping in the counseling relationship.

An elementary illustration of a self-defeating pattern of behavior re-created in counseling is the client who, without awareness, frequently offended his friends and spouse because he seemed uninterested in what they said. Instead of listening, he was busy dwelling on what he was going to say next, only partially attending to the conversation. This ingrained interactional pattern manifested itself in the counseling relationship when the client only barely attended to the counselor, resulting in occasional misunderstandings, the need to repeat messages, and the counselor's gradual awareness that he was being "tuned out" by his client. Awareness of the pattern fostered by the counselor's feedback helped the client change.

Many schools of psychotherapeutic thought use the concept of transference to explain the appearance in therapy of feelings and behaviors paralleling those from the past or from current relationships outside therapy. Traditionally, transference has referred to the displacement onto the therapist of feelings, attitudes, or conflicts involving significant past figures (mother or father) in the client's life. The existentialist psychologist Rollo May offers a different conceptualization: "What really happens is not that the neurotic patient 'transfers' feelings he has toward mother or father to wife or therapist. Rather, the neurotic is one who in certain areas never developed beyond the limited and restricted forms of experience characteristic of the infant. Hence in later years he perceives wife or therapist through the same restricted, distorted 'spectacles' as he perceived father or mother. The problem is to be understood in terms of perception and the relatedness to the world" (May, Angel, and Ellenberger, 1958, p. 79).

In the family constellation, the child is perceptually conditioned, arriving at convictions and conclusions about the nature of the world, men, women, authorities, life, and the self. Thus, early in life, many clients erroneously generalized one set of circumstances to all related circumstances. Although such generalizations aid in simplifying, organizing, evaluating, and classifying experience and thus lend some predictability to life, they tend to create problems by "programming" interpersonal perceptions with "fictions," or expectancy sets, as well as with behavioral game plans and rules for coping. Later in life many clients cannot discriminate their current worlds from their earlier experiences, thus overgeneralizing and oversimplifying life and using dysfunctional, habitual problem-solving methods for coping and for defending against threat. To illustrate, one of the authors counseled a young man from a deprived and chaotic early background involving unpredictable, alcoholic parents who could not be depended upon except, perhaps, to disappoint him. Later, juvenile arrests led him to a state correctional institution. Now he came for therapy with marital problems. Considerable effort was spent exploring his lack of trust in his spouse and helping him see the difference between his wife and his parents. In time he came to see how he had overgeneralized from his early experiences, assuming that since no one could be trusted then, no one could be trusted now either. He gradually learned to distinguish caution based on specific relationships and circumstances from blanket distrust.

Lacking awareness, many clients operate on conditioned, unquestioned assumptions and perceptual stereotypes. They may actually attempt to structure their current worlds in dysfunctional but familiar ways. Thus they may try to elicit behaviors and reactions from the counselor that conform to and confirm their perceptions—for example, conclusions about what authorities or men are like, or self-definitions as rejected persons of little worth. Such perceptions are often maintained because they are useful to the client's current life. For example, if the client expects all people to be hostile or rejecting, his conviction at least protects him from the pain of rejection by attributing such rejection to the hostile nature of others rather than to his own undesirability. The function of safeguarding self-esteem is thus served. Regardless of the particular purpose served by the perceptual set, it can be assumed in general that the more disturbed the client, the more unrealistic, inappropriate, and overgeneralized are his perceptions and behavioral reactions. A goal of counseling, therefore, is to facilitate finer, adaptive discriminations that increase flexibility and situational adaptability. The client must learn to differentiate and deal with people as unique individuals, rather than responding, in effect, to fictional mental images.

Perceptual and interpersonal patterns that appear to have been transferred from past relationships also occur in counseling because the factors involved in the establishment and growth of the therapeutic relationship resemble those in any significant personal relationship. Such factors include issues of power and control, autonomy, trust, intimacy, and the manner in which differences, conflict, and disagreement are handled. The client will generally perceive these issues through his conditioned "spectacles" and attempt to cope with them in his usual overlearned ways, thus re-enacting his conflicts and troubles. Thus, the counselor-client relationship may become like a play that has been given day after day for years; the cast may change, but the script stays pretty much the same.

What, then, is the role of the past in counseling? Exploration of the past is not an end in itself. The past is important only as it relates to and affects present difficulties. In other words, the past influences present behavior only to the extent that past experience has shaped current perceptions. Thus behavior, though derived from the past, may be "functionally autonomous" in the present (Allport, 1960). Still, knowledge of significant past relationships and childhood perceptions may alert the counselor to what might recur in the counselor-client relationship and in the client's other current relationships. The counselor can listen for those needs the client has been unable to gratify and can assess their impact on the client's development and growth. As the counselor listens to the reconstruction of past scenes and frustrated needs, valuable clues may emerge about the needs the client is trying to satisfy in current relationships.

Once counselor and client discover such recurrent styles, however, it is generally more beneficial to conceptualize, reexperience, and resolve conflicts in the here-and-now than to safely "talk about" remote, vague, and possibly distorted conflicts of a similar nature in the past. Historical information may provide clues about self-defeating patterns of behavior and perceptual distortions, but "archaeological expeditions" aimed at gaining insight into the origins of patterns and conflicts are often only unproductive, intellectual pastimes and defense mechanisms. It is important to recognize that although patterns may have evolved from past situations, the client lives in the present and defeats himself in current relationships, not historical ones. As Strachey phrases it: "Instead of having to deal as best we may with conflicts of the remote past, which are concerned with dead circumstances and mummified personalities, and whose outcome is already determined, we find ourselves in an actual and immediate situation in which we and the patient are the principal characters" (1934, p. 132).

The therapeutic encounter involves and intermingles the totality of both participants, both their healthy and their unhealthy aspects. Thus the counselor's objectionable characteristics, distortions, and errors are part of the encounter, and the client reacts to these as well as to the counselor's desirable qualities. Therefore, not all conflicts in the helping relationship stem from the client's unrealistic reactions, and his feelings toward the counselor may be quite justified. The counselor should nurture an atmosphere in which such feelings may be openly expressed and understood. He should not simply dismiss the client's experiences in the immediate relationship as inappropriate or distorted. The fact is that at times the counselor may react in nontherapeutic ways that may resemble the reactions of significant others in the client's life, thus stimulating strong affect and reinforcing his old perceptions. However, all is not lost if the counselor becomes a participant in such conflict, provided he grasps what has happened, maintains rapport, and uses the experience as a springboard for mutual exploration of the nature of the current relationship and of other problems.

Responses stemming more from the therapist's own past than

from the current counseling situation are treated in the literature as problems of countertransference. The therapist is cautioned to be sufficiently aware of his own psychological makeup to keep the treatment focused on the client's perceptual and behavioral distortions. Countertransference detracts from therapy and may cause the client new problems.

Focusing on the transactions of the immediate relationship serves a number of purposes. First, such a focus demonstrates self-defeating patterns to the client far more forcefully than does the intellectually sterile analysis involved in "talking about" remote, bygone experiences. Additionally, concentrating on current experiences in the helping relationship shows the client how to be "fully present," a quality transferable to other relationships. The counselor's interpersonal skills and the interactional experience serve as models of effective interpersonal functioning and problem solving for the client. The client experiences firsthand how to deal with interpersonal friction and conflict, as well as warmth and caring, openly and productively.

Focusing on the immediate counseling relationship may be especially productive at those times when it serves as a catalyst for the client's self-exploration and insight. In fact, Fromm-Reichmann (1959) sees the relational immediacy process not only as productive, but as essential in certain situations, taking precedence over all other aspects of the patient's communication. In listing priorities for therapeutic focus, Wolberg (1967, pp. 425, 703) reinforces Fromm-Reichmann's view, according highest priority to transactions involving the immediate relationship. Focusing on the immediate interaction and relationship seems particularly indicated when: (1) the client has negative or unrealistic and unwarranted feelings toward the counselor or counseling (for example, anger, fear, distrust, dependency, sexual desires); (2) resistance or defensiveness is sufficiently strong to block progress; (3) significant conflicts over interpersonal issues in the counselor-client relationship occur; (4) the client's manipulative or dysfunctional style of relating or perceiving is manifested in the interview; (5) the counselor has strong, persistent feelings toward the client; and (6) the client is already referring to or discussing the current relationship.

When these conditions exist, focusing on these factors and the immediate relationship should take priority over dealing with such matters as pressing environmental concerns or sources of stress, past relationships or experiences, or other of the client's feelings.

Exploring the Client's Current Behavior

The counselor may use ongoing counseling interaction to assess the client's dysfunctional and manipulative behavior and his perceptual patterns, which may be reserved for later interpretation. Generally, if such patterns are acted out in the immediate relationship, similar patterns appear or have appeared in other relationships. Once the client becomes aware of the nature and ramifications of his current interactional behavior, he can be assisted to determine whether such patterns do indeed appear elsewhere.

When the client discusses conflicts experienced in other relationships, the counselor is advised to ponder the questions, "Are there any parallels in our relationship?" and, "Is the client really talking about our relationship and his reactions, feelings, fears, or anticipations regarding me?" Conflicts outside therapy may reflect interpersonal patterns that the client might later act out in therapy, or they may at times be a displacement of feelings toward the counselor. That is, the client may displace feelings toward the practitioner onto someone else and act them out for fear that broaching these feelings to the counselor might lead to rejection or censure. An example is an attractive, twenty-year-old female college student who had been seen in counseling for about a dozen appointments with a male counselor. Early in the interview she began talking about a recent date in which she found herself very attracted to her companion and so sexually aroused that she felt vulnerable and panicky. In previous interviews the counselor had noted that the client felt quite warm and close to him. Therefore, after empathically listening for a time, he inquired whether she had ever experienced such arousal and alarm in their relationship or in other relationships with men. This question led to her disclosing that she had panicked at the intense feelings she was developing toward the counselor and of the sexual dreams she was having. Further discussion enabled the client to learn more about her sexual feelings and to manage these feelings in the relationship with the counselor and other men. Often the discussion of outside conflicts will have no parallel to the current relationship, but occasionally they may forecast something to come or be a displacement, symbolizing reactions to the counselor.

The counselor must listen to more than the obvious content of the interview. He must evaluate the interaction between himself and the client, periodically taking time to ponder the norms that have developed for interaction, the roles each takes in the relationship, and the topics that are emphasized. For instance, an over-emphasis on either the past or the present to the neglect of the other could signal defensive avoidance. The counselor should also consider the current goals and the purposiveness of the client's behavior in the interview. In this regard, the reader may find it helpful to review the material presented in Chapter Six about the purposiveness of symptomatic behavior. An important question for the counselor to consider is, "What is the purpose of the client discussing this topic in this way at this time?" Particularly when the interaction becomes sterile, frustrating, or emotionally detached and intellectualized, the counselor should disengage and look beyond the immediate content to examine the process and the possible relationship messages implied by the client's communications. It is often illuminating to ask oneself such questions as: "What is being avoided by talking about this or by acting in this way at this time?" and "What is the purpose of this behavior, right now?" and "What would the client be doing (or discussing) if he were not doing (or discussing) this right now?"

The counselor should frequently assess the possible dynamic functions served by the client's here-and-now behavior. The client's interaction with the counselor may serve to safeguard self-esteem or to provide an excuse for postponing constructive action. Discussion of trivial events, for example, may avert the feared catastrophe of condemnation by distracting the counselor and leading him away from areas where the client feels vulnerable or threatened. Excessively seeking advice or professing inadequacy may be ways of transferring responsibility for self to the counselor, thereby gaining immunity or special consideration. Feelings may also serve purposive functions (Dreikurs, 1967). People have often been well conditioned to regard feelings as the result of some external act and to believe that behavior is largely governed by feelings beyond control. This is, of course, somewhat valid, but feelings may be goal-directed as well. Thus, similar to other behaviors, emotions may serve as an excuse or as a safeguard. For instance, some alcoholics may drink not only because they are tense, or "nervous," but may actually, without awareness, seek out situations that provoke the anxiety they need to excuse their drinking.

Feelings may also serve to demonstrate strength, heroism, or superiority or to justify retribution and retaliation. Horney identifies a pattern of "functional suffering," wherein one uses self-imposed "suffering" to manipulate others, to justify having one's own way, or to glorify oneself as a martyr, thus permitting secret superiority. A client's "conflict" over feelings that pull him in opposite directions may be less a "problem" than a purposive compromise that justifies indecision and inactivity. The person is willing to pay the price of being "in conflict" because it typically purchases either protection from a loss or retention of a gain (Mosak and Gushurst, 1971). Still other feelings or responses in counseling may function to create a safe distance in the relationship, to bid for attention or sympathy, to gain power or control over the counselor, to punish or seek revenge (for example, by making the counselor feel guilty), or to excuse retreat or failure in counseling. Thus the counselor is advised not merely to look for the "cause," or precipitant, of the client's feelings, but also to observe the consequences of the emotion by asking himself what such feelings accomplish for the client. It should be remembered, however, that the counselor's awareness of the interaction does not necessarily mean that the time is appropriate for interpretation to the client. Later in this chapter, the timing of immediacy interpretations will be considered.

The client can change the topic for reasons other than avoiding conflict or anxiety, but such a change of topic may well be much more than a random occurrence. Rather, seemingly disconnected topics can in fact be dynamically associated by some underlying relatedness or connection. For example, feelings toward a parent whom a client has been discussing may be similar to those towards a boss who is mentioned next. Thus the counselor must learn to pay attention to the process of the interaction and attempt to discern whether themes connect seemingly different topics, for if he interprets every change to a different and apparently unrelated thought as an avoidance, he may miss many opportunities to understand the broader nature of conflicts or of more underlying difficulties. To illustrate further, if a client shifts from exploring intruding sexual fantasies to mentioning some occurrence in the counseling relationship, the fantasies and the relationship may be psychologically associated.

In observing the nature of the client's immediate behavior, it is useful to form an impression of the client's typical interview behavior by observing his repetitive patterns of relating in counseling sessions. Deviations from these usual patterns may be cues to underlying relational issues that need to be resolved, such as distrust, resistance, or negative feelings toward the counselor. (Resistance will be considered in more detail below.) For example, the counselor might begin by saying, "I'm uncertain what's happening, but I notice some unusual or different things occurring today," and then proceed to wonder about the meaning of the client's unusual quietness, tenseness, distance, preoccupation, reluctance to talk, or the tendency to focus on distant and safe topics.

Using the Counselor's Current Experience

In addition to observing and raising questions about the client, the counselor must also maintain awareness of his own experiencing in the relationship. The counselor can learn to use himself as an instrument for assessing the client's dynamics. We pointed out above that when the client describes symptomatic behavior, the counselor listens to determine the impact of that behavior on other people and to deduce the goals and the purposes the behavior serves. Similarly, in the interview the counselor can attend to his own emotional response, observing personal reactions to the client's expressions and behavior. The counselor should ask himself, "What effect does this behavior have on me and on what occurs?" Awareness of personal reactions provides hypotheses about what reaction the client may be trying to evoke from the counselor. As mentioned earlier, clients without awareness frequently anticipate certain reactions from others and then by their own behavior provoke precisely those anticipated reactions. Thus they may be unconsciously seeking to produce the very feelings the counselor is experiencing, either to maintain and reinforce their perceptions of themselves or others or to serve any of the various purposes discussed above. A client may, for example, attempt to avoid closeness in the counseling relationship by being angry with the counselor and thus keeping him at a distance. Similarly, another client may test the counselor to assess the latter's competence, to see whether he can be trusted, and to determine whether the counselor will respond "like all the others." Such a client may experiment by behaving with aggressiveness, criticism, or provocation or by presenting unrealistic expectations and demands. Whatever the client's implicit strategy, it is quite likely a representative behavioral sample of his everyday patterns.

Any hypothesis that the client is trying to stimulate the counselor's inner reactions should be held tentatively, especially if based on a single event, until further experience shows it to be valid or invalid. An accurate assessment of the client's dynamics, however, requires that the counselor listen to more than the client; he must also listen to himself. If a client subtly attempts to elicit a specific reaction, and the counselor responds "naturally" in the intended manner, it follows that the counselor may unwittingly reinforce the client's behavior by responding just as most people would be expected to. For example, if a counselor personalizes a client's reaction of disappointment and anger and becomes guilty and threatened, he will probably confirm the client's anticipations and thus be responding much as the client's significant others would. When the counselor experiences strong feelings of anger, anxiety, fear, attraction, inadequacy, guilt, or confusion, a definite likelihood exists that the client may have been unconsciously seeking to stimulate these feelings for a definite purpose. This is another vital reason why the counselor is encouraged to explore his feelings further, seeking to understand them better, rather than responding impulsively.

To be a therapeutic agent, the counselor often needs to respond differently from others in the client's life, disconfirming his expectations. A response that contrasts strikingly with what the client anticipated throws him into disequilibrium, forcing him to differentiate the counselor from past figures and from mental images and stereotypes. The client must deal with a unique, real, and to some degree different and unpredictable individual rather than continuing to relate to his stereotype of the counselor. An example would be a client who attempts to provoke the counselor to become critical, judgmental, and angry, but elicits instead an empathic, accepting response. Such an unanticipated reaction will probably help the client distinguish his distorted inner assumptions and constructs from the external reality experience. Subsequently, the counselor could assist the client in developing awareness of his behavior, the "private logic" and motivations behind it, and its usual self-defeating consequences.

In the middle phase of counseling, one of the important roles the counselor often plays is that of a "frustrator." A client who is able to continue to manipulate and respond in counseling in the same self-defeating ways that typify life outside has succeeded in defeating himself and his counselor. The counselor, therefore, must gently frustrate the client's maladaptive ways of coping as they appear in therapy. It is crucially important to responding therapeutically that the counselor be able to determine the purposiveness of in-therapy behavior. Otherwise, the counselor might be entrapped and seduced into responding nontherapeutically. The counselor's awareness and use of self-experiencing, thus, is of vital importance in discerning the client's immediate interactional goals.

Determining which of the client's reactions are realistic and which are distorted requires the counselor to develop self-insight. The counselor must be aware of his impact upon others in order to distinguish inappropriate, irrational responses from appropriate and justified reactions. To help counselors evaluate their feelings toward the client and to increase their awareness of the interactional process and their part in it, the authors have compiled a list of questions that can be considered from time to time with each counseling case, particularly while reviewing audio- or videotapes of interviews. Most of the questions are adapted from Johnson (1946), Brammer and Shostrom (1968), and Wolberg (1967):

1. Was that response made to satisfy the client's needs or mine?

2. What was the purpose or goal of that intervention? Was it really to assist the client? What was I trying to convey to this client? What was I reacting to when making that remark? What did that do for me?

3. How do I feel about the client? Do I anticipate seeing him? Do I feel sorry, resentful, jealous, bored, or sleepy? Do I want to protect, reject, punish, or impress this client? Does this client impress me? Do I tend to feel guarded, become defensive or tend to

argue? Do I dream or fantasize about this client between interviews?

4.   Why do I have such attitudes or feelings? Is the client doing something to stir up such feelings? Does the client resemble anyone I have known in the past or know now? If so, are my attitudes or feelings being displaced onto the client, or am I reacting in an overgeneralized pattern?

5.   Was my response a mirror reaction, for example, rejecting in the client a part of myself, oversympathizing, or doing something of a similar sort?

6.   Why did I feel impelled to give advice at that point? What was my purpose and goal? Was it because I felt that the client expected me to have all the answers? And did I respond by being the all-wise sage or guru?

7.   Why did I become so emotionally involved with the client who felt _____? Could it be that I have similar feelings?

8.   What was the purpose of my talking so much in this interview? Was it because I felt I needed to impress the client with my own knowledge?

9.   Am I reluctant to let go when the counseling with a person has reached a good termination point or when I know he should be referred for a different kind of help? What is the purpose of my reluctance?

A further aid in discriminating the client's distortions is the early negotiation and structuring of the definition of the relationship, the counselor's role, and the goals of treatment. If such structuring was done properly in the early interviews, the counselor can review these factors to assist both himself and the client to see distortions for what they are. To illustrate, a client of one of the authors expressed resentment and irritation with his counselor for not providing answers and advice. Because the nature of counseling and the counselor's role was explicitly defined in the first interview, the counselor could review the agreement and point up the discrepancies between that agreement and the client's expectations. Thus the counselor responded: "I sense your aggravation at my not giving you more answers or telling you what to do. But you will recall that when we first talked, we mutually agreed that my role would not be to dispense solutions or direct your life for you. So I'm wondering if you might be angry at me for another reason, or if at other times you find yourself feeling disappointment and resentment towards someone who hasn't given you advice or direction. You know, I'm wondering if perhaps you associate caring with doing more for you in the way of telling you what to do."

Resistance and Defensiveness

Positive affective reactions by the client are generally helpful to counseling, and usually they warrant special attention only if they become unrealistic or reach such a magnitude that they constitute a therapeutic roadblock. Moreover, the counselor generally does not focus on or interpret the client's positive feelings toward the counselor (unless they have become a roadblock) because the client may perceive the counselor as romantically interested or as seeking to ridicule the client for his attraction to the counselor. Negative feelings toward the counselor or toward counseling, however, or defensive resistance to self-examination or behavior change require immediate attention from the counselor. If a client is already reacting negatively, the potential loss in exploring these feelings is minimal. Empathic recognition of the negative feelings that are impeding counseling and their possible subsequent interpretation and working through may increase the client's self-understanding as well as reestablish the therapeutic relationship, thereby allowing counseling to proceed productively. It is a basic rule that whenever discernible negative feeling or resistance disrupts counseling, the exploration of such roadblocks must take precedence over other content areas. If, however, a client vaguely alludes to some ambivalent feeling toward the counselor, such as distrust or annoyance, but immediately continues with productive self-exploration, the value of interpreting or focusing on such feelings is questionable, for the feelings seem not to be strong enough to interfere with the task of therapy. In fact, focusing on such feelings might hinder the client's self-initiated exploration. Moreover, interpretations founded on trivial manifestations and resistances may elicit untoward reactions from the client, such as the feeling of being scrutinized under a microscope or of being used to document the counselor's clinical acumen and brilliance.

One of the most common manifestations of resistance is silence, particularly when it is preceded or followed by cues indicating that the silence is a mechanism for avoiding the discomfort of self-

exploration. Another cue of a related type of resistance is superficial talk or intellectualization, which, because the client avoids
relevant material and personal feelings, involves very little self-
exploration. If the counselor attempts to channel the discussion
toward something more personal and emotionally alive, the client
may simply ignore the counselor's statements, respond mechan-
ically without affective involvement, or respond with a different
type of superficiality. Similarly, the client may avoid a personal
focus by persistently discussing "problems," other people, referral agents, or other topics without examining the personal significance or feelings these topics involve. Typically, the counselor
can take his own feelings of boredom or sleepiness as a cue to such
resistance.

Another indication of resistance, frequently motivated by
either fear or anger, is a pattern of arriving late for appointments
or forgetting them altogether. Repeated requests to change the
appointment time may also indicate resistance. The counselor's
natural response is to grant such a request, but acquiescence may
be counterproductive. Rather, the counselor should seek to discover the meaning of the client's behavior and also set some limits
on how much he is willing to be inconvenienced. With the client
who begins to arrive late or to forget appointments, the counselor
should similarly seek to explore the meaning or purposiveness of
this behavior and of any related implicit relationship messages. He
should not, however, extend the length of appointments to make up
for lost time, for that may reinforce the client's tardiness and invite
similar behavior in the future.

Resistance may appear as hostility or negative feelings toward
the counselor or as competitiveness. The client may manifest competitiveness by reading psychology books and testing the counselor's knowledge. He may attempt to put the counselor on the
defensive and raise his anxiety through such ploys as critical and
provocative challenges, questions, or attacks on the counselor's
shortcomings or flaws. For example, a client might remark, "I notice you keep playing with your ring. Do I make you nervous?"
Still other clients resist by displaying what Wolberg (1967) labeled a
"contempt for normality," challenging the predominant values
and norms as an excuse for not accepting responsibility, thereby
maintaining the status quo and avoiding needed changes.

Propositions, sexual seductiveness, and other attempts to redefine the helping relationship as a social-sexual one are still other resistances, and they too require immediate attention. When such situations arise, the counselor is wise initially to examine whether he might have somehow subtly invited such a response. If he rules out such a possibility, he might next ask the client, "How would that help you?", encouraging exploration of the purposiveness of the behavior. In such situations the counselor is well advised to clarify further his role, to redefine the limits of the relationship, to re-examine the mutual goals of counseling, and to show the client how his "game plan" defeats those goals. However, the counselor must be very sensitive and empathic in situations that leave the client very vulnerable to rejection, as abrupt or unskillful handling may result in embarrassment and termination. Thus, besides redefining limits and roles, one might share such personal feelings as, "I experience some real discomfort with that. If I responded in that manner, I'd be doing you a real disservice because we couldn't possibly reach the goals that we've been working towards. In fact, I'm afraid our relationship would just be a repetition of other relationships you've had. At the same time I'm concerned that you may feel pushed away or think that I don't like you. And I want you to know that that is not my feeling at all."

Resistance may also be manifested through "filibustering"—that is, using a flood of words to control the interview and keep the counselor at a distance. Acting-out outside the therapeutic hour has also been traditionally regarded as resistance to talking about feelings. Other common signs of possible resistance include failure to follow through on homework assignments and waiting until the end of the hour to bring up important material.

The client's negative feeling or resistance signals the counselor to attend to the immediate state of the relationship and to focus on here-and-now experiences. The counselor may intervene with relational empathic responses, with more interpretive additive empathic responses, with respect, with authentic sharing of his experiencing of the client or the relationship, or with confrontation. The appropriate response varies with the situation, a topic to be discussed later, but all such responses, no matter what the particular type, share a common focus on the current relationship experience.

Some general procedures regarding the therapeutic handling of resistance can be suggested. In those situations where the resistance appears to derive from heightened anxiety about the topic under discussion, the counselor might consider alleviating the anxiety by temporarily diverting the subject away from the threatening area to a neutral topic or by reducing the pace and intensity of the exploration. Otherwise, the first line of response to resistance or negative feelings is to recognize the feelings empathically and acknowledge the presence of the resistance. The resistance may be resolved by little more than calling attention to it, accepting the feelings, and listening empathically. This type of response is generally a unique and unanticipated experience for most clients—witnessing another person who is unafraid of acknowledging such feelings and who, rather than becoming defensive, remains respectful and seeks to understand. If these measures do not resolve the client's feelings and resistance, the counselor must help the client analyze the possible reasons for resisting and, if necessary, actively interpret the possible purposiveness of the resistance, tentatively examining the function of the behavior or feelings and perhaps comparing interview behavior with styles of relating outside counseling.

An example will illustrate a few of these procedures. If a male client verbalizes anger that the counselor is interested not in him but simply in the fee, the counselor can initially respond by empathically recognizing the client's anger and his feelings of being exploited. He may then respond authentically, explaining that rather than feeling uninterested (assuming that this is the case), he has been feeling quite warm toward the client and was growing increasingly close to him. If these responses seem to have little impact on the client's perception of the counselor, a number of alternatives are open. The counselor can openly encourage the client to specify what led him to conclude that the counselor had no personal interest in him (a respect response). The counselor may also encourage the client to interpret the possible purposes served by his own anger. If that response is unproductive, the counselor may offer tentative interpretations, including: "My actual feelings differ so much from your perceptions that I'm left wondering what your anger might be about?"; "Since those aren't my feelings

at all, I'm questioning if perhaps you might often feel that way—
that no one is truly interested or cares about you?"; "My actual feelings of closeness to you recently are in such contrast to the feelings
you describe that I wonder if the increased closeness between us
might be so uncomfortable for you that you'd like to push me back
and create some distance with your anger?"

The counselor may also attempt to create incentive and motivation for the client to proceed. One method is to use encouragement and to cite the positive gains that might accrue from continued exploration. The counselor, for example, can try to stimulate interest in continued self-exploration by defining it as a painful
but effective way of alleviating distress and of reaching the goals
sought in therapy. Another approach is to redefine a burdensome
difficulty as an intriguing challenge and an opportunity for growth
and mastery. One might also seek to motivate a resistant client by
showing care and concern and by providing encouragement, telling him in effect, "You are already halfway there, and I feel sad
to see you progress so well and then, when the going gets tough,
put on your track shoes and run backwards." Such a statement can
be followed with an expression of concern that such a flight might
simply repeat past performances of avoiding similar painful feelings. Then the counselor might add, "You have a choice of coping
with these feelings that way again or of taking a risk and struggling
with them." The counselor can further encourage the client by
affirming his belief in the client's capacity and strength to cope with
the difficult feelings.

Still another method for encouraging movement through
resistant impasses is to help the client save face by finding with
him an acceptable way of disclosing himself. The counselor can
often help the client give his problems, feelings, or behavior more
palatable and acceptable labels. Too frequently, the client (and the
counselor) attributes problems to internal psychopathology and
views himself as abnormal, underestimating the influence of a lack
of knowledge of productive alternatives and of the deleterious impact of environmental, contextual, and external stresses. An alert
counselor can often neutralize a conflict and reduce the client's
defensiveness through reinterpreting problems in a more sensitive
way. One method of doing this is to attribute positive intentions to

the client despite his apparently undesirable actions. This technique often defuses the situation, freeing the client from defensively justifying himself and thus protecting an already precarious self-esteem. The counselor can explain past "failures," for example, as the result of ignorance of alternatives, yet simultaneously credit the client with positive goals. By helping the client save face at critical and difficult times and see himself as human and imperfect rather than sick, we are enhancing internal motivation instead of using external leverage. At critical impasses, the counselor too often reacts as significant others have, by criticizing and focusing on deficits rather than providing the client with face-saving alternatives. Helping the client improve his crippling self-definition as a "bad" person afflicted with a malady tends to break an impasse and to foster additional movement.

Gendlin seems to present a similar view when he states, "The therapist must first and foremost respond to the positive tendency which needs to be carried further from out of the negative pattern" (1968, p. 224). Often, however, the "positive tendency" may not be readily apparent, especially to counselors trained to be "pathologists" and primarily concerned with ferreting out the unsavory. Some imagination may be required. Thus, to use part of an example cited by Gendlin, if a client were manipulatively pressuring the counselor to aid in some unrealistic enterprise, the counselor might choose to respond to the constructive component of the plan, that is, that the client is trying to help himself. As Gendlin further explains: "There is always a positive tendency which we can 'read' in the negative behavior. Such reading isn't a Pollyanna invention of ours. It is, rather, that something of importance is always just then being defeated, making for a problem" (1968, p. 224).

An example from the author's practice will shed further light on the therapeutic use of positive reinterpretation. In the third interview, which included both marital partners, the wife expressed ambivalent feelings about continuing marriage counseling. At times she was unsure whether she wanted to remain in the marriage, and she found herself having daydreams about being free and able to do what she wanted, including dating other men. She explained that because she married at an early age, she had never really dated anyone other than her husband. Now she felt trapped with three small children, and she was unsure whether she wanted to be married. Recognizing a veiled, yet positive thrust for change in the woman's ambivalence, the counselor responded, "I can see something positive in your daydreams because they reflect your desire to achieve greater personal fulfillment than you're presently receiving. That unwillingness to settle for an unfulfilling marriage is the very thrust that can help you to explore your situation more deeply and to think through the alternatives you have."

In this example, the wife's reluctance to continue counseling and her contemplation of moving out of the marriage are reconceptualized as a thrust toward constructive action, a thrust compatible with the purpose of counseling. The counselor's response likewise interprets counseling as directed not necessarily toward maintaining the marriage but toward helping her decide for herself what is best for her. The client is much less likely to resist counseling when it is so interpreted, and the opportunities for exploring the marital difficulties are enhanced. Confronting her with her resistance, by contrast, would probably strengthen her opposition to counseling.

There is an old saw that the pessimist says the bottle is half empty, but the optimist says it's half full. The difference is not the amount in the bottle, but the point of view of the observer. Perhaps resistance and defensiveness are often encouraged unwittingly by pessimistic therapists who never think of alternative views that might allow clients to save face and preserve what little self-esteem they have.

When other methods of resolving resistance have failed, the counselor may try the strong tactic of confronting the client with the undesired consequences of clinging to current behavior instead of exploring and working through his problems. The client might also be confronted with the discrepancies between his original goals and his current self-defeating behavior. If the roadblock remains despite all attempts to move it aside, the counselor may consider still other possibilities, such as consulting with another therapist to gain a fresh perspective of the dynamics of the impasse, inviting another professional to serve as a co-therapist (multiple therapy), and renegotiating the treatment contract and goals, and redefining the roles of counselor and client. Renegotiation may be necessary, for example, with "scalp collectors," those clients who approach therapy as a fencing match. When all other methods have failed, the counselor might consider using the technique of paradoxical intention (Fay, 1976), or he might discuss termination or referral to another counselor.

Relational Issues or Conflicts

As was pointed out earlier, the major factors in the development of the treatment relationship resemble those present in any significant, personal relationship. Furthermore, events in the relationship are channeled through the client's personal "perceptual filter," sometimes producing distortions that the client attempts to deal with in his usual, overlearned way. The result may be the re-enactment in the therapeutic relationship of many of the client's conflicts and problem styles. We will now highlight some of the most common developmental issues involved in counseling. When conflicts develop with regard to these relational issues, the counselor should focus on the current interaction both to facilitate the progress and growth of the treatment relationship and to utilize these dynamics as a fruitful source of learning for the client.

An issue often important early in the counseling relationship, and critically important with some clients, is trust versus distrust and fear. It is certainly natural to experience some hesitancy and anxiety at disclosing very personal experiences and feelings early in any relationship. Normally trust increases only gradually as a relationship grows and as the client senses the counselor is a person who genuinely seeks to be helpful, empathic, nonevaluative, and respectful. However, many clients have had life experiences wherein they have trusted, only to be emotionally wounded again and again, with the result that they have intense fears of relating to others. Still others have such low self-esteem and so many chronic doubts about their worth and adequacy that they are easily threatened, dreading exposure of their feared identities. Common fantasies and fears that assume catastrophic proportions in the minds of some clients include the fear of being exposed as deficient and inadequate; the fear of being ridiculed; the fear of being disapproved of or being disliked; the fear of being exploited, taken advantage of, or controlled; and the fear of facing the unpleasant consequences of certain acts. Many of these common fears, which cause problems in everyday relationships (for example, distrust of a spouse), may be detected by carefully observing the manner in which the client responds in the here-and-now with the counselor. It can be a powerful growth experience for a distrustful client to have his fears recognized empathically, examined, and gradually worked through in a relationship.

Closely related dynamically to patterns of distrust are those patterns involving covert longings for intimacy and closeness opposed by overt displays of self-isolation. When counseling proceeds effectively, it is natural for feelings of warmth, care, and closeness to develop between client and counselor. Since personally relevant and deeply emotional topics are discussed, the client often comes to feel better accepted and more fully understood by the counselor than by any other person. It may be anticipated that the client will respond in his usual pattern to the conflicting pulls toward intimacy on the one hand and isolation on the other. Thus a client may panic when he senses a feeling of closeness developing, and he may react defensively by responding in some manner that will increase the emotional distance between him and the counselor. As a sense of warmth evolves, an opposite-sex client may become threatened or may attempt to "sexualize" the relationship, having never learned how to handle emotional closeness or intimacy in male-female relationships without acting out such feelings sexually.

Issues of power, control, and competition versus cooperation often appear in the counseling relationship. If a client typically reacts to others as competitive rivals or plays such roles in daily interaction as the "bully," "dictator," "Mother Superior," "boss," "high-pressure salesman," "seducer," "know-it-all," or "con man," these same reactions and roles will likely be acted out with the counselor. Many clients implicitly operate on the fiction that they can best control their own impulses and destiny and avoid catastrophe by controlling other people. Thus, when threatened by possibly losing control in counseling, such clients will try to take charge of both the counseling process and the counselor. The strategy could be to outmaneuver verbally and filibuster, for example, or perhaps to disarm, control, and defeat through seductiveness.

If the client usually responds to authority with competitive fighting and rebellious resistance, submissiveness, or dependency, the probability is high that these styles will be reenacted in the relationship with the counselor. Thus, the relational issue of dependency versus autonomy must also be managed in counseling. Will the client seek simply to maintain autonomy and individuality, strive to overpower and dominate, or try to be led, taken care of, and protected like a child by placing the counselor in a parental role? The issue of agreement versus disagreement in handling differences, making decisions, and resolving conflicts also appears in the counseling relationship.

Techniques for Handling Relational Immediacy

Generally, focusing on and interpreting relational immediacy should wait until rapport and trust have developed. These two factors are crucial in helping the client endure the vulnerability, threat, and psychological pain at times associated with such an intense personal encounter. When strong, unyielding resistance is encountered early in therapy, however, an essential precondition to effective counseling may be to focus on the feelings that apparently derive from the immediacy of the relationship.

Fully experiencing the immediacy of the relational encounter can be powerful indeed. Focusing on feelings that flow from the encounter may, for example, take the client beyond talking about his fears of allowing friends to be close, to the experiencing, acknowledging, exploring, and resolving of his current fears in relating deeply to another human being—namely, the counselor—in the here-and-now. Such an example is the difference between the lived past and the immediate, living present. Therefore, the immediate interactional process can be used first for expanding the client's awareness and later for modeling, rehearsing, and acquiring new skills. We agree with Fromm-Reichmann's (1950) conclusion that the patient needs an experience, not an explanation.

An important principle for timing interpretations of relational immediacy is: *Experiencing precedes conceptualization.* The client must first be allowed to experience conflictual feelings before interpretations are offered. Allowing problem patterns to be reenacted, emotionally relived, and experienced in the current relationship before conceptualizing them creates a context wherein a powerful corrective emotional experience can occur. More is required, however, than simply eliciting current experiencing and affective expression (Lieberman, Yalom, and Miles, 1973). If conceptualization of meaning does not follow experiencing, there is the risk that the emotional experience will be merely emotional, not corrective. May, Angel, and Ellenberger express a similar belief about timing: "Furthermore, the only thing that will grasp the patient, and in the long run make it possible for her to change, is to experience fully and deeply that she is doing precisely this to a real person, myself, in this real moment. Part of the *sense of timing* in therapy . . . consists of letting the patient experience what he or she is doing until the experience really grasps him. Then and only then will an explanation of *why* help . . ." (1958, p. 83).

An example will clarify these ideas further. Suppose that a client is displacing feelings of fear in the counseling relationship by discussing those feelings in the safer context of relationships with *others*. Irrespective of whether the feelings are rationally justified or are inappropriate and distorted, the therapist's initial goal is to redirect the feelings to their actual source and to assist the client to own them before proceeding to examine and to explore them. Therefore, the therapist first interprets the safeguarding mechanism of displacing the feelings to the client, and then he channels the experiencing and expressing of the feelings to the current relationship. When the feelings are expressed, the counselor can respond by empathically recognizing and accepting them, fostering further expression or ventilation. If the counselor "deflects" the feelings, for example, by interpreting them as transferred from past relationships, he would deny their current validity and sacrifice the client's opportunity to experience and to explore the conflict in the present. Deflection to the past may serve primarily to protect both the therapist and the client, substituting a cognitive exercise and game for a significant emotional experience.

The guidelines for choosing and timing immediacy interpretations are similar to those for additive empathic responding (Chapter Six). Immediacy interpretations should be aimed at meanings just below awareness, rather than at deep meanings well beyond awareness. Although immediacy interpretations are often indicated when resistance develops, each and every hint of resistance or distortion need not receive attention. Such interventions should be made selectively when resistance, displacement, conflict, or distortion in the current relationship poses a barrier to progress and when adequate evidence of these problems has been provided through repeated manifestations of the behavior. Interpretations are not appropriate when based on weak inferential hypotheses supported only by indirect expressions or hazy connections to the current relationship. Rather, interpretations should be made only when they can be justified by specific and repeated referents in the client's behavior. Even in these instances, the interpretation should be tentative, not authoritative. Thus slips of speech, postures, and gestures may be taken as evidence along with other information or content, but all by themselves such indirect expressions are rarely enough to justify interpretations about current processes. Likewise, focusing attention on determining the meanings of isolated nonverbal interview behaviors, as gestalt therapists frequently do, may be unproductive; frequent interventions of this nature can in fact create excessive self-consciousness and thus inhibit spontaneity. Similar to additive empathic responses, interpretations of relational immediacy should not be offered rapid-fire, one after the other. Time must be provided for the client to assimilate each interpretation.

In exploring impasses in the helping relationship, it is crucial that the exploration not assume a win-lose flavor or evolve into a contest of personal power. Rather, the client needs to be helped to perceive that the therapist intends not to condemn or disparage, but to enhance his understanding of self-defeating perceptual and behavioral patterns manifested in the relationship. If the client feels disparaged, defeated, or threatened with the loss of self-esteem or the counselor's caring, the conflict will likely escalate. By contrast, the client will probably reciprocate the counselor's empathic sensitivity, warmth, and respect.

In working with the immediate relationship, the counselor should not merely offer his interpretations, but should also invite clients to summarize and conceptualize for themselves what has occurred. It is often productive for the counselor to inquire about his impact on the client, requesting feedback and responding to it with openness. It is also most productive for the counselor to present his observations and interpretations as his own opinions and perceptions, not as pronouncements of indisputable fact.

Counseling often has a particularly forceful impact when the counselor brings the client (and the subject matter) to the present. Responses directed to the here-and-now often affect awareness potently. Responses such as, "In fact, you seem to be feeling that right now," and "Perhaps you're afraid that is happening between us right now," tend to elicit reactions free of the censoring, distortion, and withholding common in exploring less immediate material more influenced by the client's defense mechanisms.

Another way of working with immediacy is to conduct here-and-now experiments with clients. The selective application of encounter techniques, such as the trust fall, in individual therapy is discussed by Gerber (1972). An illustration from the author's practice of a here-and-now experiment is given in the following case example.

> After a number of interviews with a divorced man in his late twenties, one of the authors had become aware that the client was distrustful and fearful of emotional closeness. Rather than discuss this problem at a distance, it was more powerfully examined in the immediacy of the counselor-client relationship. He was asked if he would be willing to try an experiment, to which he hesitantly consented. The counselor then explained, "I would like you to simply be aware of what you are currently feeling and of how your experiencing changes from moment to moment as I do something." The counselor then rolled his chair forward until he was at almost knee-to-knee closeness with the client and leaning forward. The client became visibly shaken and nervous, pushing his chair back a foot. Discussion then followed about his current feelings. The counselor then asked the client to be aware of his feelings and comfort level as he shifted his chair back, away from the client a few feet. This elementary exercise evoked powerful feelings and stimulated productive exploration of the client's conflicts about trust and intimacy and stimulated an examination of the current relationship.

Malamud (1973) uses an innovative technique for examining the immediate relationship when a session is at an impasse. In the middle of a session hampered by strong resistance and evasiveness, Malamud "scraps" the session. He announces (with a twinkle in the eye) that the session is over and asks the client to step out and sit in the waiting area. After a few minutes the counselor comes out as if beginning all over, greets the client, and starts a new session. The therapist opens the "new" session by asking for the client's reaction to the "previous" session. Yalom suggests a similar technique (1975, p. 138). In a session dominated by strong resistance, avoidance, and much left unspoken, the therapist stops in midsession and says, "We still have about twenty-five minutes left. I'd like you to imagine for a moment that our hour is already over and that you are on your way home. I wonder what disappointments you would have about our time together today."

Yalom, Brown and Block (1975) propose a "written-summary" procedure for therapy groups that can be applied to individual therapy and which in fact has been used by Yalom and Elkin (1974). In the written-summary technique, either the counselor or both the counselor and the client write a summary of each therapeutic session and then either mail the summary to the other participant or exchange it after a prescribed period of time.

The gestalt-therapy technique of "presentification," or use of the empty chair, might also be employed to advantage in helping the client differentiate the counselor from past figures or stereotypes. For example, if a female client is reacting to a male counselor much as she reacts to her father or to "men" in general, she might be encouraged to put her father or her stereotype of men in an empty chair and asked to discuss with her father, with men, and with the counselor the differences among them. When there is strong emotional "unfinished business" with a past figure, like the father of this hypothetical client, we have also instructed the client to close his eyes, picture the significant other in fantasy, and then in the present tense (as though the significant other were here now) to tell this person how he feels, what he experienced in the past, and, finally, how he wished their relationship could have been different. If the client has previously experienced any similar feelings toward the counselor, he might then be encouraged to contrast the past figure with the present counselor to facilitate differentiation and to distinguish realistic from unrealistic and distorted reactions.

Communication Exercises with Modeled Responses

The following exercises help in developing skills in responding with authenticity and in responding to situations involving relational immediacy. These exercises can be used for self-instruction or for instruction in a classroom. You should consider each statement and determine whether it requires an authentic response and whether it involves relational immediacy. Then write your response and compare it with the modeled response provided at the end of the exercises. Keep in mind that the modeled response is only one of many possible appropriate responses. Your goal is to achieve the ability to respond at the same moderate and high levels incorporated into the modeled responses.

CLIENT STATEMENTS

1. *Situation:* The client is a nineteen-year-old male who barely graduated from high school (taking special-education classes) because of learning difficulties associated with mild brain damage. He had particular trouble with subject matter requiring abstract reasoning such as mathematics and English. The youngest in a family of intellectually gifted children, he was referred by his parents because of inferiority feelings and the need for vocational guidance. He made the following statement in the ninth session.

Statement: "My brother is a chemist, you know. I don't think I'd like chemistry, but I've been thinking I might like to be a nuclear physicist. My brother says you can be anything you want if you apply yourself. I've never really applied myself. What do you think about me becoming a nuclear physicist?"

2. *Situation:* Mrs. S has come to see the therapist after a series of abortive efforts with other reputable therapists. The present therapist has the impression she has been "shopping around," as though seeking someone who can offer a magical solution to her problems. The following statement comes in the initial interview after the client has recited her problems and blamed her previous therapists for the failure of earlier therapeutic endeavors.

Statement: "Well, I've pretty well laid out my problems before you. Do you think you can help me?"

3. *20-year-old male referred by his father, a physician, during early portion of an initial interview:* "Dad said I should see you, that you're an expert in working with the kind of problem I have. A couple of my friends told me to see you, too, that you'd helped a couple of their fraternity brothers."

4.   *40-year-old mother receiving counseling for problems with adolescent children:* "It'd sure be nice to be a psychologist like you. Then I'd know just what to do with my kids instead of having such a constant hassle."

5.   *Situation:* The following statement is made during an individual interview with a marital partner one week after an interview with both partners. The couple had been seen for a total of eight interviews, including four individual and four conjoint.

Statement: "I found myself feeling angry with you all week. I felt you were siding with my husband last week and didn't understand my side at all. I almost decided not to come today."

6.   *Situation:* The client is a delinquent seventeen-year-old female who has been confined in a juvenile correctional institution. The counselor is a graduate student who has only recently begun her practicum assignment in the institution. The trainee has just introduced herself to the client and is somewhat apprehensive, and the client responds with contempt and anger.

Statement: "You mean I've got *another* counselor? What happened to the last one, did she get scared away? Are you another one of those students? You look pretty scared to me."

7.   *Situation:* The child-welfare protective-services worker is interviewing a twenty-eight-year-old divorced mother regarding a complaint that she has been neglecting her three small children, leaving them alone at home while she is drinking with friends. The worker has just explained his function of investigating the complaint to ascertain whether the children are being adequately provided for and to offer help if needed.

Statement: "You say you want to help me. Well, I don't need any help. Somebody's just trying to make trouble for me. My children get cared for all right. Say, you're not thinking of taking my kids away, are you?"

8.   *Situation:* The client is a forty-six-year-old female who was referred for therapy (with some pressure) by her husband because of excessive drinking and involvement with another man. She has been guarded in the first three interviews and has revealed little of her deeper feelings about her situation. The therapist has seen her as lacking motivation and coming chiefly to placate her husband. The statement comes early in the fourth session.

Statement: "Do you think I'm making any improvement?"

9. *Situation:* This statement takes place in the closing portion of the fourteenth and final session of marriage counseling. The counseling has been successful, and the counselor feels considerable regard for the couple. The wife is speaking.

Statement: "I really want to thank you for helping us work out our problems. Things have never been better between us. We can talk to each other openly, and we share so much together now. We are both just thrilled about our marriage now, and about life."

10. *19-year-old college student, tenth interview:* "Gee, I think I must be hopeless. I get so disgusted with myself. The instructor asks a question and I know the answer, but I just sit there like an imbecile, afraid to raise my hand. I think I'm a lost cause."

11. "We have seven children in our family, and I've felt that was too many for my parents. They couldn't spread themselves around to all of us. I'm very much in favor of planned parenthood. Don't you agree?"

12. *At conclusion of the sixth interview, as the client is leaving:* "I want you to know how much I appreciate you. Things have gone a lot better since I've been seeing you. I feel a lot better after our appointments."

13. *23-year-old female to female counselor:* "I've been afraid I might be a homosexual, and that's pretty heavy. I've been afraid to tell you because I've thought you'd think, 'Wow, on top of everything else she's a damn fag.'"

14. *18-year-old college male to male counselor, looking down:* "This is, uh, hard to talk about. I, uh, always sit close to the door in your office." He pauses. "Sometimes when I say things, uh, I'm afraid. I, uh, sit close to the door,"—he pauses again—"so I could get out quick if you, uh, got up to hit me."

15. "I've felt uneasy during the week about coming to see you after our last session. It's very awkward coming after I told you my deep feelings last week."

16. *Female client to male therapist:* "I don't trust any man; I feel I can't even trust my husband."

17. *23-year-old female to female therapist:* "Sometimes I've thought how neat it would have been if I could have had a mother like you."

18. *40-year-old female:* "I need help desperately. Tell me what to do, and I'll do anything you suggest if it'll help Karl (16-year-old

son)." She pauses, smiling, and says, "You be hard on me. I need someone to straighten me out."

19. "I got to feeling so down during the week—like I had to talk to someone. I wanted to call you so bad. I picked up the phone, but then I thought, 'He's real busy and wouldn't want me to bother him.'"

20. "When I told you how sick I was last time, I had the feeling you really didn't believe me."

21. "I've found myself wondering what you think about me. I want you to be impressed with me. I guess I want to be your favorite."

22. "I didn't really want to come today. Actually, it has been an eventful week." The client hesitates. "But I haven't felt I wanted to tell you about what was happening."

23. "I've had a feeling of your being present with me at home. It's a warm, reassuring feeling. And I find myself wanting to please you." The patient hesitates. "I'm finding it very difficult to talk about."

24. *Sixth interview with a client in his twenties who spends most of his time staring at his hands, rarely looking the therapist in the eye:* "I find I avoid people, avoid contact with people in a lot of ways. And yet, I'm so damn lonely. It's stupid."

25. *Situation:* A fearful and very inhibited opposite-sex client is in a therapy-group session. The client has a long and well-established relationship with both the group and the therapist. The client has just finished a tearful and emotional statement about how hard it was to lose a parent through death in the past week. The therapist is experiencing very warm, positive, close and caring feelings toward the client. The client concludes tearfully.

Statement: "I'm really glad I have this group to turn to, to talk about my feelings with. I know I'll be all right, but I sure needed someone to talk to tonight."

26. *19-year-old student in a trade school, third interview:* "I hope that between these tests I took and all your training and experience that you'll be able to tell me what I can do and what job I ought to go into."

27. *Minority group member:* "Hell, I just want to be accepted as myself, as a person, for what *I'm* capable of doing. I don't want to just be hired because of my skin color. That's as phony and degrad-

ing as being excluded because of my color. Why can't they just accept me for who I am."

28. "I learned something from a very early age. I got the message in one way or another from my mother that my ideas and feelings weren't right. If I ever really told her what I felt or thought, she'd correct me and find something wrong with it. I learned to protect myself and play-act. I just act like I believe I'm supposed to in a situation—tell 'em what they expect to hear so they won't disapprove."

29. *A middle-aged American Indian in the third interview:* "I don't like people who stereotype Indians. A lot of people think we are either all drunks, lazy, or that we still wear feathers."

30. *Situation:* A couple is in their seventh conjoint session of marriage counseling. There seems to be a warm and solid relationship between both partners and the counselor, and they both actively participate in exploring their problems. The counselor has just now become aware of a pattern, wherein the husband seems to keep cutting his wife off in her interactions with the counselor. She typically withdraws and allows her husband to talk for her. (Having just observed this situation, write an appropriate counselor response.)

31. *Situation:* In recent interviews and earlier in this interview, a thirty-three-year-old married client has been disclosing experiences and feelings he believes repulsive and shameful.

Statement: "You know, I really question if my wife could still care for me if she knew what I'm like."

32. *Client in early twenties, third interview:* "I went over to my parents' house for dinner yesterday. What a disaster! My father is so critical of me. I'm never good enough at anything for him. Whatever I wear, say, or believe, he'll find fault with."

33. *Tenth interview:* "I really got in touch with something this week. Because of what happened with Susan, I became aware that I've really had a tendency to stereotype people and file them away in a pigeonhole based on my first impressions of them."

34. *Married client, after critically describing recent interactions with his wife and his father:* "I guess I really expect a lot of people to have higher standards for them than they ever seem to have for themselves. I feel very disappointed with people. They never seem to follow through."

MODELED RESPONSES

1. "In all honesty I don't believe you could make it in physics. Physics requires a lot of math, and that's been one of your toughest subjects. Frankly, I don't agree with your brother. I know there are a lot of things I couldn't succeed in. I'd rather see you consider a vocation where you'd have a good chance of succeeding."

2. "That's a tough question to answer because the outcome to a great extent depends on you. You've seen some capable therapists previously, and it hasn't worked out. My impression is that your lack of success with other therapists may be rooted in the expectations you've had. I'd like to talk more about that with you."

3. "Well, I hope I can be helpful to you. But whether I am or not will depend on how *you* feel about seeing me and how we're able to work together. I'd like to give you an assurance I can be helpful, but that would be unrealistic because we hardly know one another at this point. I'd like to know more about *your* feelings about seeing me."

4. *The counselor chuckles:* "You know, it *would* be nice to know just what to do all the time. But being a psychologist doesn't make it any picnic. My wife and I have struggles with our children, too, as do all parents. In fact, sometimes it seems even tougher because I'm supposed to have all the answers. Well, I don't know *anyone* who has smooth sailing with adolescent children."

5. "I sense you're feeling some of that anger even now, and I appreciate your sharing it with me. It must have been very frustrating for you to feel I didn't understand your position. It's quite possible you're right about that. I'm human and sometimes assume I understand when I don't. Let's talk more about what you feel I failed to understand."

6. "You know, you've tuned in to my feelings pretty well. I guess I am a little scared. I'm new here and just feeling my way around. You sound pretty upset about having a new counselor. As a matter of fact, I am a student, but I'll be working with you until June. I gather you have some feeling about having a student for a counselor. Could you share some of those feelings with me?"

7. "Right now I'm more interested in talking with you further about you and the children so I can see the situation more clearly. Actually, I don't know enough at this point to make any recommendation. The court takes custody of children to protect them

only as a last resort. I'm here to get better acquainted with you and your situation and to determine if any course of action is needed to assure that the children receive adequate care."

8. "I'm glad you asked that because I've been asking myself the same question. Actually, I've felt some frustration because I've felt we haven't been making any progress. Probably you've had similar feelings, or you wouldn't be asking the question. My impression has been that you've been struggling with whether you really want to get very deeply involved with therapy. I'd appreciate hearing where you are in that regard."

9. "I really feel great about that. I'm excited hearing how things are going between you. I've seen a lot of strength in both of you as you've worked to resolve your conflicts and want you to know I've enjoyed watching the two of you grow closer together. In the process I've come to feel close to both of you."

10. "Craig, I want you to know that you're far from a lost cause. You may find it hard to believe, but I can remember when I was struggling with a lot of the same kinds of feelings, being afraid to speak up. I can remember being shortchanged in stores several times and never saying anything because I was afraid and didn't want to cause any trouble. It was a real struggle for me to overcome those fears and to learn to face situations. I often thought of myself as hopeless, too. Many people struggle with similar fears, and some people go through life apologizing for themselves. But you don't have to be that way if you're sufficiently determined to overcome those fears. I'm wondering what was going on inside of you, your thoughts and feelings, as you struggled with the issue of answering the instructor's question."

11. "I guess I believe it's really an individual matter. Planned parenthood seems to fit for many people, and with the population problem it makes good sense. Still, some people are morally opposed for religious reasons. I can respect both points of view. But I guess you're saying that a large family caused some real frustrations for you. You seemed to be saying your parents weren't as available as you'd have liked, as though you had a longing for a closer relationship with them."

12. "Thank you. You know, I'm really pleased that things are going better for you and that I've been able to play a part in your progress."

13. "So you've really been living with the fear you might be homosexual. And on top of that, afraid I'd condemn you if I knew. Ginny, whether you're homosexual or not wouldn't be the determining factor in my feelings toward you. I've come to know you as a warm, sensitive, worthwhile person, and whether or not you're homosexual isn't going to change your value in my eyes."

14. This interchange is taken verbatim from an interview of one of the authors.

Therapist: "I wonder if that's what you're feeling just now, afraid of me."

Client: "Yeah, how'd you know?"

Therapist: "Your hesitancy in expressing the feelings tells me you're uncomfortable and that you're really risking yourself now."

Client: "Yeah, that's for sure!"

Therapist: "I'm wondering where that fear comes from, if I say or do anything that makes you afraid."

Client, pensively pausing: "No, not really."

Therapist: "Well, I'm glad about that. I honestly haven't been aware of any angry feelings toward you, and it wouldn't be at all like me to want to hit you. That fear must come from somewhere else."

Client: "Yeah, when I think about it, I don't really believe you'd hit me. I think I'm just afraid of older men. I know it's crazy. I was always afraid of my dad. He had an awful temper." The client continues self-exploration.

15. "I feel bad about your uneasiness because it occurred to me after our interview that you'd really shared some deep and personal feelings. I thought afterwards that you might have these feelings. I'm sorry I overlooked talking with you about that last week. It may have eased some of your discomfort."

16. "I can understand then that you might also be having some feelings of distrust for me. Could you tell me about the feelings you're experiencing in our relationship?"

17. *The counselor smiles warmly:* "Thank you for the compliment. It sounds as though you're feeling some real closeness in our relationship and experiencing my feelings of care for you, the kind of feeling you longed for as a child but never received from your

stepmother. I appreciate your feelings keenly and I value you as a person."

18. "I can sense the desperation you're feeling and the urgency of your desire to be helped with Karl. I sincerely hope I can be helpful. But as for my being hard on you and straightening you out—well, I'm not sure that would be helpful. It would be like putting me in the driver's seat and would be demeaning to you. I'd like to think of our relationship as more of a partnership with the two of us searching together for some better ways of relating to Karl."

19. "You know, I have some mixed feelings about what you just said. I'm pleased you see me as someone you'd want to turn to when you feel as badly as you did. But I feel bad that you thought I wouldn't want to be bothered. I want you to know that if you get to feeling desperate, I am someone who cares and that it's okay to call me. On the other hand, unless you're really desperate, it's usually better to tough it out until our appointment. Though it can be very painful to wait, you may find you have more strength to draw from than you might believe. Part of our task together is to help you to find that strength within yourself."

Explanation: Situations like this one have to be handled delicately. The client may feel overwhelmed by his problems and, if a positive relationship with the counselor has evolved, will feel a natural inclination to depend upon the counselor when under stress. Although the client needs to experience the caring and commitment of the counselor and derives a sense of strength therefrom, offering oneself too readily may foster dependency and prevent the client from activating latent strengths. The counselor should convey his availability in bona-fide emergencies but should always bear it in mind that his responsibility is to help the client to discover and to use his own personal resources.

20. "You know, that really makes me feel bad for a couple of reasons. It must have been very distressing to you to think I didn't believe you. Actually, I accepted what you told me at face value. If I'd had any questions, I'd have let you know. I guess I'm feeling some concern, too, that you didn't share your feelings *last* week because that, too, suggests you're feeling some uncertainty in our relationship. Tell me, what are you feeling just now as we discuss this?"

21. "So it's important to you that I have a favorable impression of you. But I gather the feelings go beyond that. It's as though you find yourself wanting to be very special to me, as though being less than favorite might leave some doubt as to how you stand with me. I wonder about that feeling of wanting to be the favorite, if perhaps you've experienced it in other relationships."

22. "So your reluctance to come has to do with your feelings about sharing with me what is happening. I gather you may have been feeling apprehensive about how I might respond if you shared what is happening. I wonder what you're experiencing right now, as we talk about it."

23. "So you're feeling very uncomfortable about sharing your feelings of closeness with me. I'm sensing that you would like me to have similar feelings of care for you, but you're perhaps afraid that I might not accept your feelings and desires. I do appreciate the courage it took for you to share these feelings with me and want you to know that I too have feelings of care for you. Considering how lonely you've been in your life, letting yourself feel closeness with me represents a major step in learning to feel closeness with others."

24. This exchange is an excerpt from an interview of one of the authors.

Therapist: "You really frustrate yourself." He pauses. "And are you aware of how you're avoiding contact with *me* right now?"

Client, looking up: "Huh?" He pauses. "Well, I guess one way I avoid everybody and push them away is by not looking at them." He looks back down at his hands.

Therapist: "I wonder if we could try a little experiment right now and just see what happens. I'd like you to try something." As the therapist points back and forth between his eyes and the client's, he says, "I want you to look up at me and just try remaining in contact with me, for a minute." There is a pause. "What do you experience as we do this?"

25. "While you were talking, my spontaneous impulse was to reach out and touch you on the arm or take your hand. I didn't because I was concerned I might frighten you if I did that. But I'd like you to know how very warm and close I feel to you and that I really wanted to give you some support and to let you know I was with you as you were struggling with those painful feelings."

26. "I need to share with you that I'm feeling very uncomfortable with the idea that I'd be able to tell you what to do with your life. As I tell you this, I'm also aware of feeling quite concerned that you may be disappointed or upset, and yet I honestly don't believe that I could know what would be best for you. I wouldn't want to make such an important decision for you. But the tests may give us some ideas to consider, and I'm surely willing to help you think through some of your alternatives."

27. "It's damn aggravating to not be seen or valued for yourself. A number of years ago when I was a student, I remember being hired for a job by a family friend because of who my father was, and on that job I was always just seen as his son and never accepted as me, for who I was or what I accomplished. That was so frustrating and degrading for me that I found another job as soon as possible. But I guess you're saying you feel that way *frequently* because of your skin color."

28. "Guess I'm wondering if you might be fearful that I'm finding fault with you too. And if you're feeling some need to protect yourself with me and play-act at times so that I won't be critical."

29. "I'm wondering if you might also be expressing some hesitancy and concern about me, wondering if *I* stereotype you like that?"

30. "I just noticed something occur between the two of you that I've observed a number of times previously. John, as Alice was talking, you cut in, sort of took over, and spoke for her. Then you, Alice, just kind of pulled back and let him do the talking for you. I can't help wondering if this doesn't happen often between the two of you. As that happened just now I found myself imagining that because of that you, John, must surely miss out on sharing a lot of what Alice has to offer but likely keeps shut up inside while you take the ball and run with it. And it's sad for you also, Alice. I'm wondering if when you allow him to take over in this way, it doesn't leave you feeling terribly frustrated, overlooked, and lonely."

31. "I'm wondering if you're also experiencing some fearfulness about our relationship right now and if you're questioning whether *I* could still respect and like *you*, knowing so much about you."

Explanation: This response assumes that the client is experiencing feelings of uncertainty in the relationship with the counselor and that this was, therefore, checked out. In such situations, however, the primary feelings may be toward another person, in this case, the wife. The counselor will also need to check this out.

32. "Have you ever been fearful that I might be responding similarly to you—finding fault and judging you as not measuring up?"

33. "I'm curious how you might have stereotyped me."

34. "I gather you may also have set some high standards for me and perhaps have experienced disappointment that I haven't measured up to your expectations."

Practicum Exercises in Authenticity and Relational Immediacy

It is, of course, one thing to compose good responses with paper and pencil and quite another to respond facilitatively in an actual interview. The following exercises help the reader bridge the gap.

EXERCISE ONE

The reader should recall relationships in his personal life in which there are unresolved issues or emotional "unfinished business." When the reader has pinpointed such a relationship, he should close his eyes and mentally picture the person involved as clearly and in as much detail as possible. It seems preferable to visualize the person, but if this proves extremely difficult, the reader can open his eyes and sit directly across from an empty chair, imagining the other person seated there. Speaking in the present tense, as though the individual involved were actually present, discuss your feelings about and perceptions of the relationship and the other person. Struggle to share authentically and constructively the range and complexity of your feelings.

EXERCISE TWO

This exercise is designed for practice groups in a classroom or workshop setting. Ask the group to write their authentic, immediate impressions of each member. These impressions are not necessarily meant to be openly shared, but rather to stimulate trainees to become more fully aware of their own current impressions, feelings, and relationship states. Next, divide the group into pairs, and have each individual sit facing his partner. The partners are to alternate speaking and at least initially to begin each sentence with the statement "Right now I'm aware of _____," saying what they are aware of in the here-and-now within themselves and in their interaction with each other. For example, one participant might begin, "Right now I'm aware of feeling very nervous and awkward and of noticing how you keep looking at your hands rather than at me." After two or three minutes, the partners move closer, take each other's hands, and continue the exercise. This procedure is not particularly intended to facilitate closeness—indeed, it may cause anxiety or embarrassment. The intent of this procedure, as of the entire exercise, is simply to provide an interpersonal context wherein the trainee may focus on current feelings and relational immediacy. During the exercise, participants might share feelings of discomfort, apprehension, irritation, or fear; strengths perceived in the partner or things they like about the partner; and feelings about where they might like the current relationship to go in the future. All communications should focus on here-and-now experiencing.

EXERCISE THREE

In a classroom or workshop setting, participants form triads. One member role-plays a client, another role-plays a counselor, and the third acts as a rater-observer. During a role-playing sequence, the counselor should seek to convey, as appropriate, all the therapeutic dimensions discussed thus far: empathy, respect, authenticity, and relational immediacy. Afterward, the client and the rater-observer give the counselor detailed feedback and rate his performance on those dimensions. The participants then exchange roles.

Chapter 10

ⱩⱩⱩⱩⱩⱩⱩⱩⱩⱩⱩⱩ ⱩⱩⱩⱩⱩⱩⱩⱩⱩ

Using Confrontation
to Remove Barriers
to Communication
and Change

It is fitting that confrontation be the final therapeutic dimension discussed in this book, for using it effectively demands high levels of all of the interpersonal skills we have treated. In this chapter, we will detail the why, what, when, and how of confrontation, building upon relevant information provided in Chapter One. The Confrontation Scale will be introduced, and its levels illustrated. Exercises in discriminating different levels of confrontation will be omitted, however, for the different levels are easily discerned without practice. In the final part of the chapter, exercises and modeled responses will be provided to assist the reader in advancing his skill with this potent technique.

It will be recalled from Chapter One that the fundamental purpose of confrontation is to facilitate change by expanding the client's awareness and motivating him to action in those aspects of living in which growth has been impeded by some barrier. Counseling and psychotherapy are commonly thwarted by an impasse that impedes progress until the sources of the impasse are identified and the impasse surmounted. Confrontation is an important tool in the therapist's armamentarium, employed to help the client achieve essential awareness of the forces blocking the thrust toward growth and change and to enhance the client's motivation to undertake remedial actions.

An adequate understanding of the purpose of confrontation requires a more thorough familiarity with the nature of the dynamic forces opposing change than we have provided thus far. The common barriers to growth and change essentially fall into two categories: (1) defense and adaptive mechanisms, and (2) natural human inclinations to perpetuate the status quo.

The defense mechanisms, of course, serve to safeguard self-esteem, maintain equilibrium, and protect the individual from becoming overwhelmed by anxiety associated with painful memories, unacceptable impulses and longings, guilt feelings, and other powerful emotions. Defense mechanisms and other adaptive patterns evolve early in life and are vital in helping the individual cope with the stresses and vicissitudes of existence. Certain mechanisms that serve vital defensive functions in childhood may, however, retain their full power and become dysfunctional or maladaptive later in life. The defense mechanism of denial, for example, keeps problem situations or feelings from consciousness, thereby precluding efforts to solve problems. Projection and rationalization, used to some extent by everyone, externalize responsibility for problems, emotions, and motives that, in fact, originate within, thus causing problems to be defined erroneously and hindering appropriate remedial actions. Isolation of affect and the related obsessive-compulsive patterns produce rigidity in behavior, constrict emotions and inhibit spontaneity, all effects inimical to emotional growth and change. Displacement, acting out, and conversion mechanisms are avoidance patterns that divert the person from facing problems directly and thus serve to perpetuate troubles.

Of the natural human inclinations that impede growth and change, the first relates to what might best be characterized as inertia. Many emotional, cognitive, and behavioral patterns are deeply entrenched and are, therefore, notorious for their tendency to persist despite vigorous efforts to change them. Consequently, major changes in these patterns are rarely achieved without a difficult, painful, and often prolonged struggle. Moreover, many people, particularly those with marked defects in character, tend to follow the path of least resistance even when confronted with exigencies that demand change, such as the threat of divorce or of the loss of custody of children.

Another major barrier to change, alluded to in Chapter Two, is the tendency of many troubled people to cling tenaciously to familiar ways of coping, however inadequate they may be, rather than face the unknown or feared consequences of unfamiliar ways. On the basis of logic, one would conclude that troubled people would welcome new approaches to coping with difficulties and would apply them without delay. Logic, however, is notoriously unreliable as a predictor of human behavior. Unfamiliar coping patterns bring people face to face with the unknown, and for many troubled people, confronting the unknown is tantamount to risking some vaguely defined disaster. Rather than take that risk, many people relegate themselves to the sidelines of life, secretly longing for life's potential successes and joys, but fearing catastrophe too much to do more than watch and wish.

This painful dilemma is well illustrated in the following poem, written during psychotherapy by a former patient of one of the authors:

Potato Bug
I'm a little potato bug.
Deep down in the dark I've dug.
It's snug down here and safe, too.
I'm all alone and hidden from view.

It's a long, long ways to the light above
Where the world sings and lives and loves.
The earth grows heavy over my head,
Here in my dark, sheltered bed.

The cold creeps up and chills my toes.
There's not a soul to hear my woes.
Hmmmm, this snug, sheltered cave
Is nothing but a deep, dark grave.

It's a long, long ways to the spinning world
That gives and takes with arms unfurled.
If I in warmth am to delight
I'll have to learn to bear the light.

From the poem, it is apparent that this patient is painfully aware of the discomfort she must bear and the direction she must take to overcome her self-imposed isolation. This awareness, incidentally, was reached with a minimum of confrontation by the therapist. Indeed, many clients gradually yield their defense mechanisms and surmount other barriers to change as their self-confidence, courage, and self-awareness increase in a therapeutic relationship characterized by high levels of the facilitative conditions. It will be recalled from Chapter One that confrontation is no substitute for these vital interpersonal ingredients. Respect fosters trust, self-respect, confidence, and courage. Authenticity encourages the client to take risks in relating with increased openness and spontaneity. Empathic communication, particularly at additive levels, enhances self-awareness and the conscious experiencing of emotions and thoughts. However, even though confrontation does not replace these interpersonal skills, it is sometimes an essential tool for correcting the refractory blind spots in the self-perceptions of some clients. Such blind spots may occur for many reasons, but all humans suffer from the limitation of being unable to step outside one's own perceptual field to look at the self. This reality sharply constrains our capacity to view ourselves objectively, a major cause of distorted self-perceptions and of the barriers to change.

Blind spots are also caused by the need to protect the self against the possible effects of receiving information about the self that is ego-alien and may destroy self-esteem. The need to protect, it follows, is the greatest for those who have weak self-concepts and are therefore most vulnerable to verbal assaults. Ill-timed and poorly handled confrontations are not unlike verbal assaults, and therefore may be deleterious or, at best, ineffectual. Premature, excessive, and otherwise bungled confrontations may precipitate psychic decompensation in the form of regressive dependency, psychotic reactions, or other psychological casualties. If the individual's protective mechanisms are functioning adequately, however, the patient may simply fail to comprehend a confrontation or reject it because he is unready to accept and integrate the input. In this regard, May cogently argues, "The act of perceiving also requires the capacity to bring to birth something in one's self; if one cannot, or for some reason is not ready, to bring to birth in himself some position, some *stance* toward what he is seeing, he cannot perceive it. . . . It is clear that the patient cannot get insights, perceive truths about himself and his life until he is ready to take some stand toward the truths, until he is able to conceive them" (1969, pp. 236–237). For this reason, keen timing is of the essence in confrontation, a subject reserved for later in the chapter.

That the therapist occupies an external vantage point and possesses a frame of reference different from the patient's is of strategic significance. This should not be construed to mean that the therapist's perceptions are always accurate, since his own perceptual screen may get in the way. The therapist's external position, however, makes it possible for him to offer fresh perspectives and corrective feedback in those instances when lack of self-awareness, distorted perceptions, irrational fears, and dysfunctional adaptive patterns are impeding the client's growth and change. Indeed, it is this very need for new perspectives and corrective feedback that motivates most people to seek help from another person when their usual coping patterns are unsuccessful. This, then, brings us to the essence of confrontation: to help the client face or achieve awareness of some aspect of his thoughts, feelings, or behavior that is contributing to or maintaining the difficulties. Confrontation thus aims at creating a moment of truth, which enables the client to assume responsibility for changing problem feelings, thoughts, or behavior that have been heretofore unrecognized, denied, ignored, or evaded.

Although empathic communication, particularly at additive levels, serves the same purpose as confrontation, the two processes are qualitatively different. Empathic communication is responsive in nature—that is, empathic responses reflect and add to the patient's feelings. In short, the direction of the therapist's response is predetermined to a great extent by the feelings the client expresses. In confrontation, however, the therapist's response emanates from the therapist's external frame of reference. Moreover, confrontation is aimed at helping the patient to understand aspects of himself that have for some reason escaped awareness, whereas empathic communication, particularly at the intermediate level, conveys the therapist's understanding of the client's expression or experience.

Yet empathic communication and confrontation do have much in common. Additive empathy depends on the therapist's external frame of reference, since it goes beyond the client's expression of feelings to draw on the therapist's understanding of the psychodynamics involved in the situation under discussion. Similarly, confrontation, like additive empathy, involves feelings at the edge of the client's awareness. In helping clients work through or surmount barriers to change, for example, it is a rule of thumb that the feelings underlying the resistance must be brought to light and resolved. As explained in Chapter Nine and earlier in this chapter, resistance is rooted in fear of the unknown and in emotions experienced in the immediacy of the therapeutic relationship. Confrontations that exclude these underlying emotions are usually ineffective and may, in fact, produce negative consequences. Because emotions are invariably associated with resistance to change, it follows that skills in relating with high levels of empathy are prerequisite to effective confrontation. Carkhuff (1969) and Egan (1975), in fact, take the position that confrontation at its best is an extension of accurate empathy, because the unmasking is based on a deep understanding of the client's feelings, experiences, and behavior.

Therapists who make frequent use of confrontation generally are those who have failed to master the other facilitative dimensions. The skillful use of the facilitative conditions, particularly additive levels of empathy, diminishes the need for confrontation, because the client tends to engage in self-confrontation increasingly as counseling progresses. Self-confrontation is preferred to therapist-initiated confrontation for two vital reasons: (1) self-confrontation is less risky; and (2) the client's readiness to integrate insights is assured in self-confrontation, whereas the therapist always faces the danger of initiating a confrontation before the client is ready to integrate the new insights. Clients, of course, vary widely in the extent to which they engage in self-confrontation. Emotionally secure, psychologically minded, introspective persons with strong self-concepts engage in self-confrontations quite readily. Most such individuals, however, are well adjusted and usually have little need for counseling or therapy. Thus those people least likely to engage in self-confrontation are those most likely to need therapy.

The readiness of some clients to engage in self-confrontation develops only gradually, at best, and with these clients, therapist-initiated confrontations often are essential to progress in counseling. Clients with certain character disorders, for example, tend to live on the surface, out of touch with their deeper emotions and with the impact of their behavior on others. Similarly, many of these clients are also prone to externalize responsibility by blaming others and circumstances for their difficulties. A common example is the antisocial personality who has frequent brushes with the law, culminating in periods of incarceration. Typically, such persons disavow responsibility for their difficulties, attributing them instead to a "bum rap" or a "snitch" (stool pigeon). These clients, who frequently are referred for professional help because of the trouble they cause others, are notoriously impervious to insight-oriented approaches, and in working with them confrontation plays a greater role than it does with other types of clients. Confrontation and type of client will be discussed later.

The Confrontation Scale*

Having defined confrontation and established its significance in therapy, let us turn to the how of confrontation. The Confrontation Scale delineates five levels of skill in employing confrontations. The reader is encouraged to study the scale carefully in conjunction with the brief examples of the five levels that follow. Further examples of effective confrontation appear in the text below and in the exercises with modeled responses in the final portion of this chapter.

LEVEL 1.0

The therapist ignores, overlooks, or passively accepts the client's inconsistencies, discrepancies, and dysfunctional behavior. Thus, potentially productive areas for confrontation are neglected.

*This scale is adapted from a similar scale developed by Carkhuff (1969).

Also included in this level are confrontations that are abrasive, critical, or blaming or that otherwise demean the client.

LEVEL 2.0

Fertile areas for confrontation are not overlooked, but the therapist does not overtly identify discrepancies, inconsistencies, and dysfunctional patterns. Rather, the therapist responds with silence or simply reflects the client's reactions to the problem behavior. Also included are those confrontations that are premature and poorly timed but which otherwise adhere to the guidelines for effective confrontation.

LEVEL 3.0

The therapist draws attention to discrepancies, inconsistencies, or dysfunctional behavior by questioning the behavior or identifying it as dysfunctional. Confrontations at this level tend to be speculative. Efforts to facilitate self-confrontation fall into this category. Timing is appropriate, and the client is not demeaned.

LEVEL 4.0

The therapist directly and specifically focuses upon and identifies discrepancies, inconsistencies, and dysfunctional behaviors. The timing is appropriate, and the client is challenged to modify the dysfunctional behavior. The dignity and self-esteem of the client are protected.

LEVEL 5.0

The therapist confronts discrepancies, inconsistencies, and dysfunctional behaviors directly and with a keen sense of timing. A high level of respect for the client's growth potential and self-esteem is conveyed. The confrontation embodies caring and helpful intent.

Examples of the Levels of Confrontation

The Brown family was referred for therapy by a school counselor because Richard, a fifteen-year-old, had been fooling around in school and doing poorly despite excellent potential. The parents had also expressed concern because Richard was associating with undesirable companions, staying out late, and using force to dominate the other children in the family. Mr. Brown, a successful businessman, spent little time with Richard, who resented his father for his authoritarian approach to discipline. The father, however, expressed a strong desire to have a better relationship with Richard, the other children, and his wife. He demonstrated some awareness of his tendency to exercise power excessively and requested help in learning to communicate more effectively. The following excerpt is taken from the fifth conjoint family session following a discussion of improvement in the communication between Richard and his father.

Mother: "The problem this past week hasn't been between Richard and his father. That's been better. But when his father is out of town, Richard tries to be the boss, and he orders the other kids around. He hit Bruce so hard it left a deep bruise on his arm."

Richard (defensively): "Well, if you'd ever get after the kids when they're being obnoxious, I wouldn't have to."

Mother: "But it isn't your place, Richard. It just makes it harder for me, and the kids resent you. You can't expect them to respect you when you bully them around."

Richard: "Well, if you'd. . . ."

Father (interrupting angrily): "Richard, I've told you a thousand times to leave the kids alone. When are you going to wise up?"

LEVEL 1.0 RESPONSE

"Sounds like there's a real problem when Dad's out of town."
Explanation. This response ignores the discrepancy between the father's hostile message and his expressed goal of improving his relationship with Richard. Thus, an opportunity for helping the father recognize his dysfunctional behavior is neglected.

LEVEL 1.0 RESPONSE

(To father): "Hey, look what you're doing. You're interrupting Richard and putting him down. How do you ever expect to have a better relationship when you do that?"
Explanation: A confrontation is appropriate, but this one is

abrasive and blaming. The father will feel put down by the therapist in the same manner that Richard feels put down by the father. Moreover, the father will feel demeaned in the eyes of the family members. The father can be expected to respond by withdrawing or by arguing defensively.

LEVEL 2.0 RESPONSE

(To father): "You're feeling angry at Richard right now."

Explanation. This response conveys empathy for the father's expressed feeling, but fails to identify the inconsistency between the father's behavior and his expressed goals. The ensuing interaction may be expected to elicit feelings but not get to the dysfunctional communicational patterns.

LEVEL 3.0 RESPONSE

(To family): "I wonder if we could stop just a minute and look at what happened. What do you think just happened?"

(Or, to father): "What did you do just now?"

(Or, to Richard): "Richard, would you tell your father your feelings about what he just said."

Explanation: In each of the above responses, the therapist intervenes actively, drawing focus to the destructive impact of the dysfunctional communication. The goal of the intervention is to facilitate self-confrontation by stimulating the family members, especially the father, to examine the dysfunctional behavior.

LEVEL 4.0 RESPONSE

"Hey, let's stop a minute and talk about what just happened. Dad, you were starting to get angry with Richard, and you cut him off in the middle of what he was saying. It's like what was happening is what you're all wanting to change. It just results in your pushing each other further apart. Richard, Mother, and Dad, I'd like you to share with each other what you were beginning to feel, but this time try to hear each other out and understand why the other might feel as he or she does."

Explanation. This discrepancy between the expressed goal and the immediate behavior is confronted on the spot, and the probable consequence of the behavior is highlighted. The therapist gives the participants responsibility for altering their behavior by asking them to discuss their immediate feelings.

LEVEL 5.0 RESPONSE

"Let's stop for a moment and analyze what just happened. I'm concerned about the direction you were moving because you cut Richard off, Dad, and you were starting to get angry with each other. I don't want to see that happen, because you push each other away and can't achieve your goals that way. Let's see if you can understand more what each of you is feeling right now about the problem we were discussing, but this time listen carefully to each other and try not to blame anyone for the problem."

Explanation. The dysfunctional communication is confronted directly, and the discrepancy between the behavior and the expressed goal is highlighted. The therapist gives suggestions for more effective communication and points the participants in that direction. Concern for the destructive impact of the behavior of the participants is given as the reason for the confrontation.

Guidelines for Confrontation

Emanuel S. Hammer says, "It's important not to get so used to tearing away people's masks that you no longer hear the rip" (1968, p. 150). Confrontation is an intense and potent method that may be psychonoxious rather than therapeutic. Some therapists routinely operate in a confrontive and highly intrusive style, justifying their approach as a "high-risk but high-yield" method. Lieberman, Yalom, and Miles (1973), however, discovered that this justification is a myth. Their findings demonstrate that destructive group leaders are often highly confrontive and challenging individuals, who frequently attack or reject members and seemingly ignore the concept of gradual change, impatiently pressuring clients for instant change. These leaders view therapy as unvarying and fail to differentiate individuals. Rather than responding to personal dynamics and tailoring treatment to the particular person, they often develop a format consisting of a "hot seat with no escape hatch" and pressure everyone to be more spontaneous, emotionally expressive, and less inhibited (Yalom and Lieberman, 1971; Lieberman, Yalom and Miles, 1973). Parloff critically warns against this type of therapeutic approach: "Leaders must also be willing to accept the assumption that not everyone is benefited by the opportunity to 'let it all hang out.' Some may, indeed, need help 'tucking it all in'" (1970, p. 203).

Confrontation is a tool and method, not a style of therapy. It is potent medicine to be used judiciously and in tolerable doses, not dispensed in an indiscriminate manner that can overwhelm the client with excessive stimulus. Borrowing an analogy that Lazarus applies to encounter groups, confrontation for some patients is about as helpful as surgery without suturing (1971, p. 186). Lieberman, Yalom, and Miles conclude that "*High* challenge or confrontation by the leader is not only unnecessary for change but is negatively correlated with outcome. . . . From the point of view of the individual, our data could give no support to the adage that a person must first be shaken up if he is to change" (1973, p. 435, emphasis added). They emphasize even more forcefully that a therapist or leader "must have a deep appreciation for the tenacity and the self-preservatory function of defense mechanisms. They cannot be battered down; patience, working through, and time are essential companions of change. . . . To attack an individual in an effort to dislodge him from familiar defensive niches is crude and often counterproductive; to attack him punitively because he refuses to comply with the leader's timetable and route for change is ignorant and censurable. . . . Timing, patience, resistance, and transference have been overlooked in the avalanche of new enthusiastic change efforts" (p. 436).

The therapist should not expect sudden or dramatic changes from a single confrontation. To expand awareness and to motivate the client to take remedial action are, of course, the primary goals of confrontation, but it would be naive to expect a single insight to produce change. Immediate change occurs but rarely. Even when a client accepts a confrontation fully, change generally requires a subsequent process of digesting, integrating, and evolving new, functional behaviors. This process of working through involves repeated reviewing of the same conflicts and of the client's typical reactions to them, but from fresh and ever-broadening perspectives. Fromm-Reichmann explains the process as follows: "Any understanding, any new piece of awareness which has been gained by interpretive clarification, has to be reconquered and tested time and again and in connections and contacts with other interlocking experiences, which may or may not have to be subsequently approached interpretively in their own right" (1950, p. 141). Raimy shows that this process, which he terms "the principle of repeated cognitive review," is an integral part of most, if not all approaches to therapy (1975, pp. 68–75).

As a general rule, confrontation is contraindicated until a good therapeutic relationship has been established. It is crucial that the client trust the counselor and perceive his helpful intent, caring, respect, and empathy. The relationship helps establish the counselor as a significant other in the client's life, adding credibility to his perceptions and increasing his reinforcing value. Even strength confrontations are generally inappropriate early in counseling. Until rapport is established, the client may interpret a strength confrontation as insincere or unempathic and out of tune with his turmoil and pain.

Early in therapy the focus is on seeing the client as he sees himself and acknowledging this view, not on sharing the counselor's differing perceptions. Understanding is a prerequisite for confrontation. Empathic responsiveness early in counseling maximizes the accuracy of later confrontations. Additionally, when the client feels understood, he is more willing to tolerate challenge and the introduction of the counselor's frame of reference. A relevant general guideline is: *Precede and follow confrontations with empathic responsiveness.* This procedure lowers threat, minimizes defensiveness, and increases receptivity to the confrontation. Furthermore, empathic responding immediately following confrontation makes the counselor aware of the effect of the intervention on the client.

The goal of confrontation is to expand the client's awareness through the counselor's feedback about discrepancies, but the client must assume the responsibility for change. His right to self-determination should always be respected and preserved. Although the counselor may at times present his frame of reference forcefully, the goal of confrontation is not to impose his views on the client. The counselor should not violate the client's autonomy, become coercive, or use confrontation to dominate the client. The client needs to sense that although the counselor is willing to be candid and authentic in sharing his perceptions of inconsistencies, he will respectfully accept the client and not infringe on his right to choose his own direction.

Confrontations should be delivered in an atmosphere of warmth, caring, concern, and understanding, not in a cold, impersonal, and uncaring way. All too often, the client perceives confrontation as a disparaging attack. The counselor is simply acting out in a destructive and hostile manner when he punitively belittles, reproaches, or tears the client down. The counselor should not play prosecuting attorney, confronting and accusing in order to evoke a confession of guilt. Berenson and Mitchell (1974) report that forty-three counselors rated low in empathy, respect, and genuineness used over fifteen times as many confrontations focused on weakness and deficits as did thirteen highly facilitative counselors. Furthermore, the thirteen facilitative counselors used over twice as many confrontations concentrating on the client's assets and strengths as did the forty-three low facilitators. Thus, in addition to being cold and abrasive, destructive counselors focus on the unsavory and pathological, regarding it as Pollyanna-like to credit the client's strengths. Confrontation to call attention to assets is particularly called for with self-effacing clients whose character style is to play the weakling. Similarly, confrontation focusing on perceived similarities to other "normal" people may be very beneficial with self-critical clients who have difficulty accepting their humanness and mistakes. The keys to facilitative confrontation are to learn to confront without affronting, to be sensitive enough to time interventions carefully, and to convey caring and regard in the confrontation.

Confrontation is widely misused, however. It is not uncommon to find counselors who confront in an impatient and demanding manner, expecting the client to be superhuman and "leap tall buildings in a single bound." Such impatience and pressure reflects the counselor's magical thinking and his need for immediate gratification, which is not dissimilar from the unreal expectations of many clients. Shaping should not be ignored in confrontation; when small changes and improvements are made, they should be acknowledged and recognized. Pressuring the client for immediate change often results in psychological casualties and deterioration, rather than improvement. Confrontation is generally contraindicated with severely disturbed and psychotic clients who have difficulty tolerating pressure and tend to misinterpret confrontations, withdrawing even further from interpersonal contact as a result.

There is a danger that confrontations may emanate from the counselor's narcissism or his unconscious goal and fantasy of being a guru or magical healer. Confrontation is meant to be a type of authentic disclosure motivated by the counselor's caring and involvement. For some counselors, however, confrontation serves as a proving ground for neurotic personal goals. A highly confrontive style may be a clue to the counselor's need to establish his "rightness," to validate his perceptions as superior, or to overpower, control, and manipulate. Therapists should always remain aware of the temptation to use confrontation to validate one's sense of power.

Another problem is the use of confrontation as a vehicle to ventilate anger with a client under the pretense of being therapeutic and helpful. In this case, the counselor takes on the role of either the prosecutor or the critical parent, with the neurotic goal of retaliation and retribution motivating the confrontation. Confrontation might be used in retaliation to an attack by the client or to prod the client when he is not progressing rapidly. In striving to be successful and to feel competent, the counselor can easily misuse confrontation to push clients too fast or to subtly punish unsuccessful clients. In all these instances, we observe the paradox of the counselor busily confronting self-defeating patterns in clients, while unaware of his own self-defeating style of confrontation. Confrontation should remain descriptive, not evaluative or judgmental. It should specifically describe and document the client's behavior and the counselor's reactions instead of overgeneralizing and pasting some ill-defined label on the client. Thus, rather than confronting a client with how "passive" he is, one might document the inconsistency between what the client says he wants and how little he has done to get it.

One risk with forceful confrontation is that a client may change for the wrong reasons—namely, submissive compliance and dependency. If a counselor continually pressures a client to change, he may convey a lack of acceptance of the client or perhaps even outright rejection. A client may respond to such disapproval or punitiveness by temporarily modifying his behavior to meet the counselor's expectations and please him. Such a shift of the locus of self-evaluation from within the self to an outsider is particularly possible with clients whose life style consists of subtly inviting coercion, pressure, demands, or attack from others and then complying. A compliant response to confrontation may be defensive. As an example, fearing the loss of the counselor's approval, a client might compliantly agree with a statement from the counselor and by that agreement evade self-examination and exploration. When a counselor senses that a client may be responding compliantly, he would be wise to follow the confrontation with the inquiry, "What do you think or feel about what I just said?"

Frequent confrontation also involves a risk directly opposite to compliance—that is, rebellion against pressure or perceived authority. When a client is already in crisis in his life, the counselor is advised against adding the therapeutic crisis of confrontation. Anxious, neurotic clients who are self-dissatisfied, pressured, and feeling inner conflict and guilt over their behavior generally are not in need of nor receptive to confrontation. In addition to being anxious already, such clients are prone to be overly sensitive to the views and perceptions of others. With these neurotic clients, the goal generally is to reduce anxiety and to foster independent and assertive behavior with supportive rather than confrontive approaches. However, with other clients, confrontation is almost essential and may even be introduced at minimal levels (level 3.0) relatively early in counseling. The population with which confrontation is most appropriate comprises those subject to what have traditionally and popularly been called character disorders. These clients frequently come to therapy under external pressure from a spouse, the court, or perhaps a child-welfare agency after their behavior has brought them into conflict with others. The client, however, experiences minimal inner conflict or anxiety, and he is self-satisfied and typically insensitive to the needs, feelings, and perceptions of others. In fact, clients with character disorders commonly believe that they are entitled to life on their own terms, and they are grossly lacking in empathy for others.

Confrontation is prescribed with such individuals to induce conflict and increase their anxiety, ideally facilitating self-evaluation. Confrontation involving the counselor's perceptions is indicated precisely because these clients tend to be unconcerned about and unaware of how others feel about them and perceive them. Furthermore, since this type of client has a very resistant character style, he frequently resists meaningful involvement in therapy. At such times, when indirect methods have not facilitated involvement, confrontation may serve to motivate exploration or movement by creating a crisis in the therapeutic relationship. A very passive-aggressive individual, for example, may feign cooperation with the counselor, while his real but hidden goal is to avoid involvement. An attempt to generate some motivation to change, however, may be made by confronting the client with his hidden motive and to illuminate the self-defeating nature of his avoidance behavior. In addition to getting at the feelings behind resistance to change, confrontation is also very useful with patterns of impulsive acting-out without concern for the consequences of the behavior.

In sum, as one considers confrontation in the middle and later phases of counseling, it is helpful to recall that the counselor must commonly play the "frustrator." Confrontation, used nondestructively yet firmly, is often the tool of choice to frustrate the client who habitually uses overlearned, maladaptive modes of coping and manipulating. Thus confrontations often serve to set limits with manipulative and demanding clients. A valuable method of confrontation is silence. Silence and ambiguity, rather than a predictable response, may have a highly confrontive impact and may also be used to extinguish inappropriate behavior.

A basic therapeutic principle is to use the least directiveness and force necessary to accomplish the therapeutic objectives. The law of parsimony similarly encourages the use of simple methods before complex ones. In addition, the counselor is advised to facilitate self-confrontation whenever possible. It is highly respectful not to do for a client what the client can do for himself. Directing a client's attention or consideration to an issue is often enough to encourage confrontation of self, and certainly self-confrontation is preferable to having an all-wise and all-knowing counselor steadily spoonfeeding the client. Learning by self-discovery is to be encouraged. Confrontation and directiveness have a distinct place in counseling, especially when time is limited and when the client manifests a lack of insight into discrepancies and inconsistencies. However, besides tempting the therapist to misuse his power, confrontation and directiveness may also reinforce the basic problem afflicting many clients—the tendency to look to the environment for support and answers instead of relying on one's self and one's own strength.

The facilitation of self-confrontation is rated at level 3.0 on the Confrontation Scale. Introducing confrontation at this minimal level encourages the clients to take maximal responsibility for exploration and change. Threat is minimized when the counselor simply raises a question about a contradiction, makes tentative comparisons of inconsistencies, or reflects discrepancies. Questions encouraging self-confrontation include: "What did you just do?"; "What are you avoiding right now?" "What would happen if you did not have that symptom?"; "I wonder if _____ is inconsistent or incompatible with _____. Do you see any contradiction?"; "You see the situation that way. Could you conjure up in your mind a group of your friends (or of people off the street)? Do you think they would perceive the situation any differently?"; "Does your behavior (feeling) fit with your goals?" A particularly useful type of level 3.0 confrontation is simply to describe the client's current behavior. This is a tentative confrontation wherein the client's behavior and discrepancies are "reflected," with the responsibility for following through and elaborating left with the client. Thus a counselor might say, "I notice that you look away from me," "I was just aware that you changed the subject," "You say you want _____, and yet you _____," or "You have tears in your eyes." Without elaboration or interpretation, a counselor might simply describe a discrepancy: "You say you're angry with me, but you have tears in your eyes," or "You tell me that you love Helen, and yet you avoid her."

One method for facilitating self-confrontation is what Levitsky and Perls (1970) call repetition and what Finney (1972) describes as "Say It Again." This technique may be particularly useful when a client swiftly passes over a significant word, phrase, or sentence. The counselor can simply request, "Could you say that again?" He may encourage the repetition several times, until the client grasps the emotional impact or meaning. Repetition may similarly be used with significant nonverbal gestures, where the client is asked, "Would you do that again?"

Discrepancies and inconsistencies are the prime target of confrontation. In order to confront effectively, the counselor must be attentive to discrepancies between verbal and nonverbal expressions, between what the client says and what he does, between ideal and real selves, between how he experiences himself and how the counselor or others experience him, and between the client's feared identity and real self. Because discrepancies are the central focus in confrontation, we will now provide a framework for conceptualizing and recognizing common discrepancies.

Confronting Discrepancies and Problem Behaviors

It should be evident by now that behavioral discrepancies are inimical to constructive change and that confrontation promotes change by focusing on discrepancies. The term *behavioral* is used in a broad sense, including thoughts, feelings, and experiences besides overt behavior. The major experiential domains of discrepancies and problem behaviors are the cognitive-perceptual, affective (emotional), and behavioral. These domains are not mutually exclusive, as will become readily apparent to the reader. Moreover, specific discrepancies are not limited to one domain, but may involve interaction between them, such as discrepancies between the cognitive-perceptual and the affective or between the affective and behavioral. Similarly, some of the specific types of discrepancies subsumed under each of the experiential domains overlap. Discrepancies do not fit into neat compartments. Our typology is largely for conceptual convenience.

The reader may question why the cognitive and perceptual domains have been combined. The rationale for this decision is that perceptions do not exist independent of the personal meanings and intentions ascribed to the object perceived. Three men, for example, may perceive the same woman in sharply contrasting ways because of differing perceptual sets shaped by certain cognitive assumptions and intentions toward women, which in turn are affected by the diverse past experiences of the three men. Let the woman in this example be attractive, shapely, well-dressed, and youthful in appearance. One of the men may view her as an object to be pursued for sexual conquest. The second male may perceive her as Madonna-like, pure and virtuous, to be admired and protected, but certainly not lusted after. The third male may perceive the same woman as cold, distant, and potentially controlling—a person not to be trusted and preferably to be avoided. All three men observe the same woman, yet their perceptions of her differ remarkably because of intervening cognitive processes. Laymen recognize the inseparability of the perceptual from the cognitive, as indicated in the commonly accepted aphorism that people see what they want to see and hear what they want to hear. The reader who would like to pursue further the intertwining of cognitive and perceptual processes is referred to May's cogent discussion of this topic (1969, pp. 235–238).

COGNITIVE-PERCEPTUAL DISCREPANCIES

Difficulties rooted in the cognitive-perceptual realm are encountered very frequently, and it is important, therefore, that helping professionals be thoroughly familiar with their manifestations, dynamics, and therapeutic management. The significance of cognitive-perceptual factors is reflected in the fact that some theorists (Beck, 1976; Ellis, 1962; and Raimy, 1975) have based approaches to intervention on cognitive-perceptual conceptualizations. Cognitive-perceptual discrepancies can be divided into eleven types.

Erroneous or insufficient information. A substantial number of the problems counselors and therapists encounter appear to be associated with the client's lack of knowledge or inaccurate information. As one example, many people with drinking problems, as well as their spouses, are unaware of the indicators of alcoholism, and they struggle to no avail for long periods of time, denying the problem or attributing their difficulties to the wrong cause. Certainly, it would be naive to assume that accurate information would be accepted in the majority of cases, for denial and rationalization are employed extensively by alcoholics and sometimes by their spouses. Nevertheless, the imparting of valid information, termed "didactic confrontation" by Berenson and Mitchell (1974), may prompt many individuals to seek help, such as that provided by Alcoholics Anonymous, thus turning their efforts from ineffectual floundering to productive problem solving.

Other common areas in which lack of accurate information may cause difficulties include parent-child problems and sexual troubles. With respect to the former, many parents raise children in destructive ways simply because they do not know anything better. Other parents, unfamiliar with what can be reasonably expected of children as they develop, may have unrealistic expectations, causing undue stress for their children and perhaps producing strains in the relationship with them. In the sexual area, problems commonly exist because of ignorance by one or both partners about the physiology of sex, techniques of adequate sexual stimulation, normal sexual behavior, or other aspects of sex.

Confrontation focuses on the discrepancy between the client's information and valid information. Imparting correct information would appear to be a simple matter, and, indeed, it is. Care, however, must be taken to handle the situation tactfully and sensitively, so as not to cause the client to look foolish or to lose face because he was inadequately informed. Humility on the counselor's part is most desirable, however learned he may be, for a humble counselor will have no need to demonstrate superior knowledge or intellect and will seek to preserve and nurture the client's self-respect. A pompous or arrogant counselor, by contrast, will demean the client, who will likely respond with increasing guardedness in confiding problems that might reveal his lack of knowledge. Other clients may simply terminate counseling, demonstrating sound judgment in protecting themselves from further humiliation and possible psychological damage.

Misconceptions about the self. Central to the majority of theories about psychopathology and psychotherapy are factors related to misconceptions about the self. Raimy (1975) convincingly documents the centrality of misconceptions to client-centered therapy, Adlerian therapy, rational-emotive therapy, transactional analysis, gestalt therapy, certain behavior therapies (including modeling), and direct psychoanalysis. To these theories, we would add existential psychotherapy. The self-concept is also pivotal to the phenomenological theories of Combs and Snygg (1959), who conceive of the self as an object in the individual's perceptual field. This "phenomenal self" is composed of everything experienced by the person as "me." Inadequate individual behavior, according to these authors, is caused by an inadequately differentiated phenomenal self and by related aspects of the total perceptual field that block the basic motivation to make the self "more adequate to cope with life" (p. 46). Successful psychotherapy, it follows, is directed to bringing about increased perceptual differentiation of the self. Although these theories emphasize the cognitive dimensions and the causes of misconceptions about the self in widely varying degrees, common to all is the importance accorded to beliefs, attitudes, assumptions, and feelings about the self as the determinants of behavior and the targets of therapeutic intervention.

The client enters psychotherapy with vague, diffuse, and inaccurate perceptions of himself and his world of experience, many of which were discussed in Chapter Six. Confrontation and additive empathy are aimed at helping the client recognize the discrepancies in his self-concept and "to reorganize his self-concept in close alignment with external reality" (Combs and Snygg, 1959, p. 436). Whether or not one subscribes to the formulations of Combs and Snygg or other "self theorists," familiarity with the manifestations and psychodynamic significance of misconceptions about the self is vital, for one will encounter such problems irrespective of one's theoretical predilections.

Self-conceptions are major determinants of individual behavior, interpersonal patterns, and life styles. A person who conceives of the self as inferior and of little value, for example, may fear exposure and humiliation in social interactions. To protect the self from exposure and humiliation, such a person may go to great lengths to avoid "risky" human encounters and may adopt a seclusive "lone wolf" life style. Similarly, those with what Raimy terms "special-person misconceptions" (1975, pp. 109–116) tend to be very striving individuals whose self-esteem depends upon believing that they hold special status in the eyes of others. As such, their self-esteem may be somewhat tenuous and susceptible to others' changing impressions of them.

Misconceptions of the self may also predispose the individual to certain maladaptive patterns. Raimy (1975) identifies clusters of misconceptions of the self commonly associated with reactive depression, obsessive behavior, hysterical personality, phobia, and phrenophobia. Raimy coined that last term to refer to "the false belief, and associated fear, that there is something wrong with one's mind which may result in 'insanity'" (p. 103). As an example of the misconceptions associated with a maladaptive pattern, consider these three found almost universally among reactive depressives: "I am, have been, and will remain hopeless"; "I have no interest in anything and will never be able to regain interest in anything"; "I am not angry or hostile toward anyone. I alone am responsible for my present condition" (p. 100).

In the authors' experience, the misconceptions of the self most frequently encountered are those which we categorize as self-demeaning. The category includes misconceptions that one is inferior, inadequate, worthless, unlovable, unattractive, stupid, different, and the like. Such misconceptions predispose people to vastly underestimate their capabilities and value, thereby causing fear of failure, discouragement, indecisiveness, and social inhibition. Individuals with such misconceptions of the self may perceive opportunities as "failure traps," hesitating or declining to risk new experiences, such as training programs, learning new skills, or dating. For example, when a client of one of the authors attended a company picnic, she always stood aside and watched the others play volleyball, secretly longing to get into the game but holding back for fear that she would miss the ball and look like a clumsy fool. Another client admired a university classmate at a distance, longing to become better acquainted with her but fearing he would be disdainfully rejected. Ironically, she was equally attracted to the client and could not understand why he seemed to avoid her glances.

Self-demeaning misconceptions also pervade the counseling process, often vitiating the client's thrust for growth and change. Fears of failure and rejection by others, feelings of helplessness, and other self-demeaning reactions may present major impediments to progress in counseling. In such instances, confrontation involving the discrepancy between the client's self-perception and the counselor's perception of him is indicated. Such strength confrontations involve crediting the client's past accomplishments, realistically assessing his personal resources, and authentically sharing one's perceptions of the client's potentialities (see Chapter Nine). It should be recalled from Chapter One that research indicates that strength confrontations are prominent in the repertoires of high-facilitative therapists, while low-facilitative therapists turn frequently to weakness confrontations.

Another deterrent to counseling is the common misconception that given personality attributes or behavioral patterns are fixed and immutable. Many clients employ this misconception to avoid committing themselves to changes essential to problem resolution.

Statements such as, "That's just the way I am," "I've always been that way," or "It's not my nature to show affection," reflect this misconception and imply that change is unreasonable and contrary to human nature. Movement, of course, requires that such misconceptions be confronted and the client helped to see that change is in fact possible and that the only obstacle is his misconception.

Self-demeaning misconceptions also affect interpersonal perceptions and patterns deleteriously. Doubts of one's self-worth or the perception of oneself as stupid or inadequate color one's perceptions of how one stands in the eyes of others. Persons with negative self-concepts thus not only tend to be hypersensitive to criticism, but may also perceive criticism when none is intended. Self-doubts and conceptions of limited self-worth may also contribute to an excessive need to please others, or, more accurately stated, to avoid displeasing others. Thus obsequious, ingratiating, placating, and similar patterns may derive from the misconception that one cannot be accepted for what he is and can avoid rejection only by slavishly seeking to meet the needs of others, real or imagined.

In therapy, misconceptions about the self arise as the client explores his deeper feelings, particularly those involving the self-concept. A climate conducive to self-exploration is fostered by removing threat from therapy, which is best accomplished by high levels of the facilitative conditions. As the client increasingly explores his deeper feelings, the misconceptions in the self-concept become more apparent to him. This awareness combined with consistently high respect and corrective feedback from the therapist provides the impetus for the client to divest him of misconceptions and to evolve an accurate self-concept. A self-concept is not easily overhauled, however, and the task often requires extensive working-through.

Interpersonal misconceptions and perceptual distortions. Misconceptions and perceptual distortions in interpersonal relationships may be associated with many factors other than misconceptions of the self. Misconceptions about sex roles, authority, and human beings in general are common. An erroneous assumption held by many males, for example, is that it is unmasculine to long for dependency or to demonstrate feelings of tenderness. Likewise, some females mistakenly believe that it is not feminine to experience erotic pleasure or to make sexual overtures to a marital partner.

Also prevalent are misconceptions regarding the opposite sex, which may produce avoidance patterns or cause interactional difficulties. It is not uncommon, for example, for some females to believe that all males are immature, irresponsible, and undependable. Still others mistakenly believe that any demonstration of affection by a male is intended merely as a prelude to sexual intercourse. A corollary to this idea is the misconception that the interest of males in females is exclusively sexual. Males, on the other hand, may hold to the distorted belief that all females are golddiggers, castrating, or emotionally flighty.

Other common misconceptions for which confrontation is appropriate involve beliefs that people in authority are punitive, exploitive, and repressive. Those who harbor this misconception tend to resent authority, often openly rebelling against supervisors, police, teachers, and other authority figures. As a consequence of their antagonism toward authority, such individuals often have difficulty holding jobs. Other group misconceptions are common. Some people, for example, mistakenly believe that all businessmen are crooks, liars, and cheats. Others are convinced that all religious people are hypocrites, all politicians dishonest, and all welfare recipients lazy, conniving parasites. Still others have stereotypes about members of certain races, ethnic groups, and religions.

Common to such misconceptions are stereotyped perceptions (faulty overgeneralizations) applied indiscriminately to all members of a given group. Overgeneralization, it will be recalled from Chapter Nine, may also be involved in the helping relationship. Some clients, for example, mistakenly believe that the therapist has no personal commitment to them and is interested only in the fees he collects. Others place the therapist in the "authority" category and fear they will be controlled, punished, or exploited in some fashion. The therapist's task is to help the client make finer interpersonal discriminations, thereby aligning his perceptions with reality, as discussed in Chapter Nine.

Another common interpersonal misconception is that apology indicates weakness. This misconception received widespread circulation in newspaper advertisements for the movie *Love Story*, which depicted one of the central characters making the asinine statement, "Love is never having to say you're sorry." Related to this misconception is the myth that compromise is tantamount to surrender. This mistaken belief impairs the ability of many marital partners to solve problems because they stubbornly resist "giving in," failing to recognize that compromise involves "getting as well as giving."

Still other misconceptions relate to interpersonal perceptual distortions involving intimate family relationships. Hepworth (1964) describes perceptual distortions of the self and the partner that commonly occur in forced marriages. Laing and Esterson (1971) examine the virulent effect on children of projective identification, the mechanism by which one attributes aspects of the self to others. Mannino and Greenspan (1976) study the same mechanism between marital partners. All these authors discuss as well the therapeutic management of the perceptual distortions in question.

Misconceptions about other facets of human existence. Myriad other misconceptions contribute to human problems, but to identify each of them is not only beyond the scope of this book but impossible. A few of the common general misconceptions significant to counseling work, however, should be mentioned. One such assumption is that man is a mere pawn in life and, therefore, powerless to shape his destiny. Such a defeatist misconception is antithetical to the philosophy and purpose of counseling, leading to resignation and despair. A sharply contrasting but equally erroneous misconception is that one can be anything one desires if he only tries hard enough. This misconception is reflected in the platitude, "Where there's a will, there's a way." This misconception, of course, is both positive and action-oriented, but it errs in failing to recognize obvious human limitations and constraints. Those who subscribe to this misconception may try heroically to succeed in chosen ventures, only to fail. Given the misconception, failure can be attributed solely to inadequate effort, thus predisposing the person to self-recrimination.

Related to cognitive misconceptions are patterns of dichotomous thinking—that is, thinking that divides the world sharply into black and white. When one thinks in such extremes, one cannot be relatively successful or basically moral; rather, one is either successful or unsuccessful, either moral or immoral. There is no in-between. Thinking in such absolute terms obviously programs people to condemn themselves and others, for no one achieves absolute success or is free from occasional wrongdoing. Individuals with such thinking patterns often also mistakenly equate thoughts and actions, contributing further to their inability to measure up to their self-expectations. One of the author's clients, for example, regarded morality as complete freedom from lustful thoughts and actions, a criterion well beyond human capacity. Because occasional sexual thoughts intruded into his thinking, he was convinced that he was an immoral person.

Other misconceptions involve beliefs about the world and human beings in general. Included are beliefs that people are "no damn good" and not to be trusted. Thus the world is perceived as a hostile place where survival is a matter of dog-eat-dog. Such a misconception, of course, leads to aggressiveness, insensitivity to others, and alienation from fellow humans.

With rigid, moralistic clients, the therapist often encounters the misconception that suffering is a virtue. This belief motivates some people to adopt the role of martyr, depriving themselves, eschewing pleasurable activities, and, in general, subjugating their needs and desires to those of others. Such persons commonly lack a zest for living and suffer from depression. For these individuals, it would seem that virtue (in suffering) is not its own reward. Confronting this discrepancy is the therapist's task, as well as assisting the person to see that playing the role of martyr, in the final analysis, brings joy to no one, particularly the martyr.

Irrational patterns of conceptualization. Self-defeating cognitive patterns are often a target of confrontation. Exaggeration or magnification is one of the most common cognitive errors. A depressed client, for example, might tend to exaggerate a small reproof from his spouse and make it evidence of personal inadequacy. The same client may also maintain the depression through the cognitive pattern of selective focus, maintaining a tunnel vision fixed on personal deficits and mistakes, while minimizing and overlooking assets and positive factors. The client, after having failed at one task, may similarly overgeneralize that he is a failure, a reaction that also illustrates dichotomous thinking. A frequent variant of the overgeneralizing pattern is the tendency to make mountains out of molehills. A husband, for example, may escalate an ordinary difference of opinion with his wife over childrearing into a general test of love or power. Personalizing is another cognitive pattern, wherein a client ascribes personal relevance to statements or events unrelated to him. An example is the client who erroneously concludes that a small group of people in the same room is talking about him. An extreme form of personalizing appears in psychotic patients who manifest ideas of reference—that is, misinterpret newspaper articles or television messages as directed to them personally. Other cognitive patterns that may need to be confronted include construing thoughts as facts rather than hypotheses, lack of humor, and hypersuggestibility.

Ellis, the founder of rational-emotive therapy, says that the misconceived "necessities" people impose on themselves make up an "irrational trinity" (1973b, p. 60). The three dictates of the trinity are (1) "Because it would be highly preferable if I were outstandingly competent, I absolutely should and must be; it is awful when I am not; and I am therefore a worthless individual"; (2) "Because it is highly desirable that others treat me considerately and fairly, they absolutely should and must, and they are rotten people who deserve to be utterly damned when they do not"; (3) "Because it is preferable that I experience pleasure rather than pain, the world should absolutely arrange this; and life is horrible, and I can't bear it when the world doesn't."

Irrational fears. The discrepancy in irrational fears is between the intensity of the fear and the relatively harmless nature or mild consequences of the feared object or situation. Irrational fears can be directed toward many objects, as demonstrated by the lengthy list of phobias commonly described in psychiatric texts, including fears of dogs, snakes, insects, germs, blood, elevators, horses, barbers, physicians, open spaces, heights, closed areas, airplane travel, public speaking, crossing streets, darkness, sexual experiences, being alone, meeting strangers, and many more. Other fears not generally regarded as phobic include those, sometimes catastrophic in proportion, associated with risking new behaviors—for example, speaking one's opinion in a class, asking a boss for a raise, declining unreasonable requests for favors, refusing to talk with a telephone solicitor, asking a sought-after female for a date, and insisting that an offensive salesman leave.

Fears are much easier to identify than other cognitive misconceptions and perceptual distortions, for the client is usually painfully and explicitly aware of them. Furthermore, the client usually has some awareness of the discrepancies involved in his irrational fears, and the therapist need not rely solely on his inferences

about the client's state, as he must often do with other distortions
and misperceptions.

Several approaches have proven successful in helping clients
master irrational fears. The behavior modification techniques of
systematic desensitization (Wolpe, 1969) and of modeling (Bandura,
1971) have both been reported as effective. Implosive therapy
(Stampfl and Levis, 1967) and flooding have also been used successfully, although these procedures are regarded as controversial
and riskier and their efficacy is much less well documented (Morganstern, 1973). A simple and direct technique for changing unrealistic fears, termed "repeated review," is described by Raimy
(1975), who maintains that he and his graduate students have had
success with it. The main element in repeated review is "the repetition in imagination of the individual's interaction with the object
of his misconception" (p. 76). Raimy describes the technique as
follows: "Once the specific avoidance reaction has been isolated, I
ask the individual to close his eyes and imagine himself in a concrete
situation where he must interact in some fashion with what he fears
or avoids. He is also asked to 'describe what happens and tell me how
you feel.' He proceeds at his own pace with little interference from
the therapist unless he introduces conditions which would nullify
the imaginary interaction. No training in relaxation is given, nor
are the imaginary scenes hierarchically graded in terms of estimated
threat. If a particular scene appears to be too threatening, the
therapist can alter it instantly by changing or deleting some of the
details. The client or patient is requested to open his eyes at the
conclusion of each recital. If the avoidance reaction has not been
satisfactorily dissipated in imagination, he is asked to repeat the
task until the imagined avoidance disappears" (p. 76).

Beck (1976) also arrives at similar formulations in using techniques of cognitive reappraisal and rehearsal. Many behaviorists
have recently employed a similar technique termed covert sensi-
tization (Mahoney and Thoresen, 1974). An additional approach
to overcoming phobias, called paradoxical intention, also works
well. First described by Frankl (1962, 1967), the founder of logotherapy, paradoxical intention involves repeatedly urging the patient to deliberately induce the feared symptoms. By doing so, the
patient confronts the feared symptom head-on, rather than avoiding it. The effect is to gradually bring the symptom under conscious

control and to neutralize it. This technique has been used successfully by the authors in helping patients overcome numerous and
varied fears. It will be evident to the reader that elements of repeated review are involved in this procedure as well as in behavioral
rehearsal, the role-playing of interpersonal conflict situations before actually facing them.

Denial of problems. Not infrequently, the client denies problems
in the face of overwhelming evidence to the contrary. An alcoholic,
for example, may persist in asserting that he has control over the
frequency and amount of drinking despite frequent benders,
missed employment, blackouts, and other indications of alcoholism.
Similarly, one marital partner may deny that anything is wrong with
the marriage, while the other partner talks of their unhappiness,
gives verbatim accounts of the one's unacceptable behavior, and
threatens or initiates divorce. The discrepancies are obvious to everyone involved, it appears, except the offending person.

Certain confrontations are indicated in such instances, but
direct confrontation without focusing on the dynamics motivating
the denial is often counterproductive. One must confront not only
the alcoholism and the breaking marriage but also the alcoholic's
fear of facing the world without the false fortification of liquor and
the marital partner's strong dependency, feelings of inadequacy,
and fears of rejection by the spouse. Such motivating dynamics are
best confronted with additive empathy. By focusing on and giving
credence to the fears, the therapist may help the patient acknowledge and accept that facing the problem, although painful, is a
major step in gaining strength and preserving a cherished relationship or valued situation. Moreover, the therapist is more likely to
be perceived as an ally than as a punitive person.

Externalization of responsibility. This common dysfunctional
mechanism involves placing responsibility for difficulties outside
oneself when in actuality one is the prime cause of the difficulties.
Thus the client assumes the role of "innocent victim" and casts others or circumstances in the villain's role. An extreme example is
the delinquent who steals a car and then blames the owner for the
theft because he left the keys in the ignition. Less extreme and more
common instances involve persons whose actions are provoked to
some extent by others, but who blame those others exclusively for
the actions. One man, for example, attributed his vicious beating of

his wife to her calling him a foul name. Alcoholics are likewise notorious for attributing their difficulties to nagging spouses. "The devil made me do it," is a classical and humorous example of the externalization of responsibility.

Anytime that someone externalizes responsibility for his own difficulties, the therapist is tempted to set the offender straight summarily. Indeed, confrontation of the discrepancy between the client's attribution and reality is the therapist's appropriate task. Vigorous frontal confrontations, however, are often counterproductive, placing the client on the defensive and jeopardizing the helping relationship. The helpful intent of the therapist tends to be obscured by the "verbal blow" the client experiences.

Effective confrontations are tempered by respect, tact, and patience in helping the client accept ownership for his part in the difficulties. These qualities convey the good will and helpful intent behind the confrontation, which the client must perceive if he is to respond positively to the confrontation. The client is most likely to perceive helpful intent if early in counseling, the counselor's role in helping the client discern his part in the difficulties was clarified. This is of special importance in marriage counseling because of an almost universal tendency for marital partners to perceive (although not necessarily accurately) the partner's part in the difficulties and to have limited awareness of the role they themselves play. Smith and Hepworth (1967) delineate the "fundamental rule" to be stipulated in marriage counseling with one partner: The goal is to help the client understand his part in the difficulties, not to change the other partner. This same rule is equally applicable in many other counseling situations. Clarifying the role of the counselor, however, is not enough to assure that the client will be receptive to confrontations aimed at externalization of responsibility.

Exploring the specific details of difficulties often elicits information that highlights the client's complicity. For example, as a mother expresses her frustration with her daughter's unwillingness to discuss her social experiences, an opportunity is presented to explore specific aspects of their interactions. The mother may, for example, disclose verbal behavior that is intrusive, demeaning, authoritarian, or dogmatic. Using this new information, the counselor can suggest tentatively that the mother's behavior possibly contributes to the daughter's unwillingness to communicate. Similar approaches may be used with students who complain that their teachers dislike them or blame them unfairly for problem situations. In marriage counseling with individual partners, eliciting specific interactional information is crucial to gaining the information upon which confrontations are based. Obviously, abundant and highly specific interactional information is vital in understanding all interpersonal difficulties.

The most potent confrontations of externalized responsibility, however, do not occur in discussions of past events. Confrontations involving spontaneous behavior in the interview have the greatest therapeutic potency, for they reveal dysfunctional behavior that the counselor can observe and experience personally. Such instances enhance the accuracy of the counselor's observations markedly, for they are not subject to the usual distortions, rationalizations, and defenses. Such on-the-spot confrontations are of particular value in conjoint interviews involving parents and children, marital partners, and family groups, but they may also be employed in many other contexts, including teacher-student and supervisor-supervisee relationships.

On-the-spot confrontations involving relational immediacy have perhaps the greatest therapeutic potency of all, for in this context the counselor experiences firsthand the client's behavior. The client, for example, may distort the meaning of a counselor's message or blame the counselor unrealistically for feelings or behaviors that originate within himself. Such an occurrence presents a rich opportunity to identify patterns of externalizing responsibility and provide corrective feedback by authentically sharing personal reactions to the behavior.

Failing to see alternatives. The difficulties some clients have are either caused or perpetuated by their inability to evolve or to implement remedial action. Such clients commonly have few problem-solving skills, and, therefore, they may attempt to cope with widely different situations in habitual and often ineffective ways. Thus their approaches to problems are characterized by "tunnel vision," precluding flexible and creative responses. Some parents, for example, in dealing with their children's disobedience or rebellion are able to employ only one coping pattern—resorting to power tactics like threats, deprivation, or physical punishment. The habitual use of power may control behavior for short periods of time, but it may produce damaging side effects, such as personal resentment and mutual blaming, power struggles between parent and child, increased rebelliousness, or the development of a passive-submissive personality in the child. Others habitually cope with difficulties by such avoidance patterns as withdrawal, use of alcohol or drugs, or literal flight. Physical or verbal aggression is another way of coping with interpersonal difficulty.

Confrontation in such instances involves helping the client recognize the discrepancy between his limited way of coping and other viable alternatives. The client is likely to benefit most if the counselor involves him to the fullest extent possible in searching for other alternatives instead of singlehandedly identifying them for the client. The latter approach fosters dependency rather than autonomy and is low in respect for the client's potential to evolve creative solutions and mobilize latent strengths. Again, as alternatives are explored, it is important to let the client decide which course of action is most appropriate. The counselor may, however, assist in this process by helping the client weigh the pros and cons of each alternative.

Often the client can be helped to broaden his repertoire of problem-solving skills by introducing him to brainstorming. This tactic forestalls the client's tendency to tackle problems prematurely, without considering all possible alternatives. Brainstorming can be particularly effective in work involving pairs or multiple relationships. In marriage counseling, for example, partners often become embroiled in conflict over such matters as finances, child-rearing, or role expectations. Each may take a stance toward a given problem unacceptable to the other, and the conflict may rage for a long time with neither partner willing to yield. Since brainstorming prevents power struggles, its use in this kind of situation may not only break the present impasse but help avoid future problems of the same sort. The goal is to discover mutually acceptable alternatives with neither partner "losing" in the process. Each partner first lists his needs in the problem and next identifies all of the possible courses of action. Both partners suspend critical judgments of the alternatives identified by the other, eliminating or minimizing fruitless arguments about their merits. After the list is complete, the partners weigh each alternative against their respective needs, seeking to identify those alternatives acceptable to both. If more than one mutually acceptable alternative is discovered, the couple seeks to assess which is preferable. When used well, brainstorming often produces dramatic results in helping clients "remove their blinders" as they analyze problems.

The task of the therapist, of course, does not end with merely assisting the client to select a remedial course of action. Implementing an alternative may require identifying possible barriers to success, which most often are fears, and seeking to surmount them through further exploration and through behavioral rehearsal (Reid, 1975).

Failure to consider consequences. A related problem is acting without adequate consideration of the consequences. Some persons act impulsively, often aggravating rather than ameliorating their difficulties. Others may simply have blind spots or fail to consider adequately the ramifications of a given course of action. Impulsive behavior tends to be governed by strong emotions and desires rather than by the cognitive processes, a fact that often precludes deliberation of the available alternatives. Some people, for example, aggressively lash out at others when frustrated, often at considerable expense to everyone concerned. A client, for example, may walk off the job in the heat of anger when frustrated by a supervisor or co-worker, resulting in discharge by the employer. Another client may fail to pass a course because he yielded to a pleasurable opportunity instead of preparing adequately for a final examination. Still another client may purchase an expensive set of encyclopedias at the urging of a persuasive salesman, even though the budget is already strained to the limit. Similarly, it is not uncommon for people, especially adolescents, to submit to group pressure to steal, drive recklessly, use drugs, or indulge sexually, behaviors that may lead to serious and even disastrous consequences.

Opportunities for confrontation often emerge as the client expresses an intention to carry out actions likely to be detrimental to himself and others. The confrontation focuses on the discrepancy between the implied intention of the client to resolve his difficulties and the likely opposite effect of the planned actions. The helpful intent behind the confrontation can be explicitly stated in terms of the therapist's desire to assist the client in averting actions that may cause personal injury, hardship, loss of self-esteem, loss of love and respect by others, and even loss of personal freedom when the planned actions involve violation of a law. A marriage-counseling client, for example, may express intentions of getting even with his spouse for flirting at a party by conspicuously stepping out. The counselor may confront the client by saying, "I can see how hurt and rejected you felt at the party and are feeling now. It's natural when you feel hurt to want to hurt back. Still, I'm wondering if it's more important to you to get even than to improve your situation. Stepping out would only seem to strain your marital relationship even further. Perhaps we could think of some other ways of dealing with your situation." Similar approaches can be applied in many different situations.

When impulsive acting-out appears to be a pattern, it may be prudent to confront the client directly with his pattern rather than deal with each event as a separate entity. The goal of the confrontation is to help the client become aware of the pattern and of the difficulties it causes, with a view toward helping him supplant the dysfunctional pattern with a thoughtful and analytical approach to problem solving. It is important not to confront the pattern prematurely, waiting until substantial evidence regarding the existence of the pattern amasses. Often the client's receptivity to such a confrontation is enhanced when the therapist explains that the client appears to let himself be governed by strong emotions instead of thinking through the actions most likely to achieve the results he intends. The client may be challenged to postpone actions until the emotions subside and until he has carefully assessed the available alternatives and weighed the consequences of each.

Discrepant intentions. Of the various discrepancies, perhaps the most subtle and covert is discrepant intentions. The client's basic intentions sometimes lie outside awareness, and they may be antithetical to the conscious intentions discerned by both client and therapist. The therapist may proceed on the assumption that the client's conscious or expressed intent is a valid indicator of his basic motivation when, in fact, underlying and obscure motivations override it. May (1969) uses the term *intentionality* in a broad sense to refer to dynamic motivating forces, conscious and unconscious, that prompt and shape human behavior. *Intention,* by contrast, is used in a much narrower sense to connote only those goals of which a client is consciously aware. Thus conflicts between intent and intentionality may confuse and impede the therapeutic process unless recognized and managed effectively. May devotes an entire chapter to illustrating discrepancies between intent and intentionality and showing how to handle them clinically (pp. 246–271). The concept of discrepant intentions also plays a pivotal role in the theories of transactional analysis formulated by Berne in his now classic work *Games People Play* (1963).

Several examples should clarify further the meaning of discrepant intentions. A client may ask for help with feelings of depression, yet seemingly resist all therapeutic efforts to evolve meaning and independence in his life. The client's ostensible intent is to gain relief from feelings of depression and to attain more zest in living. Yet one hidden goal of the client's behavior may be to place responsibility for change with the therapist and to perpetuate a dependent relationship. Another client may seek help for sexual difficulties, complaining that her husband lacks tenderness and seeks only to "use" her for his own sexual gratification. Yet each time her husband expresses warmth and affection, she responds in a cold, detached manner because she is "too busy" or "not in the mood." Overtly her intention is to improve her sexual relationship. Covertly, however, she appears to be expressing hostile feelings toward her husband and may be protecting herself against facing her own fears of sexual inadequacy. Then there is the client who persistently asks for direction and advice, yet whenever advice is offered, subtly sabotages any chance of success the advice might have had. On the surface the client manifests a genuine desire for direction. Covertly, however, his motivation appears to be to discredit the therapist. Polansky (1967) identifies several other forms of discrepant intentions.

Discrepant intentions must be brought to the client's conscious awareness. The use of additive empathic responses to illuminate hidden meanings was discussed in Chapter Six. It will be recalled that feelings associated with hidden meanings must also be explored and resolved, as, in the examples above, the fear of sexuality, dependency longings, and hostility toward significant others. Hidden goals can also be brought to awareness through confrontive techniques that highlight the discrepancies. The therapist, may, for example, state his confusion over the client's expressed intent and his contradictory behavior. He may question whether the client has feelings in opposition to the expressed goals. Such questions are interpretive in flavor and should be posed tentatively, since they may be inaccurate and since the client may not be ready or able to tolerate the anxiety associated with the discovery of the hidden meanings.

AFFECTIVE DISCREPANCIES

Before we identify and discuss discrepancies in the affective (emotional) realm, it is important to note that emotions, like perceptions, are inextricably connected with cognitive processes. Emotions are experienced with and determined by the cognitive meanings attached to the various stimulus situations and memories. A person, however, may lack awareness of the meanings attached to certain stimuli, a point implied in the discussion of misconceptions. Thus a person may experience stage fright before delivering a talk because of cognitive assumptions that he will appear ridiculous or incompetent to the audience if he looks nervous, mispronounces a word, or makes some type of mistake. Similarly, feelings of anger may derive from a conclusion (cognitive meaning) that another person has deliberately ignored, insulted, or otherwise offended one. Thus, emotional discrepancies are frequently encountered in therapy, as was explained at length in Chapter Four. By eliciting and exploring emotions, the therapist helps the client to experience and understand his feelings and to test them against and align them with reality.

Discrepancies between expressed and actual feelings. Because of fears of losing face and self-esteem by acknowledging certain painful emotions, the client sometimes expresses one emotion to mask another. An extremely lonely adolescent, for example, may deny loneliness and assert that he needs no one. A spurned suitor may mask feelings of hurt and rejection by proclaiming, "It's all for the best; she'll be happier with someone else." Similarly, a client may attempt to conceal disappointment and discouragement at being passed over for a desired job promotion by rationalizing that the promotion would have meant only increased responsibility and worry. Discrepancies of this type are easily discerned because of the lack of congruence between expressed feelings and the nonverbal cues of countenance, posture, and tone of voice. Moreover, the feelings expressed and the feelings appropriate to the situation are incongruent.

Skills in empathic communication are employed in confronting discrepancies between expressed and actual feelings. The therapist will need to listen to the nonverbal cues and channel the discussion to the feelings they indicate. This is done most effectively by suggesting that the client's demeanor indicates feelings other than those expressed. The blow to the client's self-esteem may be cushioned by explaining that it would be natural for anyone in the client's situation to experience the unexpressed feelings. The client often appreciates the therapist's astuteness in recognizing painful but unexpressed feelings. The confrontation paves the way to ventilation of the troubling emotions and facilitates productive discussion of the problem. Occasionally, however, a client may be unready to acknowledge the painful feelings, and the therapist is well-advised to defer pursuing the matter. Confronting the client vigorously under such a circumstance may needlessly damage the client's already diminutive self-esteem and the helping relationship as well.

Feelings expressed verbally and nonverbally. A closely related discrepancy is the one between feelings expressed verbally and feelings expressed nonverbally. Some clients find it difficult to talk about their feelings, and exploration of their emotional realm requires that the therapist be acutely perceptive to nonverbal cues. Moistening of the eyes, clenching of the jaws and hands, sighs, trembling in the voice, blushing, sadness in the countenance, pursing of the lips, lowering of the head, slow tempo in movement and speech— these and many other nonverbal cues may need to be confronted to bring troubled feelings into the arena of discussion. In other instances, the client may verbalize only one aspect of his feelings, omitting emotions that may be even more basic. A client, for example, may express anger over being stood up on a date and neglect to mention feelings of hurt, disappointment, and rejection. In still other instances, a client may dismiss certain feelings as unimportant when nonverbal cues, in fact, suggest acute distress.

At this point the reader may question whether responding therapeutically to such situations entails additive empathy more than confrontation. Actually, both are involved. Responding with empathy on levels 4.0 and 5.0 entails definite elements of confrontation in the sense of bringing to the client's awareness feelings that he has perceived not at all or only dimly. As we noted earlier in this chapter, confrontation and additive levels of empathy are sometimes difficult to differentiate, and the skills in both are essentially the same.

Discrepancies involving intensity of feelings. There can be discrepancy between the emotional intensity the client expresses and the intensity the client actually feels. To protect against the embarrassment or guilt associated with acknowledging certain strong negative emotions, a client may express the feeling in much milder form than befits it. A parent, for example, says he is irritated with a child when he is actually furious. Another client may describe feeling "down" rather than expose profound feelings of depression.

Unless the counselor senses the intense feelings and succeeds in drawing them out, the therapeutic impact of discussing the expressed emotion may be diluted considerably. Again, skills in empathic communication are required to locate the discrepancy, which will be hinted at by the client's nonverbal behavior and by the incongruence between the expressed feelings and the feelings appropriate to the situation. The counselor must have a rich vocabulary of feelings to confront discrepancies of this sort. If the reader has not already mastered the vocabulary presented in Chapter Four, he is urged to do so now.

Caution is indicated in confronting discrepancies of emotional intensity with clients whose self-esteem would be severely threatened by having to acknowledge such powerful negative emotions as rage, hatred, panic, humiliation, and the like. Such clients may be helped to accept these emotions by applying the principle of shaping—that is, the therapist helps the client become aware of and accept emotions only slightly more intense than those expressed. The vocabulary of feelings in Chapter Four will be particularly helpful to this process.

Occasionally one encounters clients who are overly expressive emotionally. These clients tend to be dramatic and histrionic, expressing an intensity of feelings well beyond what they actually experience. The behavior of some of these clients is aimed at capturing the attention and sympathy of others, and the counselor should avoid giving full credence to the expressed feelings. Confrontation with such clients focuses on the discrepancy between the ostensible purpose of the emotional display and the actual purpose. Ultimately, such a client may need to be helped to expand his awareness of his need for attention and to evolve interpersonal skills more effective, mature, and satisfying than his present emotional displays.

Discrepancies involving unexperienced feelings. Generally, empathic communication, as discussed in Chapters Five and Six, is the major tool for expanding the client's self-awareness, while confrontation is of only minor importance in this task. With certain clients, however, confrontation in tandem with empathic communication plays a vital role in expanding awareness of unexperienced feelings. These clients have major discrepancies between the feelings they are consciously aware of and the feelings imbedded in the substrata of their awareness. Such discrepancies are not readily discernible, and they must be inferred from the client's lack of emotional expressiveness. Some clients, for example, present themselves as emotionally bland and constricted, displaying little or no emotion when discussing events or situations that would generally be regarded as emotionally charged. Such clients appear, and indeed are, emotionally detached from the experiences they are reporting. They are literally alienated from the emotional aspect of their being. Their cognitive functions, by contrast, tend to be overdeveloped, and such clients commonly seek to establish and to maintain the helping relationship on an abstract and intellectual level.

The therapeutic task of helping such clients expand their emotional awareness requires patient and persistent efforts by the therapist over an extended period. It is vital to recognize that the client's emotional detachment evolved as a protection against being overwhelmed by emotions that threatened emotional security and self-esteem in early life and that still pose a similar threat. Devastating psychic decompensation, therefore, may result from vigorous frontal attacks on the client's defenses. Again, the therapist should adhere to the principle of shaping, seeking to expand the client's emotional self-awareness only by increments consonant with the strength of the helping relationship and the client's capacity to tolerate insights without undue stress. Stripping away the client's defenses without providing coping mechanisms to take their place is tantamount to stripping a turtle of his shell and turning him loose to face the world undefended. A strong helping relationship, however, tends to buttress a client as he experiences the inevitable vulnerability associated with evolving major new coping patterns.

Techniques for assisting clients to get in touch with emotions were discussed in Chapter Six. In employing confrontation as a means of initiating self-exploration and change, however, additional techniques are needed. One such technique involves explaining to the client that for some reason the natural human emotions have been blocked and that understanding the reasons for the blockage and removing it will permit the emotions to flow naturally, enabling the client to live comfortably and to experience life fully. Such an approach is appropriate, for example, with persons who are unable to experience sexual passion or feelings of tenderness and love. The technique of "sensate focus" developed by Masters and Johnson (1970) aims at assisting in the removal of blockages to natural erotic experiencing by temporarily divesting oneself of intellectual preoccupations and channeling one's attention to physical and emotional sensation.

A technique of value in assisting a client gradually to experience and to express tender feelings is to instruct him to behave as though the feelings are actually experienced. Thus the therapist asks the client to demonstrate warm and loving feelings "as if" he were, in fact, experiencing them. Successfully used by Stuart (1976), this technique fosters the development of feelings hitherto unexperienced. The therapist should explain to the client that expressing the feelings will seem awkward and unnatural at first, but with continued practice they will become increasingly spontaneous and natural. Indeed, this change has been the clinical experience of the authors.

Finally, it is vital in working with clients who dwell on the abstract and intellectual to channel the discussion to the concrete and the immediate. Rather than accepting the client's views and conceptualizations of events and experiences, the counselor persistently probes for specific detail—that is, the specific circumstances of the event, exactly what was said by whom, and particularly the feelings the client experienced. Each time the client digresses to the remote and the intellectual, the counselor doggedly shifts the focus back to the concrete and the immediate. Specific examples of this process were provided in Chapter Nine.

Purported and expressed feelings. As the client focuses on interpersonal relationships, particularly those involving family members, discrepancies often emerge between the feelings purportedly experienced toward another person and the feelings actually expressed. A client may, for example, proclaim to the counselor his love for his spouse, yet express such feelings to the spouse rarely, if at all, maintaining that the spouse must surely know of his love anyway. The spouse understandably may feel unloved, or, at best, uncertain of the partner's love. Similarly, a parent may feel love for or pride in a child but seldom demonstrate those feelings.

In confronting such discrepancies, the counselor may explain firmly that the spouse or child cannot read the client's mind and that humans generally require frequent nurturing to maintain morale, self-esteem, and a sense of being cherished by another. Often clients will attribute their lack of demonstrativeness to inhibition or discomfort associated with emotional expressiveness. The therapist may foster efforts to change by explaining that emotional expressiveness can be learned through practice. A certain amount of discomfort and risk is involved, but the therapist can show this to be a small price to pay for the benefit to the partner and to the relationship.

Discrepancies between purported and expressed feelings also extend to other emotions. Some individuals, for example, may report feeling angry with or hurt by another but fail to express the feeling to that person. Thus the other person is unaware of the feelings and is denied the opportunity to rectify the situation. In confronting the client, it is beneficial to explain that the situation cannot be improved if the client keeps his feelings underground. As is generally true, the therapist should explore with the client the barrier to handling the situation directly and constructively. This exploration will commonly yield fears of a negative reaction from the other person—anger, criticism, or rejection, for example. Careful exploration of these fears in turn often results in discovery of the irrational assumption that it is disastrous to be criticized, disapproved of, or rejected by another. At this point, the client will often discern the irrational elements of his fear with minimal assistance from the counselor and will formulate a remedial course of action on his own. Behavioral rehearsal involving facing the problematic situation head-on may bring to light additional feelings, as well as providing valuable preparatory experience for the client.

Difficulties and discrepancies in the emotional realm are manifested in many forms other than those already described. Some clients are emotionally labile, having marked swings of mood from euphoria to melancholy within a short time. Other clients are emotionally expressive in one setting or with one person and unexpressive in or with others. An example is the person who is kind and considerate with everyone except his immediate family. Still other clients may exhibit temporally disparate emotional patterns, being irritable and grouchy in the morning and increasingly congenial and cheerful as the day progresses. Therapeutic efforts often concentrate on these inconsistencies and problematic behaviors, but confrontation per se is usually not involved because the client is already painfully aware of these patterns.

BEHAVIORAL DISCREPANCIES

Several of the discrepancies and dysfunctional patterns we have discussed involve elements of behavioral discrepancies: interpersonal perceptions and distortions, discrepant intentions, externalized responsibility, differences between purported and expressed feelings and between verbal and nonverbal behavior. This section includes only those discrepancies not already discussed. Essentially, they fall into the following seven categories:

Dysfunctional life styles or behavioral patterns. This category includes numerous behavioral patterns and life styles that impede both personal and social functioning. Discrepancies occur between life goals or values on one hand and contradictory behavior on the other. There are too many such discrepancies to enumerate all of them, but some of the common ones will be identified.

Irresponsible behavior commonly causes difficulties in living, often of serious magnitude. Undependability in reporting to work, failure to pay bills, neglect in keeping social engagements, failure to fulfill assigned responsibilities, neglect of children and property—these and many similar derelictions often precipitate financial, interpersonal, and legal pressures and entanglements. Loss of employment, of personal relationships (including marriage), of property, of child custody, and even of personal freedom may result from irresponsible behavior. Failure to anticipate consequences of behavior and externalized responsibility are commonly associated with this type of discrepancy. Typically, the client who manifests this pattern seeks counseling only when the pressures of threatened or impending losses have mounted to the breaking point.

Irresponsible behavior frequently pervades the counseling situation as well, manifested by tardiness or failure to keep appointments and pay fees. Such clients often are "slippery" and glib in rationalizing their behavior away and promising to improve it. Effective confrontations thus require a firm, reality-oriented approach tempered by expressions of good will and concern about helping the client avoid future adverse consequences. It is a tactical error and a disservice to such clients to permit them to rationalize, deceive, and evade. The behavior of these clients often is governed by a misconception that "things will work out" or by fantasies that someone will come to their rescue. The therapist's task is to confront them with the reality that only they are in a position to alleviate the pressures besetting them. Moreover, the therapist can enhance the client's motivation by construing the problem situation as a challenge and opportunity to grow and to increase self-fulfillment by adopting mature and responsible behavior. This approach often strikes a responsive chord, for many such clients are aware of their irresponsible patterns and wish to get rid of them.

Individuals who possess such common dysfunctional patterns as abusive and violent behavior, excessive passivity, and compulsive behavior often do not request help in overcoming them, but seek counseling as a result of pressure from spouses or relatives who suffer the detrimental impact of their behavior. The counselor thus must confront the discrepancy between the problem behavior and the client's urgent wish to preserve or improve a threatened but valued relationship. Because the client's motivation is largely external in origin, special skills in dealing with inadequate motivation, discussed briefly in Chapters Two and Nine, must be employed.

Considerable leverage is available to the counselor, but he must use it judiciously. The compulsive mother and housekeeper, for example, tends to be highly sensitive to criticism, although she is likely to nag and criticize considerably herself. Her striving to be a good mother opens her to appeal from the therapist. Thus she can be helped to see that her children need affection, praise, and approval more than a spotless house. The therapist, in fact, can gently confront her with the desirability of learning to relax and to engage in recreation, at the same time challenging her misconception that to be worthwhile, she must constantly be working and driving herself to keep an immaculate house. Confrontation of violent and abusive behavior and of passive-submissive patterns also involves helping the client recognize the self-defeating nature of his behavior. The passive-submissive pattern, for example, usually evolves early in life as a way of avoiding the displeasure or wrath of others. Compliant submissiveness in adulthood, however, invites personal exploitation. The confrontation, of course, is only the prelude to the work to follow—namely, working through irrational fears and evolving functional patterns.

Some individuals subscribe to life styles that they cannot reconcile with certain needs or values. In our practices, for example, we have frequently encountered persons who have eschewed marriage and elected to cohabit with the understanding that both partners are free to engage in other sexual relationships. Some individuals, no doubt, can live comfortably with such an arrangement, but many feel insecure, hurt, and rejected if the partner becomes involved with someone else. Similarly, individuals who have been drawn philosophically to communal living or to spouse swapping experience marked emotional conflicts involving jealousy, guilt, insecurity, and confusion. Confrontation in such instances entails helping the client recognize the discrepancy between his life style and his values or needs. Confronting the discrepancies and explaining the conflicts often helps such individuals see the strength of their needs or moral convictions for the first time. This awareness is invaluable to them in choosing how to proceed in the future.

Absence of direction. Some clients appear lost in the eddies and backwaters of life, drifting aimlessly without direction or purpose. Some plead confusion about goals and values or remain in continuous conflict between opposing goals. Often confusion and conflict are rationalizations camouflaging an unwillingness to make a commitment, to take chances, and to jeopardize the status quo. Some clients maintain they have "dropped out" of the mainstream of life because of the hypocrisy of those in power and the corruption of societal institutions. Although there may be truth in such assertions, many such individuals use these assertions to conceal personal inadequacies, fears of failure, and inability to form satisfying relationships. Confrontation thus helps them come to terms with the real reasons for their withdrawal from society. This involves unmasking their rationalizations and helping them accept responsibility for creating meaning in their lives rather than resorting to drugs and alcohol for a counterfeit sense of well-being. Often such clients have extremely poor self-images and consequent defeatist attitudes toward life admixed with depression. Such a psychological state is often termed "anomic depression," which connotes the lack of values and the confusion these clients manifest. Krill (1969) has written an excellent paper on the topic.

Discrepancies between goals and behavior. The counselor commonly finds the client behaving in a way contradictory to stated goals. Such behavior may occur within or outside an interview. In either instance confrontation can be employed to advantage, particularly when the behavior is confronted in the immediacy of the interview. For example, a female client of one of the authors in family therapy said it was her goal to have her husband gain respect from the children by asserting himself more. Yet, in the family interviews, she interrupted and demeaned him whenever he attempted to assert himself. An on-the-spot confrontation focusing on the discrepancy between her goal and her behavior was both enlightening and helpful to her in identifying the part she played in her husband's reticence.

A high-school student who was a client of one of the authors had aspirations of becoming a professional vocalist, and she planned to attend a renowned university to study voice. She was referred to counseling, however, because of near-failing academic performance, which she attributed to disagreements with the educational policies and procedures practiced in the high school. Confrontation of this obvious discrepancy between her goal and her behavior was couched in a genuine expression of concern that if she persisted in her behavior she was choosing to abandon her goal, because it was most unlikely she would be graduated from high school, let alone be admitted to the university. This fact, which she had somehow evaded, was instrumental in her sharply modifying her behavior.

Discrepancies between expressed intentions or feelings and behavior. People sometimes express the intention to behave one way, only to contradict their intention through their actions. Often the discrepancy will be conspicuous to observers but not to the individual himself. Awareness thus requires confrontation. One client, for example, said he intended to avoid friction over a controversy about who would use the family automobile, even if it meant his relinquishing its use altogether. He would prefer, he maintained, to ride his motorcycle if using the car meant continued squabbling.

Yet when he discussed the matter with the other family members involved, he aggressively argued for his exclusive use of the automobile, conveying the strong impression to everyone concerned that his intention was to have his way and that his way meant exclusive use of the automobile. His asserted intention of wanting peace at any price obviously was a ploy concealing from himself and others his actual intention of having peace only on his terms. Confronting the client's discrepant behavior caused him pain, but enabled him to examine his behavior in a new light.

The common incongruence between words and actions is delineated well by Beier (1974), whose phrase "the eloquence of action" is merely a sophisticated articulation of the maxim, "Actions speak louder than words." Using a fictitious example, Beier demonstrates a typical situation in which behavior belies words. A husband stumbles home from work at 9 P.M. for the fiftieth night in a row, smelling like a brewery and looking sullen. After being ignored, his wife declares, "I want a divorce." Following an interchange in which he asks her not to leave, the wife asks him to give one good reason why she should not. He clears his throat, grins, and says, "I love you." Beier observes, "The lexical meaning of 'I love you' amounted to a stupid joke in the context of his evident lack of interest" (p. 53).

Therapists commonly encounter similar situations. Often the discrepancies involve behavior in therapy. A client may, for example, convincingly express intentions of carrying out certain actions to strengthen his marriage, only to report subsequently that he failed to perform the actions or engaged in behavior apparently at cross-purposes. Procrastination, of course, may often be involved, but in other instances the declared intentions conflict with intentionality, as noted earlier. The task of the therapist in such instances is to confront that conflict and to help the client own the meaning behind his action. Such acceptance of ownership may be a significant step in matching actions to actual, stated feelings and intentions.

Manipulative behavior. As used here, *manipulation* refers to the devious maneuvering of another person to gain a given end with little or no consideration of that person's needs or welfare. Manipulation may range from charming flattery aimed at winning a favor to the outright deception and exploitation practiced by con artists. Thus a usually arrogant and rebellious teenager who turns on the charm when he wants to use the family automobile and a persuasive salesman who promises untold wealth to a gullible widow if she will invest in a secret gold mine are both manipulating others. Manipulation may also be very subtle, as with a person who uses illness to control others. Clients, too, often seek to manipulate the therapist. One client, for example, may constantly change appointment times, always for seemingly plausible reasons. Another may consistently seek to extend the interview by bringing up "urgent" problems at the end of the allotted time. Shostrom (1968) provides a comprehensive discussion of patterns of manipulation in varying social contexts.

Manipulation may appear functional in the sense that the manipulator gains his end. In the long run, however, manipulation is dysfunctional because others may become alienated as they realize the manipulator's self-centered and exploitive intentions. Skillful manipulators may project charm for a time, but it soon wears thin. Manipulation involves "getting" with little or no "giving,' and others soon tire of the lack of reciprocity. Manipulation is also dysfunctional because the person who uses others loses the personal growth of exercising greater self-responsibility and the self-fulfillment that derives from relating to others openly, honestly, and in a reciprocal, caring manner.

People, counselors included, who permit themselves to be manipulated do a disservice to the manipulator and to themselves. Thus the counselor can unmask manipulations with good will, expressing concern over the client's tendency to engage in behavior that may be expedient for the moment but self-defeating in the long run. Thus a client who professes helplessness in facing a teacher, a parent, employer, or spouse in an attempt to persuade the counselor to intervene with the other person may be helped to see that such an action would deprive the client of the opportunity to gain strength by coping with difficulties and that it would only foster dependency on the counselor. The client who manipulates habitually may be directly confronted with his pattern and helped to recognize the price he pays by being unable to form deep and lasting relationships.

Dysfunctional communication patterns. This category probably presents more promising opportunities for confrontation than any other. Communication difficulties are prominent in virtually all interpersonal problems, particularly those involving marital and family relationships. For this reason it is imperative that counselors who engage in marriage and family counseling be well-versed in communication theory and skillful in employing confrontation. Although listing all the many dysfunctional communication patterns is beyond the scope of this book, we will identify a few of those encountered most frequently.

Failure to listen fully to others is a universal interactional problem. People tend to be preoccupied with their own thoughts and views, often thinking of what to say next or, if controversy is involved, preparing a counterargument. Thus, instead of listening intently, they often interrupt, argue or change the subject, resulting in frustration, frequent misunderstandings, and sometimes bitter recriminations.

Power tactics, including shouting, threatening, physical intimidation, blackmailing, belittling, filibustering, and fouls ("hitting below the belt"), also commonly cause interpersonal difficulties. Power tactics are aimed at winning conflicts, as are many dysfunctional communication patterns. When one person wins, however, it is at the other's expense. Both combatants, in fact, are losers if the "winning" of the conflict culminates in strain, resentment, and alienation.

Interpreting messages inaccurately and sending poorly conceived or ambiguous messages also impair effective communications. Reading meanings into messages, speaking for the other person (mind reading), jumping to conclusions without adequate interaction—these and other similar patterns interfere with good exchanges of information. In more severe and pathological forms, projective identification and disconfirmation (invalidation) may completely block communication. Explanations, descriptions, and the clinical implications of these patterns are provided by Watzlawick, Beavin, and Jackson (1967) and by Laing and Esterson (1971).

Avoidance patterns are also frequently manifested in dysfunctional communication patterns. Refusing to discuss a conflict, walking out on the other person, sidetracking (bringing up topics unrelated to the one under consideration), and pouting are common avoidance patterns. Avoidance patterns may be extended over a period of time by waging a cold war, in which avoidance and power are used in tandem to inflict suffering upon the other person with long-lasting silence punctuated by nonverbal cues that convey righteous indignation, resentment, and contempt.

The most potent confrontations involving dysfunctional communication patterns occur in conjoint interviews immediately following the dysfunctional behavior. Such on-the-spot confrontations make it possible to clarify the dysfunctional communication precisely and to elicit the recipient's emotional reaction to the dysfunctional message. The emotional reaction may provide helpful feedback to the sender of the message, although it is vital that the counselor clarify that the feedback is intended to help and not to blame. Confrontations of this type become more helpful when the counselor helps the participants learn effective ways of communicating. Many clients, for example, express feelings as if they were accusations, eliciting defensiveness from the other person and creating a climate for mutual recriminations. The counselor may capitalize upon such "teachable moments" by explaining to the clients the concept of owning feelings and sending "I" rather than "you" messages. By actively involving them in a discussion of the feelings behind such messages as, "You think more of golf and your buddies than you do of me," each can learn to better identify his own feelings and to share them constructively without attacking. Thus the accusation about golf is translated to, "I'm feeling lonely and shut out of your life. You're important to me, and I need more time with you. I guess I'm feeling less important to you than your golf."

Confrontations can be similarly employed when interruptions, changes in subject, discrepancies between verbal and nonverbal messages, misinterpretations, vaguely worded messages, and other dysfunctional behaviors appear. Frequent interventions are essential when meanings are lost or misinterpreted. Thus the counselor may ask the recipient of a message to check with the sender to determine whether the meaning received was the meaning intended. Likewise, the sender may be asked to check with the recipient to ascertain that the recipient got the message the sender wanted. Both parties can be helped to recognize the responsibility each has to make communication effective. The counselor can likewise confront the communication between himself and the client. Finally, modeling effective communication is perhaps the most powerful way the therapist has of helping the client improve his skills in communication.

Resistance to therapy. Unless resistance is brought into the therapeutic discussion, the client is left to struggle with it independently, often intensifying the resistance and culminating in premature termination. Resistance to therapy may be rooted in feelings toward the therapist or associated with barriers to change, as discussed at length in Chapters Nine and Two. Some of the common manifestations of resistance to therapy include failed or canceled appointments, tardiness, discussing trivia, attempting to relate on social terms, dissociating therapy from life, flight into health, forgetting what was discussed during the previous appointment, excessive efforts to please the therapist, intellectualizing, persistent failure to translate insight into action, acting out feelings without prior discussion, sexual seductiveness, strong negative feelings toward the therapist, repeated discussions of the same topics without remedial actions, challenging the therapist's competence, failing to pay fees, and protracted silence. The therapist must accord highest priority to resolving resistance. Otherwise, progress will be impeded, at best, or termination may occur, at worst.

Some of the major guidelines about handling both resistance and confrontation bear repeating here: (1) interpretative confrontations should be offered tentatively rather than authoritatively; (2) empathic communication should be employed to assess the client's emotional reaction to the confrontation; (3) the feelings behind resistances should be explored, respected, and resolved; (4) the resolution of resistance requires considerable time and effort.

Finally, the highest level of respect conveys our expectations that the client settle for no less than he is capable of achieving. This expectation, however, is coupled with respect for the client's right to decide upon whatever course of action he chooses. In the final analysis, confrontation is aimed at helping the client to discover his potentialities for growth and at facilitating the actualization of those potentials.

Skill-Development Exercises in Confrontation

To help the reader integrate the theoretical content of this chapter and to advance his skill, skill-development exercises with modeled responses are provided to illustrate high-level confrontations. The exercises correspond with the types of discrepancies and dysfunctional behaviors presented in this chapter, and they represent diverse clinical situations.

Each exercise comprises a brief summary of the therapeutic situation followed by a verbatim exchange between the client and the therapist. After reading the interchange, analyze the situation, determine the type of discrepancy or dysfunctional behavior involved (in some instances two or more discrepancies are involved), and then respond as though you are the therapist, following the guidelines and recommendations presented earlier. Now consult the modeled response for the exercise. Check first to see whether your identification of the discrepancy is the same as the one given. Then compare your confrontation with the model, keeping in mind that there is no "correct" response and that the one provided is only one of many possible appropriate responses. Study carefully to determine whether your response adheres to the guidelines.

CLIENT STATEMENTS

1. The client is a cunning seventeen-year-old male student confined in a state correctional institution because of incorrigibility. The correctional worker is an attractive female social worker in her late twenties. Earlier in the day, the client observed the counselor in the office of a male counselor, Mr. Olsen, discussing a case and drinking Cokes. The exchange follows a heated discussion of the client's demands for a weekend home visit although he has violated numerous rules of the institution during the week and created several disturbances.

Client: "You know, it might be best for you to let me go home this weekend."

Counselor: "How do you mean?"

Client: "Look, I'm no dumbbell. I know what's going on between you and Olsen."

Counselor: "How's that?"

Client: "Don't try to put me on. I know you've been getting it on with him. If you're not a little more cooperative with me, I just might let Mr. Brandon (the superintendent) know about his darling counselor."

2. Mrs. Welby, a thirty-four-year-old divorcee with two children, is involved with a twenty-eight-year-old bachelor, who

recently proposed marriage to her. Since the failure of her first marriage, she has been philosophically opposed to marriage, and therefore she declined his proposal. She wishes to continue the relationship as a sexual friendship. She requested counseling, however, when he began dating a previous girlfriend.

Mrs. Welby: "I've really felt hurt and angry since he's been taking Ginny out again. I certainly haven't wanted to go out with anyone else."

3. The client is a sixteen-year-old male, referred to a child-guidance clinic by juvenile authorities after detention for truancy, running away from home, and smoking marijuana. The therapist has talked with the parents, who urgently requested help. They are at their wit's end, suffering not only from longstanding difficulties with their son, but also from marital disunity and sibling rivalry. The therapist is of the opinion that conjoint family therapy is indicated. The following excerpt comes from the first interview with the son, which is intended to establish rapport and prepare him for family therapy.

Client: "Boy, I've sure learned a lot this past two weeks. I've really learned a lesson. You won't need to worry about me. I'm not going to cause any more trouble."

4. Mrs. Loomis, a twenty-seven-year-old divorcee client, has been focusing on her need for a close, enduring relationship. She trusts males little, however, because her former husband was unfaithful on several occasions and because the men she has been associating with seem interested only in one-night stands. She meets men primarily in bars. In this twelfth interview, she has been discussing her latest relationship, which culminated in the typical fashion—the fellow wanted her to spend the night with him in his apartment.

Mrs. Loomis: "I've about given up on men. All they seem interested in is sex. I don't think there's a decent man in the whole damn city."

5. Sally, a seventeen-year-old high-school student, referred herself to the school psychologist because of a deep concern about being socially inept. She described feeling alienated from her peers and expressed a plaintive wish to have some friends of her own. Yet it became evident during the first five interviews that she avoids every opportunity for social interaction, rationalizing that the sit-

uation is unimportant and unworthy of her time. The following exchange comes from the sixth interview.

Counselor: "Sally, your behavior tells me you must be torn between your desire to be more involved socially with others and your hesitancy and fear in meeting with the group when they invite you to join them."

Sally: "Do you mean I have to participate in the kids' stuff they're involved in to learn to socialize?"

6. Divorced for three months, thirty-two-year-old Bill sought help to reestablish his marriage, ostensibly because he hates to see his three children reared without their father. His coping pattern has been to telephone his wife frequently, persistently criticizing her for depriving the children of their father and appealing for another chance. Her reaction has been negative, and she sees his behavior as harassment. Several days prior to this interview, his fourth, she took the children to an adjacent state to escape his harassment and to allow herself "to think things through."

Bill: "I just don't see how she can do this to those kids. She doesn't seem to care what happens to them. All she seems concerned about is herself. I guess I'll have to go to Colorado and let her know how much I miss those kids."

Therapist: "Bill, did she tell you why she was going to Colorado?"

Bill: "Yeah! She said she needed some time to herself to think things over. But I don't believe her. She just wants to keep the kids away from me."

7. Tom, a sixteen-year-old high-school student, has been referred to the counselor by his parents because of their concern over his lack of motivation in school and at home. Formerly a good student, he has frequently been lackadaisical in class, and his grades have dropped markedly. He has also been oversleeping in the mornings, causing tardiness. The parents have tried numerous approaches to motivate him but to no avail. In the two interviews prior to this one, the counselor has learned that Tom's goal is to go to college and become an accountant. Prior to this interview, the counselor has learned that Tom has skipped over one half of his mathematics classes during the week.

Tom: "Why should I bother going to class when the teacher treats me like I don't want to do anything?"

Counselor: "Sounds like you're pretty burned with the teacher and just feel, 'To heck with him. I'll show him.'"

Tom: "Yesterday he bawled me out because I didn't have the whole assignment done. He acted like I was the only one who didn't have the homework in. Gad, there were seven or eight other guys who hadn't finished as much as I had. But he has to pick on me. I can't stand him!"

Counselor: "I can understand you'd have some resentment when you feel you're being singled out."

Tom: "He isn't even half understanding about why I wasn't able to finish the homework. Jeez, I just get to feeling why try at all."

8. A married couple, both about thirty, has sought therapy because of fighting over the wife's infidelity. The wife requested counseling to begin with, and the husband came along reluctantly. From the outset, the husband made it clear that he expected quick results and that he was uninterested in any counseling extending over more than a few interviews. The therapist explained the nature of the helping process and made it clear that he would make no promises about quick results. The client acquiesced and agreed to try counseling. He has kept the appointments regularly and appears to be making conscientious efforts. The following excerpt is taken from early in an individual interview, the fifth.

Client: "Say, do you know Dr. Taylor?"

Therapist: "I'm not sure. What's his first name?"

Client: "I don't know his first name, but he's a psychologist."

Therapist: "You must mean Larry Taylor. Yeah, I know him. Why?"

Client: "A friend told me about him. Said he'd seen him about his marriage, and it had really helped him. He said Dr. Taylor told him what the problems were and what he needed to do to straighten it out. Said it was just what he needed. I wondered what you thought of him."

9. The client is a male, age thirty-one, who is on parole after serving part of a sentence for armed robbery. He has a fairly good job but budgets poorly and lives beyond his means, which has caused stress in his marriage. Referred by his parole officer to a mental health center, he has had six interviews before the one from which this exchange is taken.

Client: "What do you think I should do about this financial mess? I mean, I want some real suggestions."

Therapist: "So you're really feeling some pressure about your bills. Well, it sounds as though you can go two directions. You can either try to increase your income or lower your expenses."

Client: "Well, I'm not about to lower my standard of living. That's out. Life's too short to live like a peasant."

Therapist: "Well, if you rule that out, I guess it just leaves trying to increase your income."

Client: "Yeah, but how do I do that?"

Therapist: "I guess there would be several possibilities—work part time, get a better-paying job. What have you thought about?"

Client: "Well, I've thought about those, but there's no future in just working all the time. And I like my job. I've thought about dealing dope. You can make a lot of bread doing that. I've been wanting a new Cadillac, and I could probably make enough in just a few months."

10. The client is a twenty-six-year-old housewife, mother of two children. Her husband is a medical student. She has been receiving psychotherapy because of mild depression and anxiety. Raised in an emotionally deprived home with a cold, rejecting, and critical mother, the client has manifested marked feelings of uncertainty and a pattern of leaning over backwards to please others. Her husband, by contrast, is domineering and critical, which tends to perpetuate and magnify her doubts about her self-worth. She responds by apologizing for herself and attempting excessively to please him. The following excerpt comes from the eighth interview.

Client: "I've really been down since Tuesday. I've just felt I'm not worth anything to anyone."

Therapist: "What happened Tuesday?"

Client: "I'd been working in the backyard all day, pulling weeds, trying to make it look decent and trying to keep my eye on the children. I thought I'd accomplished a lot. Verne came home before I'd had a chance to freshen up. I was still in the backyard, and I didn't look too good. The wind had been blowing, and my hair was pretty windblown. Well, Verne looked at me and with a scowl told me I looked like hell. He could have run over me with a tank, and it wouldn't have felt any worse."

Therapist: "You really felt crushed, then."

Client: "I'll say. I just haven't felt that Verne really loves me very much. I try so hard to please him. But I can't seem to please him." She is near tears.

11. Tom, a thirteen-year-old junior-high student, was referred to the school counselor because of recent belligerency toward one of his teachers and a refusal to apply himself in that class. The first interview was spent getting acquainted with him and touching briefly on the problem. In this, the second interview, he has ventilated resentment and anger toward the teacher for being prejudiced against him. The reason for his anger is that his teacher reportedly accused him of cheating when he was innocent. The teacher also told him he was not trying when he had, in fact, been making an honest effort until he was accused of cheating three weeks ago. The counselor has been discussing with him the fact that things seem to be going worse.

Counselor: "Maybe we can think together about some way of working things out."

Student: "Naw, she's just got it in for me. She just thinks I'm some kind of hood, I guess. There's no way to work it out. I'm just going to goof off in her class. No point in trying."

12. The client is a single male, age twenty-one, a college student who has been receiving psychotherapy for mild depression, guilt associated with emerging sexual feelings hitherto repressed, indecisiveness, and shallow interpersonal relations. In this interview, his twenty-third, he has been expressing feelings of worthlessness and self-condemnation. The therapist has asked the client to specify when and under what circumstances the feelings appeared. Some unproductive exploration ensued, but persistent probing by the therapist led to the following exchange.

Client: "I think I began to feel rotten about myself in church."

Therapist: "I see. Specifically what happened that preceded the feelings?"

Client (appearing embarrassed): "Uh, well, I was trying to listen to the speaker, but I couldn't stay focused. There was this girl sitting across the aisle from me in the row behind. She was really a knockout, and her clothes really fit her. Well, uh, she had on this short skirt, and you could see just about all of her thigh, and"—he shakes his head—"even her panties. I really felt crummy about it, but I just kept turning around and looking. All I could think of was her—and sexual thoughts." He pauses, looks at floor.

Therapist: "And that's when you began to feel rotten about yourself?"

Client: "Yes. I knew I shouldn't be thinking about her—in that way. Especially in church. All I could think of after that was what an evil person I am. I think I'm a lost cause."

13. The client is a thirty-five-year-old married female who sought psychotherapy because of depression. Her husband is disabled and receives a pension. She works full time and spends most of the rest of her time meeting the demands of her husband, who expects her undivided attention. Her life has been devoid of much personal gratification because of the burdens placed upon her. Even when she has had opportunities for diversion and recreation, however, she has not taken advantage of them because there are uncompleted tasks in the home. The therapist is of the opinion that her depression is in large measure associated with a lack of reinforcement and personal fulfillment. The following excerpt is taken from the sixth interview with the client, who has developed a relatively high level of trust and confidence in the therapist.

Therapist: "We talked last week of your love for music and the possibility of your getting season tickets to the symphony. I'd be interested in hearing your further thoughts on that."

Client: "Well, I thought about it, and it really was appealing. But then I got to thinking I'm never caught up on my housework now. I couldn't feel right about going."

Therapist: "So you're feeling that you can't do something you enjoy until your work is all finished, as though you have to earn the right to enjoy yourself."

Client: "Yeah, that's right. I don't deserve to really enjoy myself until I've finished all my work."

14. A twenty-year-old college student has been receiving counseling for academic difficulties. The student seeks desperately to measure up to his parents' expectations that he complete college, but he has never performed well academically. To improve his performance, he enrolled in a program to improve his study habits. He learned earlier in the day that he failed an important examination in a required course. The following interchange occurs as he reports this to the counselor.

Client: "I really bombed out on that English test. I'd hoped I'd do better. I knocked myself out studying."

Counselor: "You must feel really let down after building up your hopes, really disappointed."

Client: "Oh, not really." His head drops perceptibly. "I guess I knew I was kidding myself. No, I'm not really upset." His chin quivers.

15.   The client is a married female, who has been receiving marriage counseling with her husband. Therapy has consisted of both individual and conjoint interviews. The couple was referred by an attorney whom the wife had consulted to initiate divorce proceedings after learning that her husband had been having an affair for several years. He terminated the affair rather than relinquish the marriage, but she remains bitter over his infidelity. Their communication is dominated by her constant references to his infidelity, and he has been at a loss in knowing how to cope with her. The following excerpt occurs in an individual interview with the wife, the fourth such session.

Client: "I find myself feeling angry with him so often for what he did. I just can't understand why he'd do it."

Therapist: "So you're finding it difficult to let go of those feelings. Still feel so deeply hurt."

Client: "Lately I've found myself feeling that if he can do it, then why can't I. I've felt like giving him a taste of his own medicine. I've thought of sleeping with a neighbor who's made overtures on several occasions. And then I'd tell Stan. Let him hurt for a change."

16.   The patient, a forty-three-year-old father of six children, has been admitted to a hospital for cardiovascular surgery. The attending physician referred him to social services to help him ventilate some of his fears about the surgery, which the patient knows involves a high risk. During some preliminary discussion, the social worker observes that the patient has a tremor in the hands, fidgets, and smokes one cigarette after the other.

Social worker: "It must be pretty scary, having to lie in bed and think about your surgery tomorrow."

Patient: "Oh, it's a little scary, I guess. But I've been through things a lot worse than this. I'm no boob."

17.   The clients are a married couple, both in their late thirties, who have had five previous conjoint marriage counseling ses-

sions. In the preceding session, each expressed feelings of being taken for granted and otherwise unappreciated by the other. This trend was arrested in the interview, and the therapist helped both verbalize their needs for "stroking messages." Reciprocal positive feelings were elicited, and they agreed to work during the week on sending more caring messages. The following excerpt comes from early in the sixth interview.

Wife: "We've done a lot better this week. We've worked on showing each other more respect, and it's really helped. Don't you think we've done better, Fred?"

Husband: "Yeah, it's been a good week."

Wife: "Things could be a lot better between Fred and Janet (their fourteen-year-old daughter), though." She turns to her husband. "I don't think you've shown Janet much respect. Remember, on Thursday you kept putting your arms around her in the store. She told me later she wished you wouldn't do that. It makes her feel, you know, uncomfortable. She's not a little girl anymore, you know."

Husband: "You know I was only teasing."

Therapist: "Teasing? I don't understand what you mean. Could you clarify that?"

Husband: "Well, we've always been close, but lately she pushes me away."

Wife: "I've wondered if you feel she doesn't love you anymore. Is that why you tease her?"

Husband: "Well, I've wondered."

Wife: "But you know, she still comes to you. Like Friday, she came and sat on your lap and hugged you."

Husband: "Yeah, that's right, I guess. But it still hurts when she pushes me away."

MODELED RESPONSES

1. a. Manipulative behavior
    b. "Look, Frank, I know you want to go home pretty bad. I want that for you too. But the only way that's going to happen is for you to show us you're ready to control yourself better. You might as well knock off that garbage about me and Mr. Olsen. We both know that's a damn lie."
2. a. Dysfunctional life style

      b. "I can see how painful that would be for you. You're really caught in a dilemma, as I see it. You don't want the total commitment of a marriage. Yet you seem to want a total kind of a commitment from him. It really hurts when you're sharing very deeply with him to know he may be sharing similarly with Ginny."

3.   a. Denial of problem

      b. "I'm glad you feel you've learned a lot, Bob. Still, I am very concerned about you. I know you want to have things better for yourself. But learning a lesson is sometimes only the beginning. I've learned from your parents that there's a lot wrong in your family. They want to make things better for all of you. But that takes a lot of doing. Today, I'd like to get your views on your family and what changes need to be made."

4.   a. Overgeneralization, discrepancy between expressed intention and behavior

      b. "I can see how discouraged and disillusioned you feel. Yet it seems to me you're generalizing about all men on the basis of the type you've had experiences with recently. It occurs to me that a lot of difficulty is caused by the fact that the type of man you're seeking and the type who frequent bars are often miles apart. The relationships formed in bars usually tend to be more of a casual and transitory nature. I think it may be helpful to ask yourself about the type of relationship you want."

5.   a. Discrepancy between expressed intentions and behavior

      b. "I can tell you feel turned off by some of the things they do. But it's your choice, of course, Sally. To be quite frank, I'm concerned because you seem to find reasons for not mixing in each time we discuss an opportunity. It's as though part of you wants to be more involved with others, but another part of you struggles hard to avoid involvement. Somehow, you're going to have to come to terms with these opposing parts. Otherwise, you're going to remain pretty much as you are. And that's okay if it's what you really want."

6.   a. Externalization of responsibility, discrepancy between expressed goal and behavior

b. "Bill, I think I understand how much you miss your children and how much you want to have Gayle back. But I think you need to consider if what you're doing is helping or hindering your chances of reaching your goal. I have the impression that you're not seeing that the pressures you're putting on Gayle are pushing her further away. In your anxiety for a reconciliation, you're doing the very things that are likely to destroy that possibility. I think you need to ask yourself how you can work toward creating circumstances that would make a reconciliation attractive to Gayle."

7. a. Discrepancy between stated goal and behavior, externalizing responsibility

b. "Tom, I can understand you might be feeling pretty discouraged and burned with your teacher. But I'm very concerned about your not getting your work in because it hurts you more than anyone. You need the credit for that course and a decent grade if you're going to accomplish your goal of becoming an accountant. And I'd like to see you accomplish that goal—it's a good one. If you let your teacher get you down, you're at the mercy of what he does. And that means you can end up working against yourself. I don't want to see you do that to yourself."

8. a. Resistance to therapy

b. This response deals with feelings behind the resistance: "It sounds to me as though what you're really wondering is whether Dr. Taylor could help you as he apparently helped your friend. That concerns me because it tells me you're not feeling satisfied with what's happening in your counseling with me. Perhaps you'd like me to just tell you the problems and what to do about them as your friend said Dr. Taylor did with him. I'd like to hear some of your feelings about that."

9. a. Discrepancy between intention and possible action or failure to consider consequences of behavior

b. "Yes, that'd be a possible way of increasing your income. But that alternative really scares me. You've been doing pretty well, all things considered, since your parole. I'd hate to see you blow it by risking getting busted. One false step, and you'd end up back in the pen to finish your sen-

tence. On top of that, they'd throw the book at you for dealing drugs. If you go back again, they'll throw away the key.
Is it worth that to you?"

10. a. Unexperienced feelings
     b. "You know, Kathy, as I listened to you describe the situa-
        tion and your feelings, I found myself feeling bad for you.
        You've really been hurting over Verne's criticism. But
        something else seems to stand out. I get the picture of you
        working hard all day, trying to get things in shape. And
        then when Verne comes, instead of some recognition for
        what you'd accomplished, you get criticized for looking
        wind-blown. You know, if I'd been in your shoes, I think
        I'd have been pretty resentful toward Verne. It just seems
        natural to me that you'd feel some anger mixed in with the
        hurt."

11. a. Failure to see alternatives, failure to consider consequences
     b. "You sound like you've given up on Mrs. Black. I feel bad
        about that because if you goof off things will only get worse.
        Besides, I'm not so sure it's as hopeless as you think it is.
        Sometimes teachers view things differently if we let them
        know our view about what's happening and what we'd like
        to happen. Mrs. Black may not really know your feelings
        that you've been blamed unfairly. All she can see is your
        goofing off right now. Let's think about some possible ways
        of making things better for you."

12. a. Misconception about self, magnification, dichotomous
        thinking, misconception about human existence
     b. "You know, Ted, I'm very concerned about the feelings
        you've described because you seem to be inflicting pain on
        yourself over behavior that's typical for any red-blooded
        male. You set almost superhuman standards for yourself
        that no one could live up to, and then you tear yourself
        down and see yourself as totally evil when you deviate even
        slightly from them. You can never feel very good about
        yourself for long with that black-and-white thinking. You'd
        have to be dead not to look at a girl under those circum-
        stances—even in church."

13. a. Misconception about self

b. "You know, I think you just said something terribly important in understanding yourself, Betty. I'm getting a fairly strong impression that it's tied in with your feelings about yourself. As though you can't feel good about enjoying yourself just for the sake of enjoyment. It's as though you have to work constantly to feel you're worthwhile, and that doesn't leave any room for your doing something just for yourself, I mean, just because it gives you pleasure."
The client appears contemplative, then declares, "Yeah, I think that describes me all right."
The therapist continues, "Well, if it does fit, then you're carrying a conception about yourself that leads to becoming a 'workaholic.' It's as though you believe you're a bad person if you engage in something for the sheer pleasure of it. The only way you can avoid that bad feeling is to push yourself constantly. I'd like to see you get more out of life than just work. Let's think together about your assumption—how you learned it and what it's doing to you."

14. a. Discrepancy between actual and expressed feelings or between feelings expressed verbally and nonverbally
b. "But knowing you were kidding yourself isn't really much of a comfort. Your facial expression tells me you're really hurting right now. You're so disappointed you feel like crying."

15. a. Discrepancy between expressed intentions and behavior or discrepant intentions
b. "It just seems so unfair to you, that you hurt so bad. And you find yourself wanting to hurt back. I guess that's what concerns me because I'm unclear about what it is you really want. If what you want most is to get even with Stan, you can probably accomplish it that way. But that concerns me because it seems in opposition to what you've said you really wanted. Rather than strengthening your marriage, you'd be tearing it down."

16. a. Discrepancy between expressed and actual feelings
b. "Of course, you're no boob. But you're probably a lot more than a little scared. You know, it's not being a boob to be darned afraid in your situation. In fact, it'd be pretty un-

natural not to be." The client nods appreciatively. "I'd be interested in hearing what's been going through your head while you've been lying here."

17. a. Lack of information

b. "You know, Fred, I have the feeling that you've felt rejected by Janet, as though she no longer loves you." He nods agreement. "I think that Janet's behavior is pretty typical for a girl her age. In the early teens, girls often begin to feel uncomfortable and confused about giving and receiving affection from their fathers. They're developing sexually and are very much aware of this sexuality. Expressing affection sometimes gets mixed in with sexual arousal, and teenage kids can't handle that kind of feelings toward the parent of the opposite sex. The only way they know how to handle it is to back off. The fact that she still comes to you, though, tells you she still has love for you." He appears relieved. "Did you know that about teenagers, Fred?" He nods negatively and adds, "No, but it's sure good to know."

Chapter 11

❦❦❦❦❦ ❦❦❦❦❦❦❦❦❦❦ ❦❦❦

Communication
Processes in Effective
Therapy: Summary

Two decades have elapsed since Rogers (1957) postulated that empathic understanding, unconditional positive regard, and congruence are essential to successful counseling outcomes. His formulation proved to be seminal. It led to the development of scales that operationalize the ingredients in slightly modified form (accurate empathy, nonpossessive warmth or respect, and genuineness) and to dozens of research studies, most of which show a relationship between high levels of these facilitative conditions and favorable counseling outcomes. Further studies demonstrated that high levels of the conditions foster self-exploration by the client. Investigations in fields other than psychotherapy also suggest that these facilitative conditions are vital and growth-enhancing in relationships generally, including counselor-client, student-teacher, parent-child, and marital relationships. Therapists who relate with low levels of the facilitative conditions tend to be psychonoxious, producing deterioration in their clients. Although diverse techniques from various psychotherapeutic schools (for example,

333

systematic desensitization, behavioral rehearsal, task assignments) are undoubtedly effective when used with specific clients and problems, the facilitative conditions appear to be critical to positive therapy outcomes.

Unfortunately, relatively few clinical training programs include systematic skill development in authenticity, empathic understanding, and respect, and many practicing counselors are functioning at low levels of these interpersonal skills. Evidence indicates, however, that a relatively short period (for example, 100 hours) of systematic didactic and experiential training can teach graduate students or lay persons to function with a relatively high level of the facilitative conditions, comparable to that of highly experienced and proficient psychotherapists.

Our purpose in writing this book was to provide the helping professional with learning materials that go beyond mere theoretical discussion to practical guidelines and skill-development exercises for enhancing clinical skills. Thus theory and skill development have been combined in a single book with a self-instructional format of relevance to practitioners from virtually all theoretical persuasions. The remainder of this chapter presents an overview of the therapeutic process and summarizes the role of each of the facilitative dimensions and the guidelines for their effective application.

The Therapeutic Process

The therapeutic process is not unitary, and it is artificial and to some degree misleading to speak of discrete phases when therapy changes markedly with the needs of a given client. Adaptability and flexibility are crucial, and individual counselors must learn to use their own unique personalities in helpful ways, rather than rigidly following the model of some theorist or school. However, all effective counseling interviews share many common and systematic elements. Generally, particular facilitative conditions and factors play a critical role early in counseling, whereas other dimensions are more significant and helpful later.

The major process goals in the early phase of counseling are to establish a working relationship with the client; to facilitate the client's self-exploration in order to clarify the nature of his problems, goals, and expectations; to assess and enhance the client's motivation; to clarify the counselor's role; and to negotiate a therapy contract. It is crucial in initial interviews to establish rapport and secure the client's trust in the counselor's humanness and competence. The most fundamental, vital, and complex therapeutic skill, and the one central to developing rapport, is empathic communication.

Empathy involves the ability to recognize the private, inner experiences and feelings of the client and to communicate this recognition to the client. Empathy refers to an intense "being with," grasping feelings and meanings as they are experienced by the client, not diagnosed and evaluated from some external vantage point. Thus empathy is understanding as if one were the client, without becoming involved to the degree of overidentification. During the early phase of counseling, empathy says to the client, "I am with you." It reduces fears, anxiety, and defensiveness and begins to establish a safe climate wherein the client can risk revealing problems and feelings. Empathy is equally important in working with resistant and involuntary clients. Empathic recognition and acceptance of their resentment is the best way to neutralize such feelings and open the possibility of cooperative work.

Early in therapy, the counselor does not seek to be deeply empathic, for this would generally be threatening in a new relationship. Instead, he conveys empathy by giving feedback that accurately and reciprocally reflects the surface, conscious feelings of the client. Deeper, or additive, levels of empathic responding, which expand the client's awareness of his underlying feelings, meanings, goals, or purposes of behavior, are generally withheld or used sparingly until the therapeutic relationship is well established. At this stage of the process, the goal is not the facilitation of deep insights.

Respect is the second attitude and skill crucial to establishing an effective therapeutic relationship. Respect refers to a nonpossessive caring for and affirmation of another as a separate individual. It involves a warmly receptive attitude whereby the client's feelings, opinions, individuality, and uniqueness are prized and preserved. Thus, in the early phase of therapy, the counselor establishes a climate wherein the client is not judged and evaluated or dominated and controlled. Rather, the counselor seeks to sensitively understand and to warmly accept the client, affirms the client's self-determination and capacity to make his own decisions, and strives never to damage a client's self-esteem. Sensitivity and respect play a vital role in winning the client's trust and in reducing his feelings of shame and failure and his fears of being perceived as weak, deficient, or worthless. Even resistant and involuntary clients may "soften" and open themselves if they discover that their integrity and personhood are respected, that negative feelings are accepted and understood, and that the counselor is not coercive, punitive, or authoritarian.

Authenticity, another central ingredient in the helping process, refers to sharing the self by behaving in a natural, spontaneous, open, and nondefensive manner. However, authenticity does not mean that the counselor overtly expresses and totally discloses his feelings at all times. In fact, authentic expression may sometimes be counterproductive. During the initial phase of counseling, authenticity should be conveyed at moderate levels as an absence of phoniness and defensiveness. Although the counselor avoids a professional facade and seeks to convey his humanness, self-disclosures of personal feelings, reactions, and experiences are kept to a minimum until trust and a good therapeutic relationship have been established. The early part of counseling is a time of relationship building and of initial exploration characterized by empathic responsiveness and respectful acceptance. High levels of authentic disclosure are inappropriate to the primary goals of this phase.

Similarly, confrontation and relational immediacy are largely contraindicated early in counseling. These are change-oriented processes, and using them prematurely may be antithetical to the initial goals of therapy. Moving too soon toward deep insights and action runs the risks of psychological damage and of premature unilateral termination. Before a foundation of trust has been established wherein the client clearly perceives the counselor's good will and helpful intent, confrontations or interpretations of relational immediacy are likely to be misinterpreted and to frighten and overwhelm the client. Confrontation and revelation of personal values and feelings early in counseling are associated with negative therapeutic outcomes. Therefore, confrontation and relational immediacy are generally deemphasized in this phase. An exception involves character-disordered clients who attempt to "con," deceive, or manipulate the counselor. With such clients, the counselor may need to use at least mild confrontation to avoid being perceived as ineffectual and gullible and to foster the development of a relationship.

Once a secure therapeutic climate has been established, the focus of counseling shifts to deeper exploration, expansion of awareness, and insight. When the client understands the interrelationship, nature, and purposes of his self-defeating cognitions, feelings, and behaviors, goals and strategies for change can be devised. Thus, expanded awareness and cognitive insight are not the final goals of therapy, but only steps toward the ultimate objective of behavioral change. Some schools of counseling and psychotherapy accord primary importance to insight, while other approaches minimize its role. The authors take an intermediate position, maintaining that insight does not assure change and is not an end in itself and that it should be pursued only to the extent necessary to remove barriers to progress and to clarify goals. Expanded awareness must be followed with techniques that foster behavioral change.

The client's insights are facilitated in the middle phase through additive levels of empathic communication, which go beyond surface feelings to illuminate underlying emotions, purposes and meanings that are only vaguely perceived and are somewhat beyond the client's level of awareness. As the therapeutic relationship deepens, the therapist also begins to offer higher levels of respect by increasing communication of caring and positive feelings, which augments the nonjudgmental attitude and acceptance already established. As counseling progresses, even higher levels of respect come into play. The counselor does not merely accept the client; instead, he encourages the client to realize his potentials as fully as he can.

In contrast to the responsive posture of the early phase of counseling, higher levels of counselor authenticity serve well the middle-phase objectives of enhancing awareness and fostering change. A well-established relationship allows candid feedback which can provide the client with helpful information about how he is perceived by others. In addition to facilitating increased awareness, authenticity models spontaneity, openness, and humanness for the client. Authenticity is also involved in facilitating insight through relational immediacy, which refers to the intensive examination of the immediate counselor-client relationship and its use as a basis for learning. The client's problems are manifested primarily in dysfunctional interpersonal patterns, and many of these over-learned and maladaptive cognitive, perceptual, and behavioral styles are reenacted in the here-and-now of counseling. Thus interpretation of the immediate counseling interaction may foster an awareness of relationship patterns that can be gained in no other way short of filming the client's daily life or spending a week by his side. Focusing on the here-and-now in counseling, however, may be extremely intense and threatening. Therefore, it should always be borne in mind that relational immediacy is generally inappropriate during the early phase of counseling.

Confrontation is a hazy concept in the counseling literature. As we define the term, confrontation refers to constructively helping the client focus his attention on growth-defeating discrepancies in and between perceptions, feelings, behavior, values, attitudes, and communications. Thus confrontation is an intensive way of giving the client authentic feedback on inconsistencies and contradictions. The goals of confrontation fit the goals of the middle and terminal phases of counseling—to expand awareness of the obstacles to growth and to encourage movement and behavioral change. A strong therapeutic relationship is a prerequisite for confrontation. Although this mode of intervention may expand awareness and accelerate therapy, it is generally threatening, and, when inappropriately (or unskillfully) used by an inexperienced counselor with a limited repertoire of skills, it may have destructive results. Confrontation, therefore, is best used discriminately, in the middle and terminal phases of counseling.

Counterproductive Counselor Communication

Therapy should be tailored to the individual. Neither the facilitative conditions nor any specific technique is therapeutic when used indiscriminately, without regard to the situation, client dynamics, or the stage of therapy. The use of empathic communication, confrontation, or other specific techniques should be based on empirical knowledge of indications and contraindications rather than a theoretical conviction about their universal applicability. Thus the authors have chosen to provide guidelines which can serve as rules of thumb for the effective and discriminate application of the facilitative conditions. We hope that our formulations will stimulate research to test their validity.

Up till now, outcome research on the facilitative conditions has not taken into account the need for differential application. This may be one of the significant reasons why a few studies fail to replicate a positive relationship between one of the facilitative conditions and successful outcomes. Since such research neglects application guidelines, it measures the facilitative conditions indiscriminately, independent of the nature or the phase of counseling, the type of counselor-client interaction, or, in general terms, the appropriateness of the situation. In other words, a research design that accords no importance to the appropriateness of the situation in which a response is made would rate a highly empathic response as highly empathic even when that response was premature and antitherapeutic. Obviously, many such antitherapeutic interventions can lead to poor counseling outcomes, with the result that a counselor rated as highly empathic by the research study is in fact doing his client little or no good. This kind of oversight, common in the extant research, confounds our theoretical understanding of the facilitative conditions in therapy and undercuts the development of precise practical guidelines for their use.

Conclusions on facilitative conditions drawn from research that disregards the situational appropriateness of their applications seem analogous to a medical investigator who concludes from inadequately controlled studies that he has discovered a drug with curative properties, which increase proportionally to the dosage, for all manner of diverse ailments. Further development, testing, and refinement of the discriminating use of the facilitative conditions are sorely needed.

The therapist must also recognize dysfunctional communication styles that can elicit defensiveness, encourage premature termination, and be destructive. It is vital to keep in mind that on the average 10 percent of clients seen in therapy are damaged by the experience and that some counselors cause even more harm.

Passivity and ambiguity may be therapeutic and indicated at specific times with specific clients. The elevation of silence and ambiguity into a counseling style, however, tends to be counterproductive. By contrast, the counselor's domination of therapy through overactivity and excessive directiveness may be equally unproductive. Such counselors frequently interrupt, lecture, advise, and move prematurely to confrontation or other action-oriented techniques. Similarly, some counselors become psychic detectives and interrogate or grill the client, relying principally on questioning as their mode of operation. Probing inquiries may be helpful in leading clients and eliciting information, but when used excessively, they restrict interaction, circumscribe responses, and encourage passivity. Appropriate personal disclosures by the counselor might model openness and be instructive. However, self-disclosures too often turn the spotlight on the counselor, thus serving primarily the counselor's narcissism. Inappropriate self-disclosure, like dominance or interrogation, responds to the counselor's needs, not the client's.

Certain communication patterns create distance between counselor and client, safeguarding the counselor against threatening emotions and experiences, reinforce the client's dysfunctional styles, block the development of trust and rapport, and inhibit spontaneous self-exploration by the client. Counselors who are themselves unable to tolerate emotional intensity or intimacy and who have unresolved personal problems are particularly apt to create distance through such strategies as limiting interaction to the merely social while skirting uncomfortable issues, providing false reassurance, or prohibiting strong emotional expression. Still other counselors avoid personal involvement and maintain emotional detachment through intellectualization, playing the role of a technical expert, or being an ambiguous blank screen therapist.

Instead of reducing defensive barriers, some counselors unknowingly confuse the client and accentuate differences between counselor and client with technical jargon. Other counselors rationalize that profanity and crude language is a good way to be "real" and to create rapport. In actuality, vulgar language may be very unauthentic for many counselors and offensive to numerous clients. It seems most realistic and facilitative for the counselor to adapt his language to the understanding and the values of the client, at the same time preserving his own integrity.

Excessive ambition and power strivings motivate some therapists to use pressure tactics. Such "pseudoshrinks" often demand immediate change from the client, abrasively challenging, confronting, and browbeating him in an effort to bring about change. The resulting change is most often devastatingly negative. Moralizing, belittling, dogmatic interpreting, and responding in a condescending and patronizing manner are other ineffective patterns discussed in Chapter Three.

Empathic Communication

Considering empathy essential to therapy does not make one empathic. Only those therapists who have been specifically trained in this skill are able to use it to any significant degree. Acquiring the ability to communicate empathy requires the kind of practice and high-level modeling found in Chapters Four, Five, and Six.

A critical prerequisite to conveying empathic recognition to the client is the ability to accurately identify and verbalize the client's emotions. Accurate perceptiveness to feelings requires both a discrimination of the general dimension of feeling and an acute sensitivity to the particular intensity of the client's feelings. A rich vocabulary of feelings is essential to accurately labeling the client's emotions and to communicating one's own feelings authentically. A Vocabulary of Feelings consisting of ten major affective dimensions at three general levels of intensity is provided as a learning resource in Chapter Four. The vocabulary is to be used with the skill-development exercises to expand the repertoire of words available for talking about emotions sensitively.

Skills in conveying empathy depend on the counselor's ability to perceive accurately the levels of empathic communications making up the Empathic Communication Scale. An initial requirement for communicating empathy is that the counselor attend to, listen to, and concentrate on the client's verbal and nonverbal behavior. Eye contact, a receptive posture, and full moment-to-moment psychological contact are important, as is the language and phrasing of empathic statements. An empathic response leads list is provided in Chapter Five to help the counselor respond in fresh, unstereotyped language. A common error in attempts at empathic responses is focusing on understanding the external, factual circumstances instead of "tuning in" to the client's internal feelings and frame of reference. Another error is to respond in an abstract or vague manner; one should instead be concrete and specific. The frequency and timing of empathic responses is significant, and the counselor must check his perceptions with the client. Empathy also requires the counselor to respond in a voice, tone, and intensity similar to the client's.

In the middle phases of counseling, deeper empathic responses are used to go beyond the client's explicit expressions to his underlying feelings and meanings. Additive empathic responses are thus mildly to moderately interpretive in nature and are intended to expand awareness. A prime method for responding with additive empathy is to identify the client's underlying feelings. Full experiencing, however, requires an integration of both feelings and thought. Therefore, additive empathic responses may also concentrate on expanding the client's awareness of underlying meanings, associations and relationships, implicit assumptions and perceptual patterns, implicit goals and ideals, and the purposes of behavior and emotions. The counselor's responses may also reach additive levels by summarizing and synthesizing previously disconnected elements or patterns, accurately identifying the implicit meanings of postural and nonverbal expressions, and helping the client internalize and accept his role and responsibility in his problems. The moment-to-moment effectiveness of interventions can be gauged by carefully watching the client's reaction to the counselor's response and his level of self-experiencing. Additive empathic responses have to be phrased tentatively and to incorporate evidence or documentation.

Even empathic responses are not helpful in all clinical situations, and, in fact, they may be counterproductive at times. Thus the therapist should follow guidelines to the proper use of empathy. Reciprocal empathic communication is particularly indicated in the early phase of counseling and in the early portions of interviews. Preceding and following additive empathic interventions, confrontations, or other counseling techniques with reciprocal empathy heightens receptivity. Empathic responses facilitate emotional expression and are therefore indicated when one must assess the role emotions play in the client's problems; when catharsis is needed; when the client is inexperienced at, inept at, or incapable of expressing his feelings; when he is emotionally constricted, underexpressive, and unaware of his emotions; when defensiveness, negativism, and hostility in the therapeutic relationship must be worked through; and when the time is right for fostering deeper insight.

Reciprocal or mildly additive empathy is considered the baseline counseling intervention. Nonetheless, even reciprocal empathic responses are sometimes inappropriate and contraindicated. For example, responding empathically is mistaken when a client realistically needs factual information essential to problem solving, when discrepancies and inconsistencies appear in the middle and terminal phases of counseling, and when the counselor experiences persistent feelings in the current interaction that detract from his ability to "tune in" with the client. Furthermore, following early contacts with clients who have chronically antisocial, nonconforming, and impulsive character disorders, confrontation or other action-oriented techniques are generally more beneficial than continued empathic responding. Additive empathic interventions are more powerful and threatening than reciprocal responses and thus must be used more discriminately. Caution is particularly called for with clients who are distrustful and paranoid, very withdrawn and schizoid, or severely depressed. Additive responses focused on underlying feelings rather than on cognitive conceptualizations, purposes, and meanings are recommended with obsessive-compulsive clients. Emotionally overexpressive, histrionic clients, on the other hand, do better with additive responses which encourage rational processes and dampen further emotional expression. Generally, the more intense the client's emotionality, the more the counselor can formulate additive responses that conceptualize purposes, relationships, and meanings without fear of encouraging overintellectualization and repression of affect.

Respect

Respect at all the levels specified on the Respect Scale comprises four vital elements. First, respect can be communicated by demonstrating a commitment to understand the client and by encouraging his self-expression. The respectful counselor signals his sincere interest by listening attentively and responding empathically. The second vital factor in respect is communicating acceptance and warmth to the client. The counselor suspends judgment and endeavors to accept the client's feelings and opinions, rather than imposing his own perceptions or value system. Instead of arguing, evaluating, belittling, or ridiculing, the effective counselor receives and accepts warmly. The third element to respect is an affirmation of the client's worth, uniqueness, and individuality. With verbal and nonverbal messages the counselor communicates, "You are significant, important, and worthwhile." The counselor conveys caring and appreciation for the other person. He desires to be sensitive and to preserve the client's individuality, rather than altering him to fit some preconceived expectations. The final vital element in respect consists of affirming and identifying the client's problem-solving capacity and his resources, strengths, and potentials for growth. A respectful counselor safeguards and accepts the client's right to self-determination, and he believes in and trusts his ability to make decisions and to be responsible for himself. This fourth element means searching together for solutions that best fit the client and working in a cooperative partnership in which the counselor does not dominate the client.

Five situations are especially challenging to the counselor's capacity to respond respectfully: provocation by the client (for example, aggressive, abusive behavior); self-effacing clients; dependency and patterns of helplessness; humiliation and embarrassment for the client; and clients with values, beliefs, behaviors and life styles quite different from the counselor's.

Authenticity

To be authentic means to be spontaneously open, genuine, and congruent with feelings, thoughts, verbalizations, and behavior. A phony or inauthentic counselor, by contrast, may respond from a contrived role or be defensive, guarded, ambiguous, and incongruent. Openness, however, does not grant the therapist license to express feelings indiscriminately, for negative feelings can be abrasive and destructive rather than therapeutic. Thus authenticity refers to a quality of constructive openness wherein the counselor's disclosures are appropriate and carefully timed to the client's needs.

Authentic responses take several forms. One common form, self-disclosure, consists of revealing to the client experiences, interests, and attitudes extraneous to the counseling relationship. A counselor might, for example, divulge selected information about his relationship to a spouse or parent or mention past experiences and personal history. Authenticity is also manifested through sharing here-and-now feelings and physical reactions to the client or the situation—for instance, warmth and care, confusion, or irritation. Another type of sharing of self consists of expressing one's personal perceptions, reactions, ideas, and formulations. Spontaneous, here-and-now associations are another aspect of the counselor's experiencing that might be shared at times with the client. An authentic response may also embody empathic understanding, which is conveyed by the counselor's sharing of some of himself. Thus a counselor may occasionally express his own feelings or reactions to a situation to determine whether the client's feelings are similar. Lastly, the counselor can express personal feelings nonverbally by, for example, employing touch very judiciously or by moving physically closer to a member of a therapy group.

Because of the potential destructive impact of indiscriminate authentic responding, it is essential that counselors observe guidelines to the effective use of authenticity. Trust and rapport in the relationship are prerequisite to authentic disclosures, and such responses, therefore, should be made only sparingly early in therapy. The counselor must assess the client's readiness to share the counselor's frame of reference. Authentic responses should have a definite goal and purpose, be relevant to the client's needs, and not serve as a distraction by placing a spotlight on the counselor. Authenticity and impulsiveness differ sharply. Furthermore, counselor genuineness beyond moderate levels is not related to increased facilitation for clients. As a general guideline, increased counselor expressiveness is appropriate when the client is focused on impersonal, superficial, and external events. However, when the client is already engaged in relevant self-exploration and is in close contact with his own experiencing, authentic responses by the counselor tend to distract, and empathic responsiveness is more appropriate to the situation.

When the counselor experiences persistent feelings toward a client, he should seek not only to understand the feelings, but to determine whether they may be constructively shared. When the counselor feels physically attracted to a client or when his reactions are strongly negative, he should explore the feelings to understand their source and range. In addition, the counselor must consider the risk of destructive impact, the potential helpfulness, and the objective of disclosing such reactions and the ways in which they may be facilitatively shared before expressing them. Positive feelings almost always underlie negative reactions to the client, and authenticity requires more than merely sharing superficial and easily identified feelings. The counselor should try to share the whole complex range of his feelings, which often are ambivalent or conflicting, not just his surface reactions. When the counselor reveals feelings, he should seek to remain experientially descriptive, not evaluative, claiming feelings as his own instead of blaming the client. Restraint and caution must be exercised in expressing feelings through physical contact. Client requests for disclosure by the counselor that seek to evade self-examination or to redefine the relationship as a social one should be explored concurrently with or prior to counselor self-disclosure.

Relational Immediacy

Closely akin to authenticity, relational immediacy involves examining the here-and-now interaction and feelings of the counseling relationship. The client often re-creates in the therapeutic relationship the very problems that plague and defeat him in his daily interactions. One of the reasons for this is that the client continues to operate in the therapeutic relationship on the same unquestioned assumptions and conditioned perceptual stereotypes that guide him outside. Furthermore, the establishment and growth of the therapeutic relationship involves factors that resemble those in any significant personal relationship, such as the issues of power and control, autonomy, trust, the degree of intimacy and the manner in which differences, conflict, and disagreement are handled. The client will generally perceive these issues through the spectacles of his conditioning and attempt to cope with them in his usual overlearned ways. Thus the counselor-client relationship is a social microcosm within which the client's problematic interpersonal behavior and conditioned perceptual sets and distortions appear.

The immediate relationship should become the focus of counseling when the client has negative, unrealistic, or unwarranted feelings or attitudes toward the counselor or toward counseling, such as anger, fear, distrust, dependency, or sexual desires; when there is resistance or defensiveness inimical to progress; when significant conflicts over interpersonal issues in the counselor-client relationship occur; when the client manifests manipulative or dysfunctional styles of relating or perceiving in the interview; when the counselor has strong or persistent problem feelings toward the client; and when the client is already referring to or discussing the current relationship on his own initiative. Guidelines in Chapter Nine cover exploring and observing the patterns and dynamic meanings of the client's current behavior, using the counselor's immediate experiencing to understand the client and the interaction and handling resistance, defensiveness, conflicts, and relational issues.

The immediate interaction can be used to expand the client's awareness and for modeling, rehearsing, and acquiring new skills. Since the patient needs an experience, not an explanation, an important principle in the timing of relationally immediate interpretations is: Experiencing precedes conceptualization. That is, the client must be allowed to experience conflicting feelings before the counselor interprets them. Immediacy interpretations should be aimed just below the level of conscious awareness, rather than at deep meanings well beyond awareness. Such interpretations should also be tentative, and they should be substantiated by specific and repetitive references to the client's behavior, not by weak inferential hypotheses based on indirect expressions only. In addition to making interpretations, the counselor may also encourage the client to conceptualize the process of the interaction, and he may work with immediacy by conducting here-and-now experiments with the client.

Confrontation

Confrontation offers the client fresh perspectives and corrective feedback when his limited self-awareness, distorted perceptions, and dysfunctional adaptive patterns are impeding growth and change. Confrontation, however, is abused by some therapists, who justify their extensive use of this high-risk technique as a way of accelerating the client's growth. Outcome research conducted on encounter groups, however, does not support this position. In fact, frequent and vigorous confrontations are associated with relatively high rates of psychological casualties. Skillful counselors use confrontation judiciously, relying more on the facilitative dimensions, especially additive empathy, to accomplish the same purposes. Indeed, additive empathy is not easily differentiated from skillful confrontation. The latter, however, emanates largely from the therapist's external frame of reference, whereas the former is directed more to the inner experiencing of the client.

When used prudently and skillfully, confrontation helps the client face aspects of his experiencing and behavior hitherto unrecognized or unacknowledged because of blind spots. Receiving information that is ego-alien or potentially destructive to self-esteem, however, may be deleterious to the client. Confrontations, therefore, are potentially destructive, and the therapist is well-advised to refrain from using this technique until he masters the other facilitative dimensions. The skillful use of the other facilitative dimensions diminishes the need for confrontation because the client tends to engage increasingly in self-confrontation as therapy progresses. Self-confrontation is preferred to therapist-initiated confrontation because its risk is negligible. Readiness to engage in self-confrontation, however, varies widely from client to client, and therapist-initiated confrontations are often necessary. This is particularly true with certain character-disordered clients who are out of touch with their emotions and who tend to externalize responsibilities for their difficulties.

Confrontation is generally contraindicated until a good therapeutic relationship has been established. The client must trust the counselor. Without this base of understanding, the counselor's helpful intent in confrontation may easily be distorted or misperceived as criticism or blaming.

Confrontations must occur in an atmosphere of warmth and caring. If the climate is cold or impersonal, the client may well consider the confrontation an attack.

Effective confrontation requires a keen sense of timing. When a client is in crisis, severely depressed, highly anxious, or experiencing strong negative feelings toward the therapist, confrontation is generally contraindicated. In these instances, the client is likely to be unreceptive or defensive.

Confrontation should not be used to push the client for immediate change. Single confrontations rarely result in major behavioral changes. The working-through process requires patience and repeated review of the problem behavior in an ever-broadening perspective. The therapist must respect the self-preserving function of defense mechanisms. Battering down those defenses may leave the client unprotected and induce psychic decompensation.

The responsibility for change resides with the client, and his self-determination should be respected. The therapist may be candid and authentic in sharing his perceptions, but the client must feel that his right to exercise choice and to determine future directions is respected.

Confrontations should be preceded and followed by empathic responsiveness. Prefacing the confrontation with empathic messages conveys helpful intent to the client. Empathic responding immediately following the confrontation helps the therapist determine the confrontation's impact and effect on the client.

Confrontations should serve the client's needs, not the counselor's. Counselors who employ confrontation to demonstrate how astute or effective they are, to overpower, to control, or to act out their anger may damage their clients or the helping relationship.

Confrontations should be descriptive, not evaluative or judgmental. The confrontation should address specific behaviors and patterns, not pin broad, evaluative labels like passive, insensitive, or domineering on the client. Focusing on behavior and its consequences suggests directions for specific behavioral changes to the client. The client will generally consider judgmental confrontations derogatory.

With certain clients, confrontation may be used even early in therapy to increase the anxiety needed to make therapy work. Thus confrontation may be appropriate with clients who manifest little or no anxiety and who are typically unconcerned about the destructive impact their insensitivity to the needs, feelings, and welfare of others has on those around them.

In deciding whether to employ confrontation, the therapist should observe the law of parsimony. The least amount of directiveness and pressure necessary to the therapeutic objectives should be used. Thus self-confrontation should be fostered whenever possible. Several techniques useful in fostering self-confrontation are discussed in Chapter Ten.

Confrontations are directed at discrepancies, inconsistencies, and dysfunctional patterns within or between the cognitive-perceptual, affective (emotional), or behavioral realms of experiencing. Twenty-three such inconsistencies, discrepancies, and dysfunctions are encountered most commonly in therapy, and they are considered in detail in Chapter Ten.

References

Alberti, R. E., and Emmons, M. L. *Your Perfect Right*. San Luis Obispo, Calif.: Impact, 1970.

Alexander, J. F., and Parsons, B. V. "Short-term Behavioral Intervention with Delinquent Families: Impact on Family Process and Recidivism." *Journal of Abnormal Psychology*, 1973, *81*, 219–225.

Allport, G. W. *Personality and Social Encounter*. Boston: Beacon Press, 1960.

Anderson, J. D. "Human Relations Training and Social Work." *Social Work*, 1975, *20*, 195–199.

Ansbacher, H. L., and Ansbacher, R. R. (Eds.) *The Individual Psychology of Alfred Adler*. New York: Harper & Row, 1964.

Anthony, W. A. "A Methodological Investigation of the Minimally Facilitative Level of Interpersonal Functioning." *Journal of Clinical Psychology*, 1971, *27*, 156–157.

Aronson, H., and Overall, B. "Treatment Expectations of Patients in Two Social Classes." *Social Work*, 1966, *11*, 35–41.

Aspy, D. N., and Hadlock, W. "The Effects of High- and Low-Functioning Teachers upon Student Performance." Unpublished manuscript, University of Florida, 1967. (Abstract in R. R. Carkhuff and B. G. Berenson, *Beyond Counseling and Therapy*. New York: Holt, Rinehart and Winston, 1967, p. 297).

Bandura, A. "Psychotherapy Based upon Modeling Principles." In A. E. Bergin and S. L. Garfield (Eds.), *Handbook of Psychotherapy and Behavior Change: An Empirical Analysis.* New York: Wiley, 1971.

Bandura, A. *Principles of Behavior Modification.* New York: Holt, Rinehart and Winston, 1969.

Bandura, A., Lipsher, D. H., and Miller, P. E. "Psychotherapists' Approach-Avoidance Reactions to Patients' Expressions of Hostility." *Journal of Consulting Psychology,* 1960, *24,* 1–8.

Banks, G. P. "The Effects of Race on One-to-One Helping Interviews." *Social Service Review,* 1971, *45,* 137–146.

Barron, F., and Leary, T. "Change in Psychoneurotic Patients With and Without Psychotherapy." *Journal of Consulting Psychology,* 1955, *19,* 239–245.

Baum, O. E., Felzer, S. B., D'Imura, T. H., and Shumaker, E. "Psychotherapy, Dropouts, and Lower Socioeconomic Patients." *American Journal of Orthopsychiatry,* 1966, *36,* 629–635.

Beck, A. T. *Cognitive Therapy and the Emotional Disorders.* New York: International Universities Press, 1976.

Beier, E. "Nonverbal Communication: How We Send Emotional Messages." *Psychology Today,* 1974, *8* (5), 53–56.

Berenson, B. G., and Mitchell, K. M. *Confrontation: For Better or Worse!* Amherst, Mass.: Human Resource Development Press, 1974.

Bergin, A. E. "Some Implications of Psychotherapy Research for Therapeutic Practice." *Journal of Abnormal Psychology,* 1966, *71,* 235–246.

Bergin, A. E. "An Empirical Analysis of Therapeutic Issues." In D. Arbuckle (Ed.), *Counseling and Psychotherapy: An Overview.* New York: McGraw-Hill, 1967, 175–208.

Bergin, A. E. "The Evaluation of Therapeutic Outcomes." In A. E. Bergin and S. L. Garfield (Eds.), *Handbook of Psychotherapy and Behavior Change.* New York: Wiley, 1971, 217–270.

Bergin, A. E. "When Shrinks Hurt: Psychotherapy Can Be Dangerous." *Psychology Today,* 1975, *9* (6), 96–100.

Bergin, A. E., and Jasper, L. G. "Correlates of Empathy in Psychotherapy." *Journal of Abnormal Psychology,* 1969, *74,* 477–481.

Bergin, A. E., and Solomon, S. "Personality and Performance Correlates of Empathic Understanding in Psychotherapy." In

J. T. Hart and T. M. Tomlinson (Eds.), *New Directions in Client-Centered Therapy.* Boston: Houghton Mifflin, 1970.

Berne, E. *Games People Play.* New York: Grove Press, 1964.

Bettelheim, B. *Love is Not Enough.* Glencoe, Ill.: Free Press, 1950.

Betz, B. J. "Studies of the Therapist's Role in the Treatment of the Schizophrenic Patient." *American Journal of Psychiatry,* 1967, *123,* 963–971.

Beutler, L. E., Johnson, D. T., Neville, C. W., and Workman, S. N. "Accurate Empathy and the A-B Dichotomy." *Journal of Consulting and Clinical Psychology,* 1972, *38,* 372–375.

Biestek, F. *The Casework Relationship.* Chicago: Loyola University Press, 1957.

Brammer, L., and Shostrom, E. *Therapeutic Psychology: Fundamentals of Actualization Counseling and Psychotherapy.* Englewood Cliffs, N.J.: Prentice-Hall, 1968.

Buber, M. *The Way of Response.* New York: Schocken Books, 1966.

Canfield, S. F., Eley, J., Rollman, L. P., and Schur, E. L. "A Laboratory Training Model for the Development of Effective Interpersonal Communications in Social Work." *Journal of Education for Social Work,* 1975, *11,* 45–50.

Carkhuff, R. R. *The Counselor's Contribution to Facilitative Processes.* Buffalo, New York: State University of New York, 1968.

Carkhuff, R. R. *Helping and Human Relations: Practice and Research.* New York: Holt, Rinehart and Winston, 1969.

Carkhuff, R. R. "The Development and Generalization of a Systematic Resource Training Model." *Journal of Research and Development in Education,* 1971, *4,* 3–16.

Carkhuff, R. R., and Berenson, B. G. *Beyond Counseling and Therapy.* New York: Holt, Rinehart and Winston, 1967.

Carkhuff, R. R., Kratochvil, D., and Friel, T. "The Effects of Graduate Training." *Journal of Counseling Psychology,* 1968, *15,* 69–74.

Carkhuff, R. R., Piaget, G., and Pierce, R. "The Development of Skills in Interpersonal Functioning." *Counselor Education and Supervision,* 1968, *7,* 102–106.

Carkhuff, R. R., and Truax, C. B. "Training in Counseling and Psychotherapy: An Evaluation of an Integrated Didactic and Experiential Approach." *Journal of Consulting Psychology,* 1965, *29,* 333–336.

Cimbolic, P. "Counselor Race and Experience Effects on Black Clients." *Journal of Consulting and Clinical Psychology,* 1972, *39,* 328–332.

Colm, H. *The Existential Approach to Psychotherapy with Adults and Children.* New York: Grune and Stratton, 1966.

Combs, A. W., and Snygg, D. *Individual Behavior; A Perceptual Approach to Behavior* (rev. ed.) New York: Harper & Row, 1959.

DeRisi, W. J., and Butz, G. *Writing Behavioral Contracts.* Champaign, Ill.: Research Press, 1974.

Dollard, J., and Miller, N. E. *Personality and Psychotherapy: An Analysis in Terms of Learning, Thinking, and Culture.* New York: McGraw-Hill, 1950.

Douds, J., Berenson, B. G., Carkhuff, R. R., and Pierce, R. "In Search of an Honest Experience: Confrontation in Counseling and Life." In R. R. Carkhuff and B. G. Berenson (Eds.), *Beyond Counseling and Therapy.* New York: Holt, Rinehart and Winston, 1967.

Dreikurs, R. *The Challenge of Parenthood.* New York: Hawthorn Books, 1948.

Dreikurs, R. "Guilt Feelings as an Excuse." *Individual Psychology Bulletin,* 1950, *8,* 12–21.

Dreikurs, R. "The Psychological Interview in Medicine." *American Journal of Individual Psychology,* 1954, *10,* 99–122.

Dreikurs, R. *Psychodynamics, Psychotherapy, and Counseling.* Chicago: Alfred Adler Institute, 1967.

Dyer, W. G. "Congruence and Control." *Journal of Applied Behavioral Science,* 1969, *5,* 161–173.

Egan, G. *Encounter: Group Processes for Interpersonal Growth.* Monterey, Calif.: Brooks/Cole, 1970.

Egan, G. *The Skilled Helper: A Model for Systematic Helping and Interpersonal Relating.* Monterey, Calif.: Brooks/Cole, 1975.

Ellis, A. *Reason and Emotion in Psychotherapy.* New York: Lyle Stuart, 1962.

Ellis, A. *Humanistic Psychotherapy.* New York: McGraw-Hill, 1973a.

Ellis, A. "The No Cop-Out Therapy." *Psychology Today,* 1973b, 7 (2), 6–60.

Ely, A. L., Guerney, B. G. Jr., and Stover, L. "Efficacy of the Training Phase in Conjugal Therapy." *Psychotherapy: Theory, Research, and Practice,* 1973, *10,* 201–207.

Eysenck, H. J. "The Effects of Psychotherapy: An Evaluation." *Journal of Consulting Psychology,* 1952, *16,* 319–324.

Fagan, J., and Shepherd, I. L. (Eds.) *Gestalt Therapy Now: Theory, Techniques, Applications.* Palo Alto, Calif.: Science and Behavior Books, 1970.

Fay, A. "Clinical Notes on Paradoxical Therapy." In A. A. Lazarus (Ed.), *Multi-Modal Behavior Therapy.* New York: Springer Publishing Co., 1976.

Fiedler, F. E. "The Concept of an Ideal Therapeutic Relationship." *Journal of Consulting Psychology,* 1950, *14,* 239–245.

Finney, B. C. "Say It Again: An Active Therapy Technique." *Psychotherapy: Theory, Research, and Practice,* 1972, *9,* 157–165.

Frankl, V. *Man's Search for Meaning: An Introduction to Logotherapy.* Boston: Beacon Press, 1962.

Frankl, V. *Psychotherapy and Existentialism.* New York: Simon and Schuster, 1967.

Fromm-Reichmann, F. *Principles of Intensive Psychotherapy.* Chicago: University of Chicago Press, 1950.

Fromm-Reichmann, F. "Notes on Personal and Professional Requirements of a Psychotherapist." In D. Bullard (Ed.), *Psychoanalysis and Psychotherapy.* Chicago: University of Chicago Press, 1959.

Garfield, S. L. "Research on Client Variables in Psychotherapy." In A. E. Bergin and S. L. Garfield (Eds.), *Handbook of Psychotherapy and Behavior Change: An Empirical Analysis.* New York: Wiley, 1971.

Gazda, G. M., Asburg, F. R., Balzer, F. J., Childers, W. C ., Desselle, R. E., and Walters, R. P. *Human Relations Development: A Manual for Educators.* Boston: Allyn & Bacon, 1973.

Gelfand, B., Starak, I., and Nevidon, P. "Training for Empathy in Child Welfare." *Child Welfare,* 1973, *52,* 595–600.

Gendlin, E. T. "Therapeutic Procedures in Dealing with Schizophrenics." In C. R. Rogers, E. T. Gendlin, D. J. Kiesler, and C. B. Truax (Eds.) *The Therapeutic Relationship and Its Impact: A Study of Psychotherapy with Schizophrenics.* Madison: University of Wisconsin Press, 1967.

Gendlin, E. T. "Client-Centered: The Experiential Response." In E. F. Hammer (Ed.), *Use of Interpretation in Treatment: Technique and Art.* New York: Grune and Stratton, 1968.

Gendlin, E. T. "Focusing." *Psychotherapy: Theory, Research, and Practice,* 1969, *6,* 4–15.

Gendlin, E. T. "Existentialism and Experiential Psychotherapy." In J. T. Hart and T. M. Tomlinson (Eds.), *New Directions in Client-Centered Therapy.* Boston: Houghton Mifflin, 1970.

Gendlin, E. T. "Client-Centered and Experiential Psychotherapy." In D. A. Wexler and L. N. Rice (Eds.), *Innovations in Client-Centered Therapy.* New York: Wiley, 1974.

Gerber, L. A. "Integrating Encounter Techniques into Individual Psychotherapy." *American Journal of Psychotherapy,* 1972, *26,* 251–262.

Giannandrea, V., and Murphy, K. C. "Similarity of Self-Disclosure and Return for a Second Interview." *Journal of Counseling Psychology,* 1973, *20,* 545–548.

Ginott, H. G. *Between Parent and Child.* New York: Avon Books, 1965.

Ginott, H. G. *Between Parent and Teenager.* New York: Macmillan, 1969.

Glasser, W. *Reality Therapy, A New Approach to Psychiatry.* New York: Harper & Row, 1965.

Goldberg, G. "Breaking the Communication Barrier: The Initial Interview with an Abusing Parent." *Child Welfare,* 1975, *54,* 274–282.

Gordon, T. *Parent Effectiveness Training.* New York: P. H. Wyden, 1970.

Gottlieb, W., and Stanley, J. H. "Mutual Goals and Goal-Setting in Casework." *Social Casework,* 1967, *48,* 471–477.

Gottshalk, L. A., and Pattison, E. M. "Psychiatric Perspectives on T-Groups and Laboratory Movement." *American Journal of Psychiatry,* 1969, *126,* 823–839.

Griffin, A. H., and Banks, G. "Inner-City Workshop for Better Schools." *American International College Alumni Magazine,* Fall, 1969.

Grinker, R. R., MacGregor, H., Selan, K., Klein, A., and Kohrman, J. *Psychiatric Social Work: A Transactional Case Book.* New York: Basic Books, 1961.

Gurman, A. S. "Couples' Facilitative Skill as a Dimension of Marital Therapy Outcome." *Journal of Marriage and Family Counseling,* 1975, *1,* 163–174.

Gurin, G., Veroff, J., and Feld, S. *Americans View Their Mental Health.* New York: Basic Books, 1960.

Halleck, S. L. "The Impact of Professional Dishonesty on Behavior of Disturbed Adolescents." *Social Work,* 1963, *8* (2), 48–56.

Hammer, E. S. (Ed.) *Use of Interpretation in Treatment.* New York: Grune and Stratton, 1968.

Hammond, D. C., Hepworth, D. H., and Smith, V. G. "Research on Central Ingredients: A Critique and Challenge for New Directions." Unpublished paper. University of Utah, Salt Lake City, 1975.

Hawkins, J. L. "Counselor Involvement in Marriage and Family Counseling." *Journal of Marriage and Family Counseling,* 1976, *2,* 37–47.

Hefele, T. "The Effects of Systematic Human Relations Training Upon Student Achievement." *Journal of Research and Development in Education,* 1971, *4,* 52–69.

Heller, K., Davis, J. D., and Myers, R. A. "The Effects of Interviewer Style in a Standardized Interview." *Journal of Consulting Psychology,* 1966, *30,* 501–508.

Hepworth, D. "The Clinical Implications of Perceptual Distortions in Forced Marriages." *Social Casework,* 1964, *45,* 579–585.

Herre, E. A. "Aggressive Casework in a Protective Services Unit." *Social Casework,* 1965, *6,* 358–362.

Hoehn-Saric, R., Frank, J. D., Imber, S. D., Nash, E. H., Stone, A. R., and Battle, C. C. "Systematic Preparation of Patients for Psychotherapy—Effects on Therapy Behavior and Outcome." *Journal of Psychiatric Research,* 1964, *2,* 267–281.

Holder, T., Carkhuff, R. R., and Berenson, B. G. "Differential Effects of the Manipulation of Therapeutic Conditions upon High– and Low–Functioning Clients." *Journal of Counseling Psychology,* 1967, *14,* 63–66.

Hollenbeck, G. P. "Conditions and Outcomes in the Student-Parent Relationship." *Journal of Consulting Psychology,* 1965, *29,* 237–241.

Hollis, F. "Continuance and Discontinuance in Marital Counseling and Some Observations on Joint Interviews." *Social Casework,* 1968, *49,* 167–174.

Johnson, D. *Marriage Counseling: Theory and Practice.* Englewood Cliffs, New Jersey: Prentice-Hall, 1961.

Johnson, W. *People In Quandaries: The Semantics of Personal Adjust-ment.* New York: Harper & Row, 1946.

Jourard, S. *The Transparent Self.* New York: D. Van Nostrand, 1971.

Kanfer, F. H. "Comments on Learning in Psychotherapy." *Psycho-logical Reports,* 1961, *9,* 681–699.

Kanfer, F. H., and Goldstein, A. P. *Helping People Change: A Text-book of Methods.* New York: Pergamon Press, 1975.

Kanfer, F. H., and Saslow, C. "Behavioral Diagnosis." In C. Franks (Ed.), *Behavior Therapy: Appraisal and Status.* New York: McGraw-Hill, 1969.

Kaul, T. J., Kaul, M. A., and Bednar, R. L. "Counselor Confronta-tion and Client Depth of Self-Exploration." *Journal of Coun-seling Psychology,* 1973, *20,* 132–136.

Kelly, B. J. "Concerned Confrontation: The Art of Counseling." *Southern Journal of Educational Research.* 1975, *9,* 100–122.

Kelly, G. A. *The Psychology of Personal Constructs, Vol. II: Clinical Diagnosis and Psychotherapy.* New York: Norton, 1955.

Kiesler, D. G. "A Scale for the Rating of Congruence." In C. R. Rogers and others, *The Therapeutic Relationship and its Impact: A Study of Psychotherapy with Schizophrenics.* Madison: University of Wisconsin Press, 1967.

Klein, M. H., Mathieu, P. L., Gendlin, E. T., and Kiesler, D. G. *The Experiencing Scale: A Research and Training Manual (two vol-umes).* Madison: Wisconsin Psychiatric Institute, 1969.

Krasner, L. "Studies of the Conditioning of Verbal Behavior." *Psy-chological Bulletin,* 1958, *55,* 148–170.

Krasner, L. "The Therapist as a Social Reinforcement Machine." In H. H. Strupp and L. Luborsky (Eds.), *Research in Psycho-therapy.* Vol. 2. Washington, D.C.: American Psychological Association, 1962.

Krasner, L. "Reinforcement, Verbal Behavior, and Psychotherapy." *American Journal of Orthopsychiatry,* 1963, *33,* 601–613.

Krasner, L. "Verbal Conditioning and Psychotherapy." In L. Kras-ner and L. P. Ullmann (Eds.), *Research in Behavior Modification.* New York: Holt, Rinehart and Winston, 1965.

Krill, D. F. "Existential Psychotherapy and the Problem of Anomie." *Social Work,* 1969, *14* (2), 33–49.

Kurtz, R. R., and Grummon, W. L. "Different Approaches to the Measurement of Therapist Empathy and Their Relationship to Therapy Outcomes." *Journal of Consulting and Clinical Psychology,* 1972, *39,* 106–115.

Laing, R. D., and Esterson, A. *Sanity, Madness, and the Family.* (rev. ed.) New York: Basic Books, 1971.

Larsen, J. A., and Hepworth, D. H. "Skill Development Through Competency-Based Education." *Journal of Education for Social Work,* 1975.

Lazarus, A. "Multimodel Behavior Therapy: Treating the 'Basic Id.'" *Journal of Nervous and Mental Disease,* 1963, *156,* 404–411.

Lazarus, A. A. "Behavior Therapy in Groups." In G. M. Gazda (Ed.), *Basic Approaches to Group Psychotherapy and Group Counseling.* Springfield, Ill.: Charles C. Thomas, 1968.

Lazarus, A. A. *Behavior Therapy and Beyond.* New York: McGraw-Hill, 1971.

Leavitt, E. E. "The Results of Psychotherapy with Children: An Evaluation." *Journal of Consulting Psychology,* 1957, *21,* 189–196.

Levitsky, A., and Perls, F. S. "The Rules and Games of Gestalt Therapy." In J. Fagan and I. L. Shepherd (Eds.) *Gestalt Therapy Now: Theory, Techniques, Applications.* Palo Alto, California: Science and Behavior Books, 1970.

Lieberman, M. A., Yalom, I. D., and Miles, M. B. *Encounter Groups: First Facts.* New York: Basic Books, 1973.

Mahoney, M. J., and Thoresen, C. E. *Self-Control: Power to the Person.* Monterey, Calif.: Brooks/Cole, 1974.

Mahrer, A. R. *Goals of Psychotherapy.* New York: Appleton-Century-Crofts, 1967.

Malamud, D. I. "Self-Confrontation Methods in Psychotherapy." *Journal of Psychotherapy: Theory, Research, and Practice,* 1973, *10,* 123–130.

Mannino, F., and Greenspan, S. "Projection and Misperception in Couples Treatment." *Journal of Marriage and Family Counseling,* 1976, *2,* 139–143.

Markowitz, J. "The Nature of the Child's Initial Resistance to Psychotherapy." *Social Work,* 1954, *4* (3), 46–51.

Martin, J. C., Carkhuff, R. R., and Berenson, B. G. "Process Variables in Counseling and Psychotherapy: A Study of Counseling and Friendship." *Journal of Counseling Psychology,* 1964, *26,* 264–267.

Masserman, J. H. "Historical-Comparative and Experimental Roots of Short-Term Therapy." In L. R. Wolberg (Ed.), *Short-Term Psychotherapy*. New York: Grune and Stratton, 1965, 44–66.

Masters, W. H., and Johnson, V. E. *Human Sexual Inadequacy*. Boston: Little, Brown, 1970.

May, R. *Love and Will*. New York: Norton, 1969.

May, R., Angel, E., and Ellenberger, H. F. *Existence: A New Dimension in Psychiatry and Psychology*. New York: Simon & Schuster, 1958.

Mayer, J., and Timms, N. "Clash in Perspective between Worker and Client." *Social Casework*, 1969, *50*, 32–40.

Mickelson, D. J., and Stevic, R. R. "Differential Effects of Facilitative and Nonfacilitative Behavioral Counselors." *Journal of Counseling Psychology*, 1971, *18*, 314–319.

Middleman, R. R., and Goldberg, G. *Social Service Delivery: A Structural Approach to Social Work Practice*. New York: Columbia University Press, 1974.

Miller, S., Nunnally, E., and Wackman, D. *The Minnesota Couples Communication Program Handbook*. Minneapolis: Minnesota Couples Communication Program, 1972.

Mitchell, K. M., and Namenek, T. M. "Effects of Therapist Confrontation on Subsequent Client and Therapist Behavior during the First Therapy Interview." *Journal of Counseling Psychology*, 1972, *19*,196–201.

Morgan, R. "Is It Scientific to be Optimistic?" *Social Work*, 1961, *6* (4), 2–21.

Morganstern, K. P. "Implosive Therapy and Flooding Procedures: A Critical Review." *Psychological Bulletin*, 1973, *79*, 318–334.

Morris, R. J., and Suckerman, K. R. "Therapist Warmth as a Factor in Automated Systematic Desensitization." *Journal of Consulting and Clinical Psychology*, 1974a, *42*, 244–250.

Morris, R. J., and Suckerman, K. R. "The Importance of the Therapeutic Relationship in Systematic Desensitization." *Journal of Consulting and Clinical Psychology*, 1974b, *42*, 148.

Mosak, H. H., and Gushurst, R. "What Patients Say and What They Mean." *American Journal of Psychotherapy*, 1971, *25*, 428–436.

Murphy, K. C., and Strong, S. R. "Some Effects of Similarity Disclosure." *Journal of Counseling Psychology*, 1976, *19*, 121–124.

Nikelly, A.G., and Dinkmeyer, D. "The Process of Encouragement." In A.G. Nikelly (Ed.), *Techniques for Behavior Change.* Springfield, Ill.: Charles C. Thomas, 1971.

Oxley, G.B. "The Methods Lab—An Experiment in Experiential Classroom Learning." *Social Work Education Reporter,* 1973, *21,* 60–63.

Parloff, M.B. "Sheltered Workshops for the Alienated." *International Journal of Psychiatry,* 1970, *9,* 197–204.

Payne, P.A., and Gralinski, D.M. "Effects of Supervision Style and Empathy upon Counselor Learning." *Journal of Counseling Psychology,* 1968, *15,* 517–521.

Perlman, H.H. *Social Casework: A Problem-Solving Process.* Chicago: University of Chicago Press, 1957.

Perls, F. *Gestalt Therapy Verbatim.* Moab, Utah: Real People Press, 1969.

Perls, F. *The Gestalt Approach and Eye Witness to Therapy.* Ben Lomond, Calif.: Science and Behavior Books, 1973.

Perry, M. "Modeling and Instructions in Training for Counselor Empathy." *Journal of Counseling Psychology,* 1975, *22,* 173–179.

Phillips, E.L., Phillips, E.A., Fixsen, D.L., and Wolf, M. "Behavior Shaping Works for Delinquents." *Psychology Today,* 1973, *7* (1), 75–79.

Piaget, G., Berenson, B.G., and Carkhuff, R.R. "The Differential Effects of the Manipulation of Therapeutic Conditions by High– and Low–Functioning Counselors Upon High– and Low– Functioning Clients." *Journal of Consulting Psychology,* 1967, *31,* 481–486.

Pierce, R. "An Investigation of Grade-Point Average and Therapeutic Process Variables." Ph.D. dissertation, University of Massachusetts, 1966.

Pierce, R., and Schauble, P. "Graduate Training of Facilitative Counselors: The Effects of Individual Supervision." *Journal of Counseling Psychology,* 1970.

Polansky, N. "On Duplicity in the Interview." *American Journal of Orthopsychiatry,* 1967, *37,* 568–579.

Poser, E.G. "The Effect of Therapist Training on Group Therapeutic Outcome." *Journal of Consulting Psychology,* 1966, *30,* 283–289.

Rachman, S., and Teasdale, J. *Aversion Therapy and Behavior Disorders: An Analysis.* Coral Gables, Fla.: University of Miami Press, 1969.

Raimy, V. *Misunderstandings of the Self.* San Francisco: Jossey-Bass, 1975.

Reid, C. *Celebrate the Temporary.* New York: Harper & Row, 1972.

Reid, W. J. "Implications of Research for the Goals of Casework." *Smith College Studies in Social Work,* 1970, *40,* 140–154.

Reid, W. J. "A Test of a Task-Centered Approach." *Social Work,* 1975, *20,* 3–9.

Reid, W. J., and Epstein, L. *Task-Centered Casework.* New York: Columbia University Press, 1972.

Rice, L. N. "The Evocative Function of the Therapist." In D. A. Wexler and L. N. Rice (Eds.), *Innovations in Client-Centered Therapy.* New York: Wiley, 1974.

Ripple, L. *Motivation, Capacity, and Opportunity.* Chicago: School of Social Service Administration, 1964.

Rogers, C. R. "The Necessary and Sufficient Conditions of Therapeutic Personality Change." *Journal of Consulting Psychology,* 1957, *22,* 95–103.

Rogers, C. R. *On Becoming A Person.* Boston: Houghton Mifflin, 1961.

Rogers, C. R. "Client-Centered Therapy." In S. Arieto (Ed.), *American Handbook of Psychiatry.* Vol. 3. New York: Basic Books, 1966.

Rogers, C. R. "Empathic: An Unappreciated Way of Being." *The Counseling Psychologist,* 1975, *5,* 2–9.

Rogers, C. R., and Dymond, R. F. *Psychotherapy and Personality Change.* Chicago: University of Chicago Press, 1954.

Rogers, C. R., Gendlin, E. T., Kiesler, D., and Truax, C. B. *The Therapeutic Relationship and Its Impact: A Study of Psychotherapy with Schizophrenics.* Madison: University of Wisconsin Press, 1967.

Rokeach, M. *Beliefs, Attitudes, and Values.* San Francisco: Jossey-Bass, 1968.

Rose, S. D., Sundel, M., DeLange, J., Corwin, L., and Palumbo, A. "The Hartung Project: A Behavioral Approach to the Treatment of Juvenile Offenders." In R. Ulrich, T. Stachnik, and

J. Mabry (Eds.), *Control of Human Behavior, II: From Cure to Prevention.* Glenview, Ill.: Scott, Foresman, 1970.

Rose, S. D. "In Pursuit of Social Competence." *Social Work,* 1975, *20,* 33–39.

Rosenthal, D., and Frank, J. D. "Psychotherapy and the Placebo Effect." *Psychological Bulletin,* 1956, *53,* 294–302.

Rotter, J. B. *Social Learning and Clinical Psychology.* Englewood Cliffs, New Jersey: Prentice-Hall, 1954.

Ruesch, J. *Therapeutic Communication.* New York: Norton, 1961.

Ryan, V., and Gizynski, M. "Behavior Therapy in Retrospect: Patients' Feelings about Their Behavior Therapies." *Journal of Consulting and Clinical Psychology,* 1971, *35,* 1–9.

Salzinger, K. "Experimental Manipulation of Verbal Behavior: A Review." *Journal of General Psychology,* 1959, 61, 65–94.

Santa Cruz, L. A., and Hepworth, D. H. "Effects of Cultural Orientation on Casework." *Social Casework,* 1975, *56,* 52–57.

Schmidt, J. T. "The Use of Purpose in Casework." *Social Work,* 1969, *14* (1), 77–84.

Schwartz, A., and Goldiamond, I. *Social Casework: A Behavioral Approach.* New York: Columbia University Press, 1975.

Seabury, B. A. "The Contract: Uses, Abuses, and Limitations." *Social Work,* 1976, *21,* 16–19.

Shelton, J. L., and Ackerman, J. M. *Homework in Counseling and Psychotherapy.* Springfield, Ill.: Charles C. Thomas, 1974.

Sherman, S. N. "The Therapist and Changing Sex Roles." *Social Casework,* 1976, *57,* 93–96.

Shostrom, E. L. *Man, the Manipulator.* New York: Bantam Books, 1968.

Shulman, B. H. "Psychological Disturbances Which Interfere with the Patient's Cooperation." *Psychosomatics,* 1964, *5,* 213–220.

Shulman, B. H. "Confrontation Techniques in Adlerian Psychotherapy." *Journal of Individual Psychology,* 1971, *27,* 167–175.

Shulman, B. H. "Life Style." In B. H. Shulman (Ed.), *Contributions to Individual Psychology.* Chicago: Alfred Adler Institute, 1973.

Sifneos, P. "Two Kinds of Psychotherapy of Short Duration." *American Journal of Psychiatry,* 1967, *130,* 1069–1073.

Simonson, N. R. "The Impact of Therapist Disclosure on Patient Disclosure." *Journal of Counseling Psychology,* 1976, *23,* 3–6.

Smith, V. G., and Hepworth, D. H. "Marriage Counseling with One Marital Partner: Rationale and Clinical Implications." *Social Casework,* 1967, *48,* 352–359.

Speisman, J. C. "Depth of Interpretation and Verbal Resistance in Psychotherapy." *Journal of Consulting Psychology,* 1959, *23,* 93–99.

Stampfl, T. G., and Levis, D. J. "Essentials of Implosive Therapy: A Learning-Theory-Based Psychodynamic Behavioral Therapy." *Journal of Abnormal Psychology,* 1967, *72,* 496–503.

Stampfl, T. G. "Implosive Therapy: Staring Down Your Nightmares." *Psychology Today,* 1975, *8* (9), 66–73.

Stark, F. B. "Barriers to Client-Worker Communication at Intake." *Social Casework,* 1959, *40,* 177–183.

Stoffer, D. L. "Investigation of Positive Behavioral Change as a Function of Genuineness, Nonpossessive Warmth, and Empathic Understanding." *Journal of Education Research,* 1970, *63,* 225–228.

Strachey, J. "The Nature of the Therapeutic Action of Psychoanalysis." *International Journal of Psychoanalysis,* 1934, *15,* 127–159.

Strupp, H. H. "Psychotherapeutic Technique, Professional Affiliation, and Experience Level." *Journal of Consulting Psychology,* 1955, *19,* 97–102.

Strupp, H. H. *Psychotherapists in Action.* New York: Grune and Stratton, 1960.

Strupp, H. H. *Psychotherapy: Clinical, Research, and Theoretical Issues.* New York: Jason Aronson, 1973.

Stuart, R. B. "An Operant Interpersonal Program for Couples." In D. Olson (Ed.), *Treating Relationships.* Lake Mills, Iowa: Graphic Publishing, 1976, 119–132.

Studt, E. "Worker-Client Authority Relationships in Social Work." *Social Work,* 1959, *4* (1), 18–28.

Subotnik, L. "Spontaneous Remission: Fact or Artifact." *Psychological Bulletin,* 1972, *77,* 32–48.

Tarachow, S. *An Introduction to Psychotherapy.* New York: International Universities Press, 1963.

Thoresen, C. E., and Mahoney, M. J. *Behavioral Self-Control.* New York: Holt, Rinehart and Winston, 1974.

Thorne, F. C. *Psychological Case Handling.* Brandon, Vt.: Clinical Psychology Publishing Co., 1968.

Truax, C. B., and Carkhuff, R. R. "For Better or for Worse: The Process of Psychotherapeutic Change." In *Recent Advances in Behavioral Change.* Montreal: McGill University Press, 1964.

Truax, C. B., and Carkhuff, R. R. *Toward Effective Counseling and Psychotherapy: Training and Practice.* Chicago: Aldine-Atherton, 1967.

Truax, C. B., and Mitchell, K. M. "Research on Certain Therapist Interpersonal Skills in Relation to Process and Outcome." In A. E. Bergin and S. L. Garfield (Eds.), *Handbook of Psychotherapy and Behavior Change.* New York: Wiley, 1971.

Truax, C. B., and Tatum, C. R. "An Extension from the Effective Psychotherapeutic Model to Constructive Personality Change in Preschool Children." *Childhood Education,* 1966, *42,* 456–462.

Tyler, L. E. "Minimum Change Therapy." *Personnel and Guidance Journal,* 1960, *38,* 475–479.

Vitalo, R. "Effects of Facilitative Interpersonal Functioning in a Verbal Conditioning Paradigm." *Journal of Counseling Psychology,* 1970, *17,* 141–144.

Wagner, H. M., and Mitchell, K. M. "Relationship Between Perceived Instructor's Accurate Empathy, Warmth and Genuineness and College Achievement." Discussion Paper No. 13. Arkansas Rehabilitation Research and Training Center, University of Arkansas, 1969.

Watzlawick, P., Beavin, J. H., and Jackson, D. D. *Pragmatics of Human Communication.* New York: Norton, 1967.

Watzlawick, P., Weakland, J., and Fisch, R. *Change: Principles of Problem Formulation and Problem Resolution.* New York: Norton, 1974.

Wells, R. A., and Miller, D. "Developing Relationship Skills in Social Work Students." *Social Work Education Reporter,* 1973, *21,* 68–73.

Wells, R. A. "Training in Facilitative Skills." *Social Work,* 1975, *20,* 242–243.

Wolberg, L. R. *The Technique of Psychotherapy.* New York: Grune and Stratton, 1967.

Wolpe, J. *The Practice of Behavior Therapy.* New York: Pergamon Press, 1969.

Yalom, I. *The Theory and Practice of Group Psychotherapy.* New York: Basic Books, 1975.

Yalom, I., Brown, S., and Block, S. "The Written Summary as a Group Psychotherapy Technique." *Archives of General Psychiatry,* 1975, *32,* 605–613.

Yalom, I., and Elkin, G. *Every-Day Gets a Little Closer: A Twice Told Therapy.* New York: Basic Books, 1974.

Yalom, I., and Lieberman, M. A. "A Study of Encounter Group Casualties." *Archives of General Psychiatry,* 1971, *25,* 16–30.

Yelaja, S. A. "The Concept of Authority and Its Use in Child Protective Service." *Child Welfare,* 1965, *44,* 514–522.

Index

A

Abusive behavior, 311–312
Acceptance, conveying, 183–186
ACKERMAN, J. M. (with SHELTON), 54
Acting out, 243, 269
Additive empathic intervention/responding/responses: communication exercises for, 157–168; confrontation and, 347–348; deep, 137–169; documentation of, 152; in early phase, 34; effectiveness of, 140–141; examples of, 101; for expanding meanings, 137–169; level of, 99; in middle phase, 55–56, 342–343; modeled responses for, 162–168; phrasing, 151–152; practicum exercises for, 168–169; timing of, 138–140
ADLER, ALFRED, 147, 229
Admonishing, 76
Adolescents, 72
Affect, isolation of, 269
Affective discrepancies, 304–310
Aggressiveness, 84
ALBERTI, R. E., and M. L. EMMONS, 54
ALEXANDER, J. F., and B. V. PARSONS, 54
Alienated clients, 32–33

ALLPORT, G. W., 231
Aloneness, 84
Alternatives, failing to see, 299–301
Ambiguity, 284, 339
Amnesia, 83
ANDERSON, J. D., 16, 32–33
ANGEL, E. (with MAY and ELLENBERGER), 230, 251
ANSBACHER, H. L., and ANSBACHER, R. R. (Eds.), 147
ANSBACHER, R. R. (with H. L. ANSBACHER), 147
ANTHONY, W. A., 21, 112
Arguing, 77–78
ARNOLD, MATTHEW, 82
ARONSON, H., and B. OVERALL, 38
ASBURG, F. R. (in GAZDA and others), 171n, 206n
ASPY, D. N., and W. HADLOCK, 17, 188
Assertiveness training, 54
Attention, guidelines for, 110–112
Authenticity/authentic responding, 336–338, 344–346; communication exercises for, 254–266; condescending violates, 76–77; during early phase, 45; emotional detachment and, 73–74; emo-

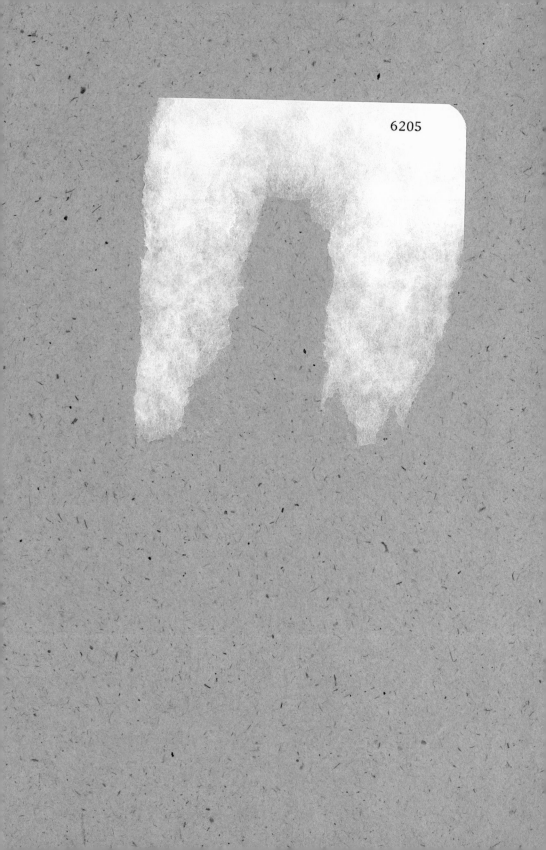

6205